NANDA Approved Diagnostic Labels*
Grouped by Human Response Pattern

EXCHANGING (Pattern 1)
Airway clearance, ineffective
Aspiration, high risk for
Body temperature, high risk for altered
Breathing pattern, ineffective
Cardiac output, decreased
Constipation
Constipation, colonic
Constipation, perceived
Diarrhea
Disuse Syndrome, high risk for
Dysreflexia
Fluid volume deficit (1)
Fluid volume deficit (2)
Fluid volume deficit, high risk for
Fluid volume excess
Gas exchange, impaired
Hyperthermia
Hypothermia
Incontinence, bowel
Incontinence, functional (urinary)
Incontinence, reflex (urinary)
Incontinence, stress (urinary)
Incontinence, total (urinary)
Incontinence, urge (urinary)
Infection, high risk for
Injury, high risk for
Nutrition, altered: less than body
    requirements
Nutrition, altered: more than body
    requirements
Nutrition, altered: high risk for more
    than body requirements
Oral mucous membrane, altered
Poisoning, high risk for
Protection, altered*
Skin integrity, impaired
Skin integrity, high risk for impaired
Suffocation, high risk for
Thermoregulation, ineffective
Tissue integrity, impaired
Tissue perfusion, altered (specify):
    cardiopulmonary, cerebral,
    gastrointestinal, peripheral, renal
Trauma, high risk for
Urinary elimination, altered patterns of
Urinary retention
Ventilation, inability to sustain
    spontaneous*

Ventilatory weaning response,
    dysfunctional*

COMMUNICATING (Pattern 2)
Verbal communication, impaired

RELATING (Pattern 3)
Caregiver role strain*
Caregiver role strain, high risk for*
Family processes, altered
Parental role conflict
Parenting, altered
Parenting, high risk for altered
Role performance, altered
Sexual dysfunction
Sexuality patterns, altered
Social interaction, impaired
Social isolation

VALUING (Pattern 4)
Spiritual distress (distress of the human
    spirit)

CHOOSING (Pattern 5)
Adjustment, impaired
Coping, defensive
Coping (family), ineffective: compro-
    mised
Coping (family), ineffective: disabling
Coping (family): potential for growth
Coping (individual), ineffective
Decisional conflict (specify)
Denial, ineffective
Health seeking behaviors (specify)
Management of therapeutic regimen,
    ineffective*
Noncompliance (specify)

MOVING (Pattern 6)
Activity intolerance
Activity intolerance, high risk for
Bathing/hygiene self care deficit
Breastfeeding, effective*
Breastfeeding, ineffective
Breastfeeding, interrupted*
Diversional activity deficit
Dressing/grooming self care deficit

Fatigue
Feeding self care deficit
Growth and development, altered
Health maintenance, altered
Home maintenance management,
    impaired
Infant feeding pattern, ineffective*
Mobility, impaired physical
Peripheral neurovascular dysfunction,
    high risk for*
Relocation stress syndrome*
Sleep pattern disturbance
Swallowing, impaired
Toileting self care deficit

PERCEIVING (Pattern 7)
Body image disturbance
Hopelessness
Personal identify disturbance
Powerlessness
Self-esteem, chronic low
Self-esteem disturbance
Self-esteem, situational low
Sensory/perceptual alterations (specify):
    auditory, gustatory, kinesthetic,
    olfactory, tactile, visual
Unilateral neglect

KNOWING (Pattern 8)
Knowledge deficit (specify)
Thought processes, altered

FEELING (Pattern 9)
Anxiety
Fear
Grieving, anticipatory
Grieving, dysfunctional
Pain
Pain, chronic
Post-trauma response
Rape-trauma syndrome
Rape-trauma syndrome: compound
    reaction
Rape-trauma syndrome: silent reaction
Self-mutilation, high risk for*
Violence, high risk for: self-directed or
    directed at others

NURSING PROCESS IN ACTION

A CRITICAL THINKING APPROACH

NURSING PROCESS IN ACTION

A CRITICAL THINKING APPROACH

Judith M. Wilkinson, MA, MS, RNC

Johnson County Community College
Overland Park, Kansas

ADDISON-WESLEY NURSING

A Division of the Benjamin/Cummings Publishing Company, Inc.

Redwood City, California • Menlo Park, California
Reading, Massachusetts • New York • Don Mills, Ontario
Wokingham, U.K. • Amsterdam • Bonn • Sydney • Singapore
Tokyo • Madrid • San Juan

Executive Editor: Patricia L. Cleary
Editorial Assistant: Bradley Burch
Production Coordinator: Megan Rundel
Cover and interior design and logo art: Irene Imfeld
Copyeditor: Nicholas Murray
Proofreader: Anita Wagner
Composition: Fog Press

Library of Congress Cataloging-in-Publication Data

Wilkinson, Judith M.
    Nursing process in action: a critcal thinking approach / Judith M. Wilkinson.
        p.   cm.
    Includes bibliographical references and index.
    ISBN 0-8053-9362-5
    1. Nursing.   2. Critical thinking.   I. Title.
    [DNLM: 1. Decision Making.   2. Nursing Diagnosis.   3. Nursing Process.   WY 100
W686n]
RT41.W57   1991
610.73--dc20
DNLM/DLC
for Library of Congress   91-25915
                                                                                 :CIP

ISBN 0-8053-9362-5
        5 6 7 8 9 10-MU-95

Addison-Wesley Nursing
A Division of The Benjamin/Cummings Publishing Company, Inc.
390 Bridge Parkway
Redwood City, California 94065

PREFACE

The nursing process is the foundation for professional practice. It is within the framework of the entire nursing process that the professional applies the unique combination of knowledge, skills, and caring that comprises the art and science of nursing. Therefore, the purpose of this book is to promote professional practice through effective use of the nursing process. To that end, the text integrates consideration of professional standards of care, ethical issues, critical thinking, wellness, and nursing frameworks into the discussion of each nursing process step. This is a serious text, with in-depth treatment of concepts, despite the fact that students find it easy, even enjoyable, to use.

It is important for nurses to have a conceptual understanding of the nursing process, as well as the practical ability to create a nursing care plan. This text balances conceptual and practical aspects (e.g., Chapter 4 explains the diagnostic process, and Chapter 5 explains how to write a diagnostic statement; Chapter 6 discusses planning, and Chapter 9 is a detailed explanation of how to create a working care plan for a real patient).

Nursing diagnosis is an important part of the nursing process, but its emphasis in this book is not meant to minimize the importance of the rest of the process. Nursing diagnosis is expanded more than other steps for the following reasons:

1. It is important in defining the domain of nursing.
2. The author believes that students should be introduced to the diagnostic *process* before attempting to write diagnostic statements.
3. The complexity of the diagnostic process requires in-depth explanation and practice to enable students to grasp the concepts.
4. Students often have difficulty writing good diagnostic statements.
5. Opportunities for ample application and practice may make this step less intimidating for students.
6. Once a good nursing diagnosis is made, the rest of the nursing process falls into place with relative ease.

The Nursing Diagnosis Guide in the back of this text includes suggestions for using problematic diagnostic labels.

In order to increase student awareness of ethical issues embedded in the practice of nursing, each chapter includes ethical considerations and principles pertinent to the nursing process step being presented (e.g., maintaining confidentiality of client data in the assessment step).

The author maintains that critical thinking should be promoted in the educational process from kindergarten through graduate school, and that it is especially important for nurses—perhaps in different degrees and for different uses, but at all levels. The nursing process provides an excellent vehicle for encouraging critical thinking; therefore, a brief chapter on critical thinking is included. In addition, the nursing process exercises are designed to foster critical thinking, and special critical thinking exercises are provided in each chapter to teach specific critical thinking skills. The critical thinking exercises are excellent for class discussion or small-group projects.

The nursing process (and critical thinking) are similar to mathematics in that they cannot be mastered merely by memorizing facts and principles. In order to remember and apply the concepts, students need practice; they need to "work problems." This text provides ample practice problems. The exercises are not just a "workbook;" they are application exercises, designed to promote high-level thinking skills. The answer keys provide the rationale for both correct and incorrect answers, and they frequently demonstrate the thinking process used to arrive at the answers. This detailed feedback provides opportunity for truly interactive learning, as well as the kind of student-instructor dialogue that is so important in learning the nursing process. Students are easily frustrated by the many ambiguities and seeming contradictions that arise when applying the nursing process. The answer key discussions are a vital because they decrease this frustration and model the thinking inherent in the process.

Wellness language and examples are frequently used in order to promote awareness of wellness as a vital part of the domain of nursing practice. Most chapters include a section in which wellness concepts are related to the chapter material, and the exercises include wellness examples where appropriate.

Regarding terminology, *client* is used to emphasize the following points:

1. Nurses have independent functions.

2. Nurses are increasingly accountable to clients instead of institutions.

3. Nursing services are not provided exclusively to ill people.

4. Clients are increasingly more active in managing their own health care.

5. Nursing is not setting-bound; for example, it is not done only in hospitals.

Most nursing, however, does occur in hospitals, where ill people are frequently in a dependent state. Furthermore, most nurses are paid by an employing health agency rather than directly by the patient. In these situations, the term *patient* seems more accurate. Because either term can be appropriate, depending upon the situation, both terms are used in this text.

A similar approach is used for words denoting gender. The author freely acknowledges and welcomes the presence of men in nursing and, further, realizes that patients are both men and women. However, terms like *s/he* or *she/he* are awkward to read, and they are not used in this text. Both nurses and clients are randomly assigned gender and referred to as *he* or *she* .

A glossary is not included because (1) this text includes only a very few terms that are suitable for inclusion in a glossary and (2) key terms in each chapter appear in bold print. The accompanying *Instructor's Manual* includes key-terms exercises that can be assigned if the instuctor wishes to reinforce key terms for each chapter.

This text is versatile; it is suitable for nursing students as an introduction to the nursing process, or for use in the continuing education of professionals who may need refresher information and practice. It is effective for students who have had nursing process early in the curriculum and who later have difficulty applying the nursing process in a clinical course. The text is organized to accommodate the instructor's professional judgment—that is, it can be used for students of different levels, depending upon what the instructor chooses to assign or emphasize. For example, if the instructor believes the concept of possible problems is too difficult for beginning students, this portion of Chapter 4 could be omitted without damaging the continuity of the material. Some instructors may choose to present Chapter 5 before Chapter 4; others prefer to use Chapter 9 just before Chapter 6. Both approaches are workable. As another example, several nursing frameworks are summarized and demonstrated, but the instructor could choose not to emphasize frameworks, or could ask students to use only one framework and assign additional readings on that framework for in-depth understanding.

This text can be used for independent study by duplicating test questions and other materials from *Instructor's Manual*, but it is in no way limited to that approach. It can be used as a text to supplement lectures, either in a discrete course or when the nursing process is integrated in the curriculum.

The author has used these chapters and the *Instructor's Manual* as learning units to teach the nursing process to students of various levels, as well as in continuing education for practicing nurses. Student response has been over-whelmingly positive. Time previously allotted to lecture is now used mainly to discuss student questions about their care plans for clinical. Even more exciting, fewer instructor comments are needed on student care plans, and fewer individual conferences are being held to help students with nursing process.

Acknowledgements

My thanks to the following people for their valuable assistance. For information on critical thinking: Douglas Martin, of Sonoma State University, and Mathew Keller, of the Cotati-Rohnert Park Unified School District. For helpful discussions about nursing diagnosis: Rose Mary Carroll-Johnson, MN, RN, Nurse Editor, and Rita Olivieri, RN, PhD, of the School of Nursing at Boston College. For permission to use portions of exercises developed while under contract to them: the Association of Independent Hospitals, Kansas City, MO. I would also like to thank my friend, Melissa Bourque, who supplied a non-nursing perspective, and my former student and friend, Trish Postier, RN, for moral support.

Reviewers

I am grateful to the following for their manuscript reviews: Ginny Adams, Tomoroh Lutz, Jeanne Stein, and Lelani Taylor, nursing students at Johnson County Community College; Donna Burleson, RN, BSN, MS, Director of Health Occupations, Cisco Junior College; Patricia Diehl, RN, BSN, MA, West Virgina University School of Nursing; and Faith M. Reirson, RN, MN, Former Coordinator, Nursing Program, Olympic College, Bremerton, WA; and to Carol Green-Nigro, MN, RN, and Penny L. Marshall, MN, RN, Nursing Department, Johnson County Community College for reviews, case studies and care plans.

Special Appreciation

Special appreciation and thanks are due to Patti Cleary, Executive Editor, for her incredible ability to provide valuable, on-target criticism without stifling creativity; to my mother, who taught me to read, and who provided a role model of a strong, assertive woman not circumscribed by her gender; to my father, who role-modeled self-confidence and taught me that all work is art if you do it with pride and care; and to Todd, Bryan, and Chris, who keep me humble.

Getting the Most from Your Reading

The following suggestions should help you get the maximum benefit from your study of this text.

1. For each chapter, begin by reading the chapter objectives. These direct your reading toward achieving particular goals.

2. The key terms are in bold print in the chapter text. Be sure you are able to recognize and define these terms.

3. Next, read the chapter content.

4. Do the critical thinking exercises. Discuss these with your instructor and/or your classmates to be sure you are on the right track. There are no answer keys for these, because that would defeat the purpose of the exercises; the emphasis is not on the correct *answer* but on correct use of the *skill*, or how you arrived at your answer. These skills can be acquired best in discussions with your peers, either individually or in class.

5. Work the application activities. The nursing process must be *applied*, not simply understood and remembered. You will be applying the nursing process in the real world, not simply recalling facts about it—so begin learning to do that now. Work the exercises before you look at the answer keys, and refer back to the chapter text as you need to. Be sure you understand the rationale provided in the answer keys.

If you have difficulty with the exercises, reread the chapter, read more of the the suggested additional readings, and try again. If you are still having trouble, your instructor may suggest additional exercises, audiovisual materials, or readings.

CONTENTS

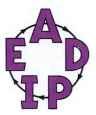

CHAPTER 1

OVERVIEW OF THE NURSING PROCESS

OBJECTIVES

Upon completing this chapter, you should be able to do the following:
* State the relationship between the nursing process and the standards of care set by the American Nurses Association.
* Define the nursing process in terms of purpose, characteristics, and organization.
* Name and describe the five steps of the nursing process.
* Explain how the nursing process steps are both sequential and overlapping.
* Describe the qualities a nurse needs in order to use the nursing process successfully.
* Explain how the nursing process can benefit the client, the nurse, and the profession.
* Discuss how the nursing process applies to both well and ill clients.

INTRODUCTION

When you first begin studying it, the nursing process may seem somewhat complicated. Because nursing process texts (and teachers) talk about *ideas* and *processes,* students sometimes wonder what all this has to do with taking care of patients. As you will learn in this chapter and throughout the book, the **nursing process** is a special way of thinking that nurses use. It is also what nurses *do* when giving patient care. In other words, the nursing process is a thinking/doing *approach* that nurses use in their work. Keeping this general idea in mind will help you as you work through the more detailed explanation developed in the following sections. The five basic steps of the nursing process are shown in Figure 1–1.

DEFINING NURSING

Nursing and the nursing process are so interrelated that it is difficult to talk about them separately. The nursing process is an essential part of nursing, but it is only one aspect of nursing. An understanding of what nursing is will help you to understand the nursing process and place it in proper perspective. **Nursing** is a unique blend of art and science applied within the context of interpersonal relationships for the purpose of promoting wellness, preventing illness, and restoring health.

Nursing has been defined by professional organizations and individual nursing leaders. The first nurse theorist, Florence Nightingale (1969 [1859]), said that what nurses do "is to put the patient in the best condition for nature to act

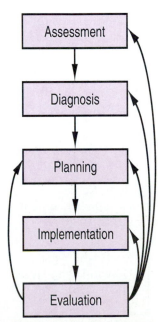

Figure 1–1. The Five Basic Steps of the Nursing Process

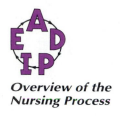

Overview of the Nursing Process

upon him" (p. 133). More recently, the American Nurses Association (ANA), the professional organization for nurses, issued *Nursing: A Social Policy Statement* (1980), which defines nursing as "the diagnosis and treatment of human responses to actual or potential health problems" (p. 9).

Nursing models and theories are based on the theorist's values and assumptions about health, the client, nursing, and the environment. Each model describes these concepts and explains how they are related. There are almost as many definitions of nursing as there have been nurse leaders and theorists (see Table 1–1 for a few examples).

Table 1–1. Definitions of Nursing by Nurse Theorists

Theorist	Definition of Nursing
Hildegarde Peplau Interpersonal model (1952)	"A significant therapeutic interpersonal process which functions cooperatively with other human processes that make health possible for individuals" (p.16). "A maturing force and educative instrument" (p.8). A practice discipline.
Dorothy Johnson Behavioral System model (1961, 1980)	Nursing is concerned with behavior rather than biological functions. It is both art and science—a profession offering a distinctive service. Nursing is an external regulatory force that reduces stress and tension, helping individuals to achieve adaptation and system stability.
Martha Rogers Unitary Man model (1970, 1980)	Nursing is both art and science; a learned profession. It promotes achievement of maximum health potential by promoting "symphonic interaction between man and environment, to strengthen the coherence and integrity of the human field" (1970, p. 122). Nurses promote health, prevent illness, and care for and rehabilitate the sick and disabled (1970, p. vii).
Sister Callista Roy Adaptation model (1970, 1976, 1980)	Nursing is "a theoretical system of knowledge which prescribes a process of analysis and action related to care of the ill or potentially ill person" (1976, p. 31). Nurses promote adaptation of the client in the physiologic, self-concept, role-function, and interdependence modes by manipulating stimuli (or stressors).
Dorothea Orem Self-Care model (1971)	Nursing is a human service concerned with the need for continuous self-care action in order to sustain life and health or to recover from disease or injury. Nursing has both health and illness dimensions. Nurses help clients (mainly individuals) to achieve self-care agency and maintain an optimal state of health.
Betty Neuman Health-Care System model (1972, 1980)	The nurse helps the client to attain and maintain system equilibrium. Nursing is concerned with all variables that affect a person's response to stressors. The nurse attempts to help the client avoid or defend against stressors. Both client and nurse are active, but the nurse is more so.
Rosemarie Parse Human-Living-Health model (1974, 1981, 1987)	"Nursing is a human science profession concerned with the care of unitary man as he evolves from conception to death" (1974, p. 7). Nursing is a science and an art concerned with exploring personal meanings of lived experiences. The nurse guides clients in assuming responsibility for their health.

Although definitions of nursing vary, there is general agreement that even though nursing is concerned with health problems, it is not limited to concern with disease processes, and its phenomena of concern are different from those of medicine. Overall, nursing models describe nursing as an art and a science with its own evolving, scientific body of knowledge; as holistic, or concerned with the client's physical, psychosocial, and spiritual needs; as involving caring; as occurring in a variety of settings; and as concerned with health promotion, disease prevention, and care during illness. It is the blending of art (caring) and science (problem solving) within the person-to-person relationship that makes nursing special and unique.

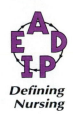

Defining Nursing

Human Responses

According to the ANA definition of nursing, human responses are the phenomena of nursing concern. **Human responses** are biological, psychological, social, or spiritual reactions to an event or a stressor, such as a disease or injury. Nurses, viewing the client holistically, are interested in responses in all these dimensions. Nurses diagnose and treat the client's *responses* to diseases such as diabetes (e.g., lack of knowledge about diet, altered skin integrity, loss of self-esteem) rather than the disease itself.

> **Nursing** is a unique blend of art and science, applied within the context of interpersonal relationships for the purpose of promoting wellness, preventing illness, and restoring health.

> *Example:* Consider the following possible responses to a heart attack:

Physical response	Pain
Psychological response	Fear
Sociological response	Returning to work before she is well
Spiritual response	Praying

There is an infinite variety of possible human responses. Note, too, that the stressors that cause health problems are not always diseases or microorganisms. They can be environmental (e.g., too much exposure to the sun produces a sunburn), interpersonal (e.g., the stress of adapting to parenthood when a new baby is born), or spiritual.

Nursing and Medicine

The American Nurses Association definition emphasizes that nursing is different from medicine. Medicine is primarily concerned with diagnosing and treating disease; nursing is concerned with giving care during the cure. This is sometimes referred to as *curing vs. caring.* Of course both nurses and physicians are capable of caring *about* patients. However, caring in this sense refers to the activities that nurses perform in *taking care of* patients; not the subjective feeling of caring *about* patients. That feeling may certainly be involved, but it does not necessarily differentiate nursing from medicine.

Medicine focuses on the pathophysiology of the disease and its physical effects on the person; nursing is concerned with the whole person, including psychosocial and spiritual responses to disease processes. Table 1–2 summarizes the differences between the concerns of nursing and medicine.

Table 1–2. Comparison of Nursing and Medical Concerns

Medical Focus	Nursing Focus
1. Diagnose and treat disease	1. Diagnose and treat human responses
2. Cure disease	2. Care for patient
3. Biological, physical effects	3. Holistic—effects on whole person

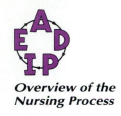

Overview of the Nursing Process

Nursing in Wellness and Illness

Nursing is concerned with the whole person, well or ill. The nurse supports ill people and helps them to solve or reduce their health problems. She also helps patients to adapt to and accept problems that cannot be treated, and helps those who are terminally ill to achieve a peaceful death. For well people, the nurse aims to prevent illness and promote wellness. This may involve a variety of activities, such as role-modeling a healthy life-style, being an advocate for community environmental changes, or teaching self-care strategies, decision-making, and problem-solving.

DEFINING THE NURSING PROCESS

The **nursing process** is a special way of thinking and acting. It is the systematic, problem-solving approach used to identify, prevent, and treat actual or potential health problems and promote wellness. It also provides the framework in which nurses use their knowledge and skills to express human caring. The nursing process can be more completely defined by explaining its relationship to the definition of nursing and its background, purpose, characteristics, and five-step organization.

Relationship to Nursing

Notice that the definition of the nursing process is similar to the definition of nursing. Nursing and the nursing process are interrelated, but nursing is more than just the nursing process. You may have an organized, systematic, deliberate approach that is, nevertheless, mechanical and lacking in warmth and caring. You may also feel deeply for a patient, want to help, and yet not have the problem-solving skills that would enable you to do so. Although the nursing process is systematic and logical, its use does not negate the caring aspect of nursing. As you master the nursing process and it becomes second nature to you, it will actually facilitate your caring.

Background

Hall (1955) first described nursing as a *process.* Johnson (1959), Orlando (1961), and Wiedenbach (1963) were among the first to use the term *nursing process* to refer to a series of steps describing the process of nursing. Since then, it has evolved from a three-step process to a five-step process.

Using the nursing process as a basis, the American Nurses Association developed standards in 1973 for evaluating the quality of care that nurses deliver (see Box 1–1 on page 13). The publication of these standards provided the impetus for a number of states to revise their nurse practice acts to include assessment, diagnosis, planning, implementation, and evaluation as legitimate parts of the nursing role. Since then, the nursing process has been accepted by virtually all nurses as the basis of their practice.

The nursing process is now taught in nearly every school of nursing and included in most state nurse practice acts. The National Council Licensure Examination for registered nurses ("state board exams") is organized around the nursing process. National accrediting bodies (e.g., the Joint Commission on Accreditation of Healthcare Organizations and the National League for Nursing) include use of the nursing process in their criteria for evaluating hospitals and schools of nursing.

Purpose

The purpose of the nursing process is to provide a framework within which nurses can assist clients in meeting their health needs. The nursing process gives deliberate direction for planning, implementing, and evaluating effective, individualized nursing care. Usually the vehicle for this is a written client-care plan. In carrying out the nursing process, the focus is always upon the client, and client input is solicited and encouraged at each step.

Characteristics

The following characteristics describe the nature of the nursing process and expand upon its definition.

1. **The nursing process is *dynamic and cyclic.*** The very concept of a process suggests change. The nursing process is an ongoing evaluation of changing client responses to nursing interventions in order to make necessary revisions in the plan of care. Previously completed steps are constantly reexamined for accuracy and appropriateness.

2. **The nursing process is *client-centered.*** The plan of care is based on the client's needs and strengths and is organized in terms of client problems rather than nursing goals. The nurse-client relationship is a therapeutic relationship, in which the client's needs always take precedence. Clients are encouraged, to the extent they are able, to exercise control over their health and to make decisions about their care.

3. **The nursing process is *goal-directed.*** Interventions are carefully considered and based on principles rather than tradition ("We've always done it that way"). The nursing orders chosen are those believed likely to bring about achievement of client goals.

4. **The nursing process is *flexible.*** The nursing process can be used with clients of any age, with any medical diagnosis, and at any point on the wellness-illness continuum. The term *client,* rather than *patient,* is sometimes used to indicate that the nursing process is not used only with ill persons. It is useful in any setting (e.g., schools, hospitals, clinics, home health, industries) and across specialties (e.g., orthopedic nursing, maternity nursing, intensive care, surgical nursing).

5. **The nursing process is *problem-oriented.*** This means that care plans are organized according to patient problems. Of course the nursing process cannot eliminate every patient problem. Some chronic health problems, such as the pain and immobility associated with arthritis, cannot be cured, even with perfect application of the nursing process. When problems cannot be eliminated, the purpose of the nursing process is to relieve them to the degree possible, to support the patient's strengths in coping with the problem, and to help patients to understand and find meaning in their situation.

6. **The nursing process is a *cognitive process.*** It involves the use of intellectual skills in problem solving and decision making. The nurse uses critical thinking to apply nursing knowledge systematically and logically to client data, enabling her to determine its meaning and plan appropriate care. This characteristic is discussed further in Chapter 2.

7. **The nursing process is *action-oriented.*** It does not stop with the plan of care, but continues on to carry out and evaluate the plan. The nurse plans, delivers, and evaluates patient care.

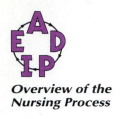

Organization: The Steps of the Nursing Process

A series of five steps makes up the nursing process. The acronym *ADPIE* may help you remember their names.

Assessment—Getting the facts

In the first step of the nursing process, the nurse collects information needed to identify client problems and plan for care. Data is collected by examining clients and talking to them and their families, and from their charts and other sources. No conclusions about the data are drawn in this step.

Example: After Maura Greenberg's baby was born, the nurse performed a comprehensive assessment upon admitting her to the postpartum unit. She recorded on the nursing history Ms. Greenberg's statements that she is often constipated, snacks frequently, doesn't drink much, and does not take laxatives.

Diagnosis—What is the problem?

During diagnosis, the nurse analyzes the collected data and then identifies the client's strengths and actual, potential, and possible health problems. Nursing diagnoses are written as precise statements of the problem situation and the etiology (or cause) of the problem. The problems identified are prioritized and provide the basis for the remaining steps.

Example: The nurse wrote the following diagnosis on Ms. Greenberg's care plan: "High Risk for Constipation related to insufficient intake of fiber and fluids."

Planning—What do you want to happen? How can you make it happen?

In the planning step, the nurse works with the client to set goals for preventing, correcting, or relieving health problems. The nurse next identifies actions that will lead to achievement of the goals. The planning stage ends when the problems, goals, and nursing orders are recorded on a care plan for the client.

Example: The nurse wrote the following on Ms. Greenberg's care plan:

Goal	Nursing Orders
Will be able to name at least six high-fiber foods before dismissal on May 16.	1. Give client the pamphlet "Fiber in Your Diet." 2. Help client fill out menu, identifying high-fiber foods. 3. Explain the relationship of fiber and fluids to bowel elimination.

Implementation—Doing, delegating, and documenting

The nurse communicates the plan of care to other members of the health-care team, for instance, at the change-of-shift report. The interventions indicated on the care plan are carried out or delegated to others. The final action in this phase is to record the care given and the client's responses on the appropriate documents (usually under "nursing progress notes" in the client's chart).

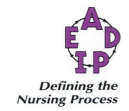

Example: The nurse took the pamphlet to Ms. Greenberg and talked with her about the importance of fiber and fluids and of preventing constipation in the postpartum period. She recorded these interventions in the nursing progress notes.

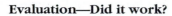Evaluation—Did it work?

In this ongoing step the nurse determines the client's progress, using the goals of care as criteria. After implementing the nursing orders, the nurse determines from the client's responses which orders were or were not helpful in achieving the goals. The nursing care plan is revised as needed. The nursing process is cyclic: the nurse must keep reexamining the previous steps of assessment, diagnosis, planning, and implementation to determine what is effective and what should be changed.

Example: Ms. Greenberg was dismissed from the hospital 24 hours after the birth of her infant. Because she had not yet had a bowel movement, the nurse advised her to continue her fluid-and-fiber regimen and to telephone her physician if she did not have a bowel movement within the next 48 hours.

Table 1–3 summarizes the five steps of the nursing process.

Sequential Steps

The steps are sequential; each step depends upon satisfactory completion of the preceding steps. For example, you must have correct data (from the assessment step) in order to make the correct nursing diagnosis (in the diagnosis step). As another example, the goals you set (in the planning step) are used to evaluate the effect of the nursing interventions (during the evaluation step).

However, the steps do not always occur in the ADPIE order; that is, you will not always perform one step completely before proceeding to the next. For example, a nurse does not always gather a complete set of data about a patient before taking action. In an emergency situation, for instance, you would quickly think of an action (planning) and implement it immediately (implementation) before doing any formal planning. Of course you would have made some observations (assessment) in order to realize that action was necessary, but the entire initial assessment step might not have been completed, and you may not have consciously formulated a problem statement. After taking action, you would evaluate whether the emergency was over, and then return to a more thorough collection and analysis of data.

Table 1–3. Nursing Process Steps	
Step	**Activities**
Assessment	Collecting and organizing data
Diagnosis	Identifying client strengths and problems
Planning	Setting goals and writing nursing orders
Implementation	Carrying out the plan of action
Evaluation	Determining if the plan was effective

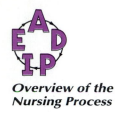

**Overview of the
Nursing Process**

Example: Carlene Collins is admitted to your unit with extreme anxiety and severe abdominal pain of unknown origin. You take whatever preliminary actions you can to relieve her pain and anxiety before attempting any in-depth data collection. When you have evaluated that her pain and anxiety are sufficiently relieved, you perform the complete admission interview and examination.

Overlapping Steps

The steps of the nursing process are distinct, and they are described separately in order to help you understand them. However, in practice they overlap a great deal. For example, even though the first encounter with a client nearly always begins with some form of data collection, assessment is actually an ongoing process. While you are bathing a client (implementation), you may at the same time be observing the condition of the skin over his bony prominences (assessment). If you observe some redness (assessment), you may conclude that the skin-integrity goals are not being met (evaluation).

RELATIONSHIP TO THE PROBLEM-SOLVING PROCESS

The nursing process is similar to the method used in making any kind of decision about a problem; the same steps are used, but in different order. In a problem-solving process, the first step is to identify the problem. The problem is then analyzed and carefully defined, and the problem statement serves as a guide for setting criteria by which to evaluate possible solutions. Data relating specifically to the problem is collected, and some solutions are generated. After considering the consequences of each, the preferred solution is put into effect, and the results are evaluated.

Example: Suppose you are on your way to an important job interview when your car breaks down. Your analysis of the situation is that your most important and most immediate need is not to repair the car but to get a job. You have specified the exact nature of your problem: Possible loss of a job opportunity caused by being late to the interview. You have the following data: (1) it is too far to walk, and (2) no one is at home to come get you. You make a quick plan. Your goal is to get there on time. You decide to walk to the nearest telephone and call a taxi for yourself and a tow truck for the car. The outcome of your plan is a fabulous job and a new car—you evaluate that the plan was successful.

Table 1-4. Comparison of the Problem-Solving Process and the Nursing Process	
Problem-Solving Process	**Nursing Process**
1. Recognizing that a problem exists	**1.** *Assessment:* Collecting all data related to the client's health
2. Analyzing and stating the problem	**2.** *Diagnosis:* Stating the problem
3. Collecting data	
4. Generating and selecting solutions	**3.** *Planning:* Setting goals, selecting interventions
5. Putting the solution into effect	**4.** *Implementation:* Taking action
6. Evaluating the results	**5.** *Evaluation:* Evaluating the results

When using the nursing process, the problem is not usually so obvious. The nurse begins with comprehensive data collection, and the data is used to identify the problem(s). The problem-solving process is slightly different, in that the problem is identified before extensive data is collected; the only information gathered is that which pertains to the problem. Table 1–4 compares these two processes.

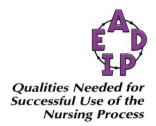

Qualities Needed for Successful Use of the Nursing Process

QUALITIES NEEDED FOR SUCCESSFUL USE OF THE NURSING PROCESS

The following qualities and attitudes of the nurse contribute to successful use of the nursing process. They are all qualities that you can further develop by awareness, effort and practice.

Intellectual (Cognitive) Skills

Nurses need to be able to think both logically and creatively in helping clients to solve their problems. Intellectual skills used in the nursing process are creative thinking, critical thinking, problem solving, and decision making.

Decision making is the process of choosing the best action to take—the action most likely to produce the desired goal. It involves deliberation, judgment, and choice. Decision making is an important skill in the problem-solving process, but not all decisions involve problem solving. Problem solving is a matter of identifying a problem from a set of data and taking steps to solve it. The problem-solving process is discussed in Chapter 4.

Creative thinking involves the ability to establish new relationships and concepts and find new solutions to problems. It is more associative than systematic. Unlike problem solving and decision making, creative thinking may not establish logical explanations for actions and may not consider possible outcomes.

Critical thinking is goal-oriented, purposeful thinking that involves a number of skills, such as evaluating the credibility of sources, making inferences, and clarifying ideas. It is an important intellectual skill and is essential to making good clinical judgments. Critical thinking is further explained in Chapter 2.

Interpersonal Skills

Interpersonal skills include the verbal and nonverbal activities used in person-to-person communication. Implementation of care takes place within the nurse-client relationship. Development of a trusting relationship depends upon the ability to communicate—to listen and to convey compassion, interest and information.

Example: Elsa is the primary nurse for a team of patients. When she notices that the nursing assistant is not using correct body mechanics to help Mr. Davis out of bed, she draws upon her interpersonal skills. She must intervene for the safety of both Mr. Davis and the assistant without embarrassing the assistant or undermining Mr. Davis's confidence in her.

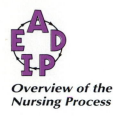

Technical Skills

Nurses use psychomotor skills to carry out various procedures and to work with high-technology equipment, such as heart monitors and respirators. They must master technical and psychomotor skills in order to bring about the desired results for clients and gain their trust.

Example: Turning a patient smoothly to minimize pain will help establish trust and rapport. If you are clumsy with this operation, the patient may not think you are competent and will be less likely to trust you in other situations. He may hesitate to ask you for information or help, and you may not be able to get important data from him.

Creativity and Curiosity

Vision and insight are needed to find new and better ways of doing things. Always ask yourself, "*Why* are we doing this? Why are we doing it *this* way?" The excellent nurse understands the rationale for every nursing activity. If she cannot find a reason for the activity or cannot show that it is having the desired effect, she works to have it discontinued.

Example: Mauricio works on a unit where most of the patients are ambulatory. One day as he was changing bed linens for a patient, he wondered, "Why am I using this draw sheet? These patients are ambulatory, and we use fitted bottom sheets." When the unit manager realized this piece of linen served no useful purpose, it was discontinued, saving both money and nursing time.

Adaptability

Always enter a situation with a tentative plan, but be flexible enough to adapt to the demands of the situation. Realize that nursing care must be adjusted as the client's needs change.

Example: According to the care plan, Mr. Akers was to be up in a chair for 15 minutes. However, as soon as he was out of bed he became pale and dizzy, so his nurse helped him back to bed instead of continuing toward the chair.

BENEFITS OF THE NURSING PROCESS

Using the nursing process as the framework for planning and giving care provides benefits for the client, the nurse, and the nursing profession.

Benefits to the Client

Because the client is the focus of nursing, the most important reasons for using the nursing process are the ways in which it benefits clients.

Continuity of Care

A written care plan provides continuity and coordination of care. Hospitals are staffed 24 hours a day, so patients are usually cared for by at least two or three RNs during a 24-hour day, depending on the staffing schedule. Each of these nurses might be competent, but if the staff does not function in a coordinated manner, patients may not perceive them as competent and begin to lose confidence that their needs will be met.

Example: Janelle Washington has just had her first baby and is having difficulty breastfeeding. The evening nurse has told her she should wake the baby up and try to feed him every two hours. The day nurse tells Ms. Washington to feed the baby on demand, because he will wake up when he gets hungry. Ms. Washington is becoming confused and discouraged. She tells her husband, "Maybe we should bottle feed the baby; this is really hard to do."

Prevention of Omission and Duplication

A systematic approach improves the quality of care by preventing omissions and duplications. Duplication of care wastes time that could be spent productively. Furthermore, it can be tiring and irritating for clients.

Example: Melissa Carpenter has just had a baby and is on a postpartum unit where the nurses use written care plans with a checklist for teaching needs. When the evening nurse arrives, she sees that the day nurse has already marked off the section on episiotomy care, so she does not reteach that information. Instead, she spends her time talking with Ms. Carpenter about care of the infant.

Individualized Care

The nursing process promotes individualized care. Each person is unique, and human responses to a disease (or any stressor) are infinitely variable. Some people are reassured by receiving a lot of detailed information; others are made anxious by it. Some people react to pain by crying and moving about; others withdraw and become very still. With a care plan to point out the client's specific, unique needs, the tendency to categorize and care for clients solely on the basis of their medical diagnosis can be avoided.

Example: On a women's care unit, the usual care of a client with a hysterectomy includes monitoring for complications and providing client teaching. Because Carol Wirth's care plan stated that she had a hearing problem, the nurses were careful to position themselves so that Ms. Wirth could read their lips and understand the preoperative teaching.

Notice that the interventions for Ms. Wirth's hearing deficit were unrelated to her most obvious stressor (hysterectomy). Because the nurses focused on the individual (Ms. Wirth) instead of the diagnosis (hysterectomy), the client's needs were successfully met.

Increased Client Participation

The nursing process encourages clients to participate more actively in their care. Clients are involved at each step of the nursing process; for instance, they provide assessment data, validate the nursing diagnoses, and give input for goal setting. Clients realize that their contributions are important and as they learn more about their bodies, they are more able to make wise health decisions.

Taking all of the above into account, you can see that the basic benefit to clients is that the nursing process improves the quality of care they receive. When the nursing process is implemented, continuous evaluation of care occurs, assuring that the client's changing needs are met.

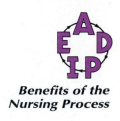

Benefits of the Nursing Process

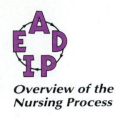

Benefits to the Nurse

The nursing process benefits not only the client, but the nurse as well.

Job Satisfaction

Using the nursing process can increase your job satisfaction. Many of the rewards in nursing come from realizing that you have helped someone. As you begin to see how the nursing process increases your ability to help, you will benefit from the satisfaction of a job well done. Additionally, good care plans will save you time, energy, and frustration, thereby increasing your ability to find creative solutions to client care. Creativity helps prevent the burnout that can result from a repetitive, "cookbook" approach to your daily work.

Continual Learning

Effective use of the nursing process fosters inquiry and continued learning by increasing your awareness of accountability to the client. As this awareness stimulates you to further develop your knowledge and skills, you will grow in your nursing role and gain pride in your professional achievements.

Increased Self-Confidence

Using care plans will increase your confidence and comfort in the nursing role. Good care plans define client problems specifically, state goals that are important to the client, and give directions for accomplishing them. This kind of specific guidance helps you to feel secure with the interventions you make.

Staffing Assignments

Nurses use written care plans when making staffing assignments. They allow quick reference to the amount and type of nursing care needed without lengthy perusal of the client's chart. This enables the nurse to assign the staff member best suited for each client. Some clients need an experienced professional nurse; for other clients an aide might provide good care with only some supervision from the professional nurse.

Standards of Practice

Successful use of the nursing process will help assure you of meeting the standards of practice for your profession. As mentioned before, the ANA has developed standards for nursing practice (Box 1–1). These are the standards to which you will be held accountable. Other organizations have developed additional standards for specialty areas of nursing. For instance NAACOG (The Organization for Obstetric, Gynecologic, & Neonatal Nurses) sets standards that apply especially to nursing care of women and infants. The ability to use the nursing process is a part of the standards of practice of all these organizations.

Benefits to the Profession

Proper use of the nursing process *promotes collaboration* among members of the nursing team as they work together to implement the care plan. Communication improves when all team members value a systematic, organized approach. As teamwork progresses, and everyone begins to feel the satisfaction of delivering effective, individualized care, the work atmosphere becomes more positive.

The nursing process *helps people to understand what nurses do*. Because of the complex nature of nursing, nurses sometimes find it difficult to define their role specifically to someone outside the profession. It is important to clearly demonstrate to the public and to other professions the contributions that nurses make to the health of individuals and to the general public. Nurses do much more than help the doctor, give medicine, and fetch the bedpan—which is how some people think of them. You can use the nursing process to show how careful assessment and problem intervention benefits clients, prevents complications, and hastens recovery.

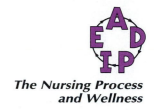

The Nursing Process and Wellness

THE NURSING PROCESS AND WELLNESS

The nursing process is applicable in health as well as illness. Under pressure for cost-containment, health care is shifting from hospitals to outpatient clinics, surgicenters, schools, the workplace, and the home. Some predict that by the year 2010 the nature of hospitals will change dramatically, and nurses will increasingly be working in nontraditional settings (Aydelotte, 1987). Nurses in such settings frequently work with well clients and focus on health promotion, health protection, and disease prevention. **Health-promotion** activities (e.g., moderate, daily exercise) are directed toward achieving a higher level of wellness; they are not aimed at avoiding any particular disease. **Health protection** focuses on activities that decrease environmental threats to health (e.g., air pollution). **Disease prevention** involves actions that help to prevent specific health problems or diseases (e.g., immunizations, prenatal care).

While most of the national health budget is still spent on care and treatment of illnesses, health-promotion initiatives are receiving increased attention from government agencies. The U.S. Public Health Service, in *Healthy People 2000* (1990), outlines a national strategy for improving the health of the nation during the coming decade. In this report, they acknowledge that health promotion and

---

Box 1–1. American Nurses Association Standards of Nursing Practice

  I. The collection of data about the health status of the client/patient is systematic and continuous. The data are accessible, communicated, and recorded.

  II. Nursing diagnoses are derived from health-status data.

  III. The plan of nursing care includes goals derived from the nursing diagnoses.

  IV. The plan of nursing care includes priorities and the prescribed nursing approaches or measures to achieve the goals derived from the nursing diagnoses.

  V. Nursing actions provide for client/patient participation in health promotion, maintenance, and restoration.

  VI. The nursing actions assist the client/patient to maximize his health capabilities.

  VII. The client/patient's progress or lack of progress toward goal achievement is determined by the client/patient and the nurse.

  VIII. The client/patient's progress or lack of progress toward goal achievement directs reassessment, reordering of priorities, new goal setting, and revision of the plan of nursing care.

From *Standards of Nursing Practice*, © 1973 by American Nurses Association, Kansas City, MO. Reprinted with permission.

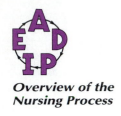

Overview of the Nursing Process

disease prevention provide the best opportunities for preserving our health-care resources. The broad goals outlined in this report follow:

1. Increase the span of healthy life for Americans.
2. Reduce health disparities among population groups.
3. Achieve access to preventive services for all Americans.

Table 1–5 is a list of specific objectives (priorities) contributing to achievement of these goals. These target areas can be used to guide nursing assessment and interventions for well clients.

Consider how the nursing process might work in the following case study. Phases of the nursing process are underlined.

Example: Judy Witkowski is a 40-year-old corporate executive. Her company requires her to have an annual physical exam, so she has come to the company nurse. The nurse takes a complete health history (<u>assessment</u>), which reveals no past medical problems, except that Ms. Witkowski's father died of a heart attack when he was 62 years old. The nurse performs a complete physical

Table 1–5. U.S. Public Health Service Priorities for the Year 2000	
Goals	**Objectives**
Health Promotion	**1.** Increase physical activity and fitness.
	2. Improve nutrition.
	3. Reduce use of tobacco.
	4. Reduce alcohol and other drug abuse.
	5. Improve family planning.
	6. Improve mental health and prevent mental disorders.
	7. Reduce violent and abusive behavior.
	8. Enhance educational and community-based programs.
Health Protection	**9.** Reduce unintentional injuries.
	10. Improve occupational safety and health.
	11. Improve environmental health.
	12. Ensure food and drug safety.
	13. Improve oral health.
Preventive Services	**14.** Improve maternal and infant health.
	15. Reduce heart disease and stroke.
	16. Prevent and control cancer.
	17. Reduce diabetes and chronic disabling conditions.
	18. Prevent and control HIV infection.
	19. Reduce sexually transmitted diseases.
	20. Increase immunization and prevent infectious diseases.
	21. Expand access and use of clinical preventive services.
Surveillance and Data Systems	**22.** Improve surveillance and data systems.

From *Healthy People 2000: National Health Promotion and Disease Prevention Objectives.* DHHS Publication No. (PHS) 91-50212. Washington, DC: U.S. Government Printing Office.

examination (<u>assessment</u>) and discovers no physical problems: Ms. Witkowski's blood pressure is 120/74 and her pulse is 84; she is 10 lb. overweight. The nurse also asks her about her health habits and life-style. He discovers that Judy works long hours and often takes work home; her only exercise is an occasional golf game; she eats a balanced diet and gets about 7 hours of sleep a day; and she smokes a pack of cigarettes per day. Ms. Witkowski's lab results and chest X ray provide no indication of an existing health problem.

If nursing were concerned only with ill persons, Ms. Witkowski's nurse would analyze this data, diagnose that no problem exists, and conclude that no interventions are needed (<u>diagnosis</u>). However, he takes a holistic perspective rather than a disease-oriented one, and understands the importance of nursing in disease prevention and health promotion. The nurse diagnoses that Ms. Witkowski has unmet health-promotion needs (<u>diagnosis</u>). Using input from Ms. Witkowski, he sets broad goals (<u>planning</u>) that she will (1) become aware of ways in which her life-style can either increase or decrease her risk of disease and (2) experience improved health status, as evidenced by quitting smoking, instituting an exercise program, and maintaining her present weight. The nurse does not include a goal that she will reduce her work hours, since Judy insists that she needs to work long hours, that she enjoys it, and that she has no interest in changing that behavior.

The nurse writes the goals on Ms. Witkowski's care plan and chooses nursing orders (<u>planning</u>) aimed at meeting the goals. To reach Goal 1, the nurse will talk with Judy about the effect of smoking on coronary and peripheral circulation, and about the relationship of exercise and diet to weight control. To meet Goal 2, he will give her printed information about the four basic food groups, a "Stop Smoking" pamphlet, and a booklet of suggested aerobic exercises. He also encourages her to attend the company-sponsored Stop Smoking Clinic (<u>implementation</u>). He does not refer her to a dietitian, since she seems adequately informed and motivated to avoid gaining weight when she stops smoking. Judy and the nurse include in the plan that she will return in a month to be weighed. At that time, they will also evaluate her efforts to stop smoking and institute an exercise program (<u>evaluation</u>). If goals are being met, the nurse plans to assess Judy's stress level and coping mechanisms to see what effect, if any, her strenuous work schedule may be having on her. At that point, modifications may be made in her care plan (<u>evaluation</u>).

Summary

The nursing process
- ✓ is a systematic problem-solving approach to delivering holistic care to well and ill clients.
- ✓ benefits clients, nurses, and the nursing profession.
- ✓ consists of five interrelated steps—assessment, diagnosis, planning, implementation, and evaluation.
- ✓ is client centered, goal directed, systematic, and flexible.
- ✓ requires special nursing knowledge and skills in order to be used successfully.

Skill-Building Activities

(Answer Key, p. 373)

1. Brian Callaway <u>has smoked two packs of cigarettes a day for the past 30 years</u>. He has just been told that his chest X ray shows some suspicious <u>lesions on his lung</u> and that he will need a <u>biopsy</u> to see if he has lung cancer. Mr. Callaway says <u>he coughs a lot</u> and that <u>he becomes short of breath when climbing stairs</u>. Which of the underlined data items are appropriate phenomena of concern to the nurse, and which ones are medical concerns?

   Nursing Concerns   *Medical Concerns*

2. What is the most important purpose of the nursing process?

3. Match each stage of the nursing process with the examples of activities that occur in that stage.

   a. Assessment   **1.** ____ Writing short-term objectives

   b. Diagnosis   **2.** ____ Conducting a nursing interview

   c. Planning   **3.** ____ Writing nursing orders on the care plan

   d. Implementation   **4.** ____ Carrying out the nursing orders

   e. Evaluation   **5.** ____ Charting the care given to the client

                              6. ____ Performing a physical examination

                              7. ____ Giving the client a bedbath

                              8. ____ Using client data to decide whether goals have been met

                              9. ____ Stating the client's problem and its cause

4. The nurse has written a care plan for his patient. The next day, after the nursing orders have been implemented by the nurses on the other two shifts, he evaluates the patient's responses, determines that some goals have not been met, reexamines the nursing diagnoses for accuracy, and writes some new nursing orders aimed at goal achievement. Check the quality (qualities) of the nursing process that this example illustrates. The nursing process is

____ dynamic/cyclic.   ____ a series of overlapping steps.
____ client-centered.   ____ a series of sequential steps.
____ goal-directed.

5. What qualities of the nurse are being demonstrated in the following examples? Choose the correct quality from the list below:

Adaptability   Interpersonal skills
Creativity and curiosity   Technical skills
Intellectual skills

a. _____ The nurse sits quietly while an elderly client reminisces about old friends.

b. _____ The student nurse practices catheterization in the school lab.

c. _____ The student nurse performs the critical thinking activities in this text.

d. _____ The head nurse works on a unit with ambulatory patients. All the beds have draw sheets on them. When he discovers no one can give a reason for using the draw sheets, the nurse has the staff stop using them, saving time and money for the hospital.

e. _____ The care plan says the patient's dressing should be changed at 0900 and 2100. At 0900, Mr. Sanchez has the first visitor he has had in his three-week hospital stay. His nurse decides to postpone his dressing change until his visitor leaves.

6. Read the following case study.

Alma Boiko had been in an intermediate care facility since having a stroke that left her unable to care for herself. When she developed pneumonia, she was transferred to a hospital. Juan Apodaca, RN, settled her comfortably in bed and briefly interviewed her about her symptoms. He obtained a temperature of 101° F, pulse 120, respirations 32, and B/P of 100/68. Juan examined Ms. Boiko's chart to obtain a history of her illness and a record of her nursing care. He applied oxygen by nasal cannula, as ordered by the physician. When performing the physical examination, Juan noticed a reddened area over Ms. Boiko's coccyx.

Because she was unable to move about in bed, he wrote a diagnosis of "High Risk for Impaired Skin Integrity over coccyx related to constant pressure to bony prominences caused by inability to move about in bed." He set a goal that the skin on Ms. Boiko's coccyx would remain intact, and that the redness would be gone within 2 days. He wrote nursing orders for skin care, a schedule for turning Ms. Boiko every 2 hours, and orders for frequent, continued observation of her skin.

Two days later, while bathing Ms. Boiko, Juan observed that her coccygeal area was still red, a small area of skin was peeling off, and there was some serous drainage. Juan concluded that the goal had not been met. He was sure his data was adequate, and he changed his nursing diagnosis to "Actual Impaired Skin Integrity over coccyx. . . ." When asked, the other staff members assured Juan that the 2-hour turning schedule had been carried out, except for 6 hours at night when Ms. Boiko was left to sleep undisturbed. Even though turning every 2 hours while awake was a standard of care on that unit and had been adequate for other clients, Juan concluded that this was not often enough for Ms. Boiko. He decided to change the order on the care plan to read "Turn every 2 hours around the clock."

a. Label the underlined activities *A, D, P, I,* or *E,* according to the step of the nursing process represented by the activity.

b. List below all the client data (human responses) Juan obtained.

c. Circle the activities that show the cyclic nature of the nursing process.

d. List all the nursing orders described in the case. (Note that some are summarized in the case study instead of being fully written out in nursing-order format.)

e. Where in the case study do you see the most obvious example of overlapping in the nursing process steps?

f. How did Juan demonstrate the nursing qualities of creativity and adaptability in Ms. Boiko's care?

g. Ordering a turning schedule that was more frequent than usual for Ms. Boiko benefited her by providing which of the following?

(1) Continuity of care
(2) Freedom from omission and duplication
(3) Individualized care
(4) Maximum client participation in care

REFERENCES

American Nurses Association. (1973). *Standards of Nursing Practice*. Kansas City, MO.

American Nurses Association. (1980). *Nursing: A Social Policy Statement*. Kansas City, MO.

American Nurses Association. (1985). *Code for Nurses with Interpretive Statements*. Kansas City, MO.

Aydelotte, M. (1987). Nursing's preferred future. *Nursing Outlook, 35*(3): 114–20.

Carper, B. (1978). Fundamental patterns of knowing in nursing. *Advances in Nursing Science, 1:* 13–23.

Hall, L. (1955). Quality of nursing care. *Public Health News* (June). New Jersey State Department of Health.

Johnson, D. (1959). A philosophy for nursing diagnosis. *Nursing Outlook, 7:*198–200.

Johnson, D. (1961). The significance of nursing care. *American Journal of Nursing, 61*(11): 63–66.

Johnson, D. (1980). The behavioral system model for nursing. In Riehl, J., and Roy, C., eds., *Conceptual Models for Nursing Practice*. 2nd ed. New York: Appleton-Century-Crofts, 207–16.

Neuman, B. (1972). The Betty Neuman model: A total person approach to viewing patient problems. *Nursing Research, 21*(3): 264–69.

Neuman, B. (1980). The Betty Neuman health-care systems model: A total person approach to patient problems. In Riehl, J., and Roy, C., eds., *Conceptual Models for Nursing Practice*. New York: Appleton-Century-Crofts.

Nightingale, F. (1969). *Notes on Nursing. What it Is, What it Is Not*. New York: Dover Publications. Originally published in 1859.

Orem, D. (1971). *Nursing: Concepts of Practice*. New York: McGraw-Hill.

Orlando, I. (1961). *The Dynamic Nurse-Patient Relationship*. New York: G. P. Putnam's Sons.

Parse, R. (1974). *Nursing Fundamentals*. Flushing, New York: Medical Examination Publishing.

Parse, R. (1981). *Man-Living-Health: A Theory of Nursing*. New York: John Wiley & Sons.

Parse, R. (1987). *Nursing Science: Major Paradigms, Theories, and Critiques*. Philadelphia: W. B. Saunders.

Peplau, H. (1952). *Interpersonal Relations in Nursing*. New York: G. P. Putnam's Sons.

Rogers, M. (1970). *The Theoretical Basis of Nursing*. Philadelphia: F. A. Davis.

Rogers, M. (1980). Nursing: A science of unitary man. In Riehl, J., and Roy, C., eds., *Conceptual Models for Nursing Practice*. 2nd ed. New York: Appleton-Century-Crofts.

Roy, C. (1970). A conceptual framework for nursing. *Nursing Outlook, 18*(3): 42–45.

Roy, C. (1976). *Introduction to Nursing: An Adaptation Model*. Englewood Cliffs, NJ: Prentice Hall.

Roy, C. (1980). The Roy adaptation model. In Riehl, J., and Roy, C., eds., *Conceptual Models for Nursing Practice*. 2nd ed. New York: Appleton-Century-Crofts.

Travelbee, J. (1971). *Intervention in Psychiatric Nursing*. Philadelphia: F. A. Davis.

U.S. Department of Health and Human Services, Public Health Service. (1990). *Healthy People 2000*. DHHS Publication No. (PHS) 91-50212. Washington, DC: Superintendent of Documents, U.S. Government Printing Office.

Wiedenbach, E. (1963). The helping art of nursing. *American Journal of Nursing, 63*(11): 54–57.

Wiedenbach, E. (1964). *Clinical Nursing: A Helping Art*. New York: Springer.

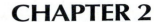

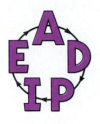

CHAPTER 2

CRITICAL THINKING AND THE NURSING PROCESS

OBJECTIVES

Upon completing this chapter, you should be able to do the following:
- Define critical thinking.
- Explain the importance of critical thinking for nurses.
- Discuss the relationship between critical thinking and the nursing process.
- Describe some important critical-thinking skills.
- Critically examine the merits of the nursing process and its use in nursing practice.

WHY NURSES NEED TO THINK CRITICALLY

Education is more than storing up facts. A truly educated person is able to use critical thinking to *do* something with the information she has acquired: e.g., solve problems, create new information, or gain self-knowledge. Nursing decisions can profoundly affect the lives of others; in fact, they may be concerned with matters of life and death. Because of the nature of their discipline and the nature of their work, nurses must be educated people—critical thinkers.

Nursing Is an Applied Discipline

A discipline is a field of study. An *applied* discipline, like music, law, or nursing, requires performance, not just knowledge of facts. If someone is an expert on music history, has memorized the scales and chords in all keys, and can even read music—you still wouldn't recognize him as a musician unless he performs his art by singing or playing an instrument. The same is true of a nurse. She is not actually "performing" until she uses her knowledge to interpret data and apply it in caring for patients. Applying knowledge is a critical thinking skill. Nurses need to think critically in order to apply knowledge of general principles to specific cases.

Types of Nursing Knowledge

Critical thinking is not exercised in a vacuum. It is used to apply a basic core of knowledge to each client situation. The nurse's fund of knowledge affects her ability to use cognitive, interpersonal, or technical skills effectively. Four "patterns of knowing" make up the basic core of nursing knowledge: nursing science, nursing art, nursing ethics, and personal knowledge (Carper, 1978; Ziegler et al., 1986).

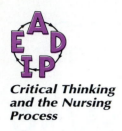

**Critical Thinking
and the Nursing
Process**

Scientific Knowledge   In the field of nursing, scientific knowledge consists of research findings and conceptual models of nursing (e.g., Roy's Adaptation model, 1980; Neuman's Systems model, 1972), as well as theoretical explanations and research findings from other fields and disciplines (e.g., physiology, psychology). It is used to describe, explain, and predict.

For example, nurses must have scientific knowledge to understand the nature of a helping relationship and know how to use verbal and nonverbal communication techniques. Because nursing takes place in the context of interpersonal relationships, nurses use interpersonal skills to interact with patients, families and other health team members (for instance, to communicate caring and support to a client during a technical procedure). Some examples of interpersonal skills are active listening, conveying interest, giving clear explanations, comforting, making referrals, and sharing attitudes, feelings, and knowledge. Other interpersonal skills, such as managing, delegating, and evaluating, are used when supervising the care given by other team members.

Another specific example of scientific knowledge is understanding the effect of sociocultural and developmental factors on client behavior. When working directly with clients or when supervising other team members who are performing delegated tasks, knowledge of change theory and motivational theory are useful.

Scientific knowledge also includes the facts and information necessary for performing technical skills (i.e., principles of the skill, steps of the procedure, knowledge of the equipment). Technical skills (also called psychomotor skills) are used in performing a variety of hands-on skills, such as changing dressings, giving injections, turning and positioning patients, attaching a client to a monitor, and suctioning a tracheostomy. They are often task-oriented and involve direct contact with the client. For well clients, the nurse might use technical skills to teach CPR (cardiopulmonary resuscitation) to a group, or use a slide projector when teaching a high school class about sexually transmitted diseases.

When procedures are done skillfully, nursing actions are more likely to be successful (e.g., if bed linens are not taut and wrinkle-free, the plan to protect the client's skin integrity may fail). Competent performance of technical skills also helps build rapport with the client. If the nurse can turn and reposition a client confidently and with minimal discomfort, the client perceives her as someone who can help, and trust is established.

The Art of Nursing   The art of a profession is the *way* in which its practitioners express their knowledge. Scientific knowledge is acquired by scientific investigation; art involves feelings gained by subjective experience. Scientific knowledge can be verified and explained to others; but nursing art is more difficult to describe. It is through the art of nursing that nurses express caring; therefore it must include affective considerations, such as attitudes, beliefs, and values.

Sensitivity and empathy are important facets of this mode of knowing. They enable the nurse to be aware of the client's perspective and attentive to verbal and nonverbal cues to his psychological state. **Empathy** is the ability to imagine what another person is feeling. A nurse who is highly skilled in empathizing with patients has a wider range of interventions available for providing effective, satisfying nursing care (Carper, 1978).

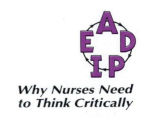

Ethical Knowledge   Ethical knowledge refers to knowledge of accepted professional standards of conduct. It is concerned with matters of obligation, or what ought to be done, and it consists of information about basic moral principles and processes for determining right and wrong actions. Nurses are accountable to clients and to each other for the ethical performance of their work. Whether developed formally or informally, the ethics of a profession represent the traditions and values of the group.

A **professional code of ethics** is a formal set of written statements reflecting the goals and values of the profession. Formal codes define professional expectations and provide a framework for making ethical decisions. Appendix A, the American Nurses Association "Code for Nurses" (1985), is an example of one formal code of ethics for nurses.

The informal ethics of a profession are based on **conventional moral principles**—those which are widely held in a profession, expressed in practice, and enforced by rewards and sanctions (e.g., approval or disapproval of fellow professionals). The conventional moral principles of nursing are those unwritten values that are rooted in nurses' more general moral views, their experiences, and the history of the profession. The following are four important conventional principles of the nursing profession:

1. Nurses have an obligation to be competent.
2. The good of patients should be the nurse's primary concern.
3. Nurses should not use their positions to exploit patients.
4. Nurses should be loyal to each other. (Jameton, 1984, p. 73)

Personal Knowledge   Personal knowing is concerned with encountering, knowing, and actualizing one's *self*. It involves knowing self in relation to another human being and interacting on a person-to-person rather than a role-to-role basis. This pattern of knowing enables nurses to approach patients as people rather than objects, and to establish therapeutic relationships. The more highly developed the nurse's self-awareness and self-knowledge, and the better her self-concept, the more attuned to the patient she is likely to be (Carper, 1978).

Practice Wisdom   Practice wisdom is acquired from intuition, tradition, authority, trial and error, and experience (Ziegler et al., 1986). It provides the basis for much of the nursing care that is given during the implementation step. As a broader, research-based body of knowledge is developed, nurses will come to depend less on practice wisdom. Meanwhile, you should refine and use your critical thinking skills to evaluate strategies based on practice wisdom, and continue to seek new scientific and ethical knowledge as it becomes available.

Nursing Draws on Knowledge from Other Fields

Some professionals, like chemists or mathematicians, are concerned almost exclusively with the single body of knowledge that makes up their field. This is not the case for nurses. Because nursing deals holistically with human responses, nurses must draw meaningful information from other subject areas (such as physiology, nutrition, psychology, etc.) in order to understand the meaning of client data and plan effective interventions. Using insight from one subject to shed light on another, as nurses do, requires critical thinking skills.

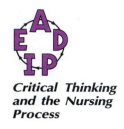

Critical Thinking and the Nursing Process

Nurses Deal with Change in Stressful Environments

The rapidly changing situations in which nurses work make it especially important for them to think critically. Treatments, medications, and technology change constantly, and a patient's condition may change from minute to minute. Therefore, routine behaviors, or "the usual procedure," may not be adequate for the situation at hand. Knowing the routine for giving nine o'clock medications may not help you to deal with a patient who is frightened of injections, or one who does not wish to take a medication. The clinical environment is fast-paced and sometimes hectic; nurses must base their decisions on knowledge and rational thinking in order to respond appropriately under stress.

Nurses Make Frequent, Varied, and Important Decisions

During the course of a workday, a nurse makes decisions of many kinds. These are not trivial decisions; they often involve a client's well-being, even her survival, so it is important that the decisions be good ones. Nurses use critical thinking skills to collect and interpret information and make sound judgments that contribute to good decisions. They must use good judgment to decide which of their many observations to report to physicians and which to handle on their own. While the level of decision-making may vary, all health-care personnel need to use critical thinking.

Example: Part of Edna Clay's assignment as a nursing assistant is to answer patients' call lights. She has been told in report which patients are on bedrest and which ones need help to ambulate. She has helped Ms. Porter to the bathroom three times in the past 3 hours. Realizing that Ms. Porter usually does not void this often, Edna decides to give this information to the RN now instead of waiting until the end-of-shift report.

THE NATURE OF CRITICAL THINKING

By now you may be wondering, What is critical thinking? Do I do it? How can I tell when others are doing it?

Definition

Critical thinking is a purposeful mental activity in which ideas are produced and evaluated and judgments are made. According to Paul (1988b), **critical thinking** is disciplined, self-directed, rational thinking that "certifies what we know and makes clear wherein we are ignorant. . . ." It is "the art of thinking about your thinking while you're thinking so as to make your thinking more clear, precise, accurate, relevant, consistent, and fair" (pp. 2–3).

Critical thinking is both an attitude and a skill. As you might expect of such a complex behavior, there is no single, simple definition for it. However, it has some characteristics that will help you to know when it is taking place.

Characteristics

Critical thinking involves conceptualization. Conceptualization is the intellectual process of forming a concept. A **concept** is a mental image of reality. In conceptualization, an abstract idea is generalized from particular instances, and exists as a symbol in the mind. Concepts are ideas about events, objects, and properties, as well as the relationships between them. Nursing uses concepts about two kinds of reality: (1) **properties**, or the way things are; and (2) **processes**, or the way things happen. A property concept, for example, might be about the patient's level of anxiety, or whether his incision is infected. A process concept might be about how morphine works in the central nervous system, or what the patient experiences when he is in pain (Kim, 1983, pp. 8–10).

Critical thinking is rational and reasonable. This is the most obvious feature of critical thinking. Reason and **rationality** refer to the fact that the thinking is based on reasons rather than prejudice, preferences, self-interest, or fears. Suppose you decide to vote for the Democratic candidate in an election because your family has always voted for Democrats. That decision is based on preference, prejudice, and, possibly, self-interest. On the other hand, suppose you had taken time to reflect on what the candidate said about the issues in the election, and had based your choice on that. In that case, even though you might still have voted for the Democrat, you would have been thinking rationally, using facts and observations to draw your conclusions.

Critical thinking is reflective. This means that the person who thinks critically does not jump to conclusions or make a hurried decision, but takes the time to collect data and then think the matter through in a disciplined manner, weighing facts and evidence.

Critical thinking is, in part, an attitude. It is an attitude of inquiry. A critical thinker examines existing claims and statements to see if they are true or valid rather than blindly accepting them. In response to a claim like, "Fords are better than Chevrolets," a critical thinker might ask: (1) What do you mean by "better than"; better in what ways? and (2) What information do you have that this is so? Critical thinkers are skeptical, but constructively so. They ask, "Why?" and "How?"

Critical thinking is autonomous thinking. A critical thinker thinks for himself. He does not passively accept the beliefs of others, but analyzes the issues and decides which authorities are credible. For example, he uses critical thinking to examine beliefs acquired as a child, accepting them for rational reasons or rejecting those he has been holding for the wrong reasons. Because they will not accept or reject a belief they do not understand, critical thinkers are not easily manipulated.

Critical thinking includes creative thinking. Creative thinking is a productive intellectual skill that creates original ideas by establishing relationships among thoughts and concepts. It involves the ability to break up and transfer a concept to new settings or uses. For example, the concept of *brick* could be thought of along the lines of its molecular structure, its dimensions, its color, its effect on the economy, its hardness, its ability to transfer heat, and so on. Whatever the idea is, the creative thinker is able to transfer it—to find it again in other settings (e.g., a remembered smell, a relationship, a psychomotor

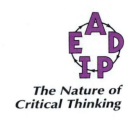

The Nature of Critical Thinking

25

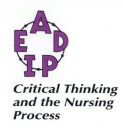

Critical Thinking and the Nursing Process

procedure). The creative thinker does not simply memorize and evaluate existing knowledge; she creates alternative courses of action, makes reasonable hypotheses and finds new solutions to problems.

Creative thinking involves more or less random thought and occurs at different levels of consciousness. It may not establish logical explanations for actions, especially when the problem is unusual; nor does it necessarily consider possible outcomes in forming the new idea. Creative thinking, however, is directed, even though it is more random than systematic. **Directed thinking** is purposeful and goal-directed, unlike **associative thinking**, which involves random, unstructured thoughts (for example, daydreaming).

Critical thinking is fair thinking. The critical thinker attempts to remove bias and one-sidedness from his own thinking and to recognize it in others. This requires him to examine the reasons for his choices and decisions. It also requires an awareness of his own values and feelings and a willingness to examine the basis for them.

Critical thinking focuses on deciding what to believe or do. Critical thinking is used to evaluate arguments and conclusions, create new ideas or alternative courses of action, decide upon a course of action, produce reliable observations, draw sound conclusions, and solve problems. The critical thinker uses accepted standards to examine her own views as well as the views of others; she does the following (Paul, 1988a):

1. Explores the thinking that underlies her emotions and feelings.
2. Suspends judgments when she lacks sufficient evidence.
3. Develops criteria for evaluation and applies them fairly and accurately.
4. Evaluates the credibility of sources used to justify beliefs.
5. Makes interdisciplinary connections and uses insights from one subject to illuminate and correct other subjects.
6. Distinguishes facts from ideals and what she would like to be from what she is.
7. Examines assumptions that underlie thoughts and behavior.
8. Distinguishes the relevant from the irrelevant, and the important from the trivial.
9. Makes plausible inferences and distinguishes conclusions from the reasoning that supports them.
10. Seeks out evidence and gives evidence when questioned.

Necessary Traits of Mind

Seven interdependent traits of mind are essential to becoming a critical thinker (Paul, 1988b), and they are best developed simultaneously. It may take *courage,* for instance, to become aware of the limits of your knowledge and develop *intellectual humility.* The seven traits follow.

1. **Intellectual humility.** Humility involves being aware of the limits of your knowledge and sensitive to the possibility of self-deception. It includes being sensitive to the bias and prejudice in your views. This trait is based on the recognition that no one should claim more than he really knows. Humility does not imply submissiveness or false modesty, but absence of intellectual conceit.

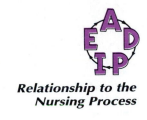

2. **Intellectual courage.** This involves the willingness to listen to and examine fairly ideas to which you may have a strong, negative reaction. This type of courage comes from recognizing that the beliefs of those around you, or your own beliefs, are sometimes false or misleading. Inevitably, you will come to see some truth in ideas you had considered dangerous, and some falsity in ideas strongly held in your social group. Courage is needed to be true to your thinking in such cases, especially as social penalties for nonconformity may be severe.

3. **Intellectual empathy.** You must be aware of the need to imagine yourself in the place of others in order to understand them. This trait requires that you recognize the human tendency to identify as "truth" our own longstanding beliefs or immediate perceptions. Intellectual empathy gives you the ability to reason from the viewpoints of others.

4. **Intellectual good faith (integrity).** This means that you apply the same rigorous standards of proof to your own evidence that you apply to the evidence of others. It requires that you honestly admit inconsistencies and error in your own thought and actions.

5. **Intellectual perseverance.** You must be willing to seek intellectual insights and truths in spite of difficulties and frustrations, even when others oppose your search. You may need to struggle with unsettled questions over a long period of time to achieve understanding and insight.

6. **Faith in reason.** Be confident that it is in your own best interest, and in the interests of others as well, to develop in yourself and in others the ability to think rationally. This implies faith that people can learn to think for themselves and become reasonable, despite deep-seated tendencies of the mind to do otherwise.

7. **Intellectual sense of justice.** This requires that you assess all viewpoints with the same standards and do not base your judgments on self-interest or the interests of your friends, community, or nation. It implies that you will hold to intellectual standards without seeking your own advantage.

RELATIONSHIP TO THE NURSING PROCESS

Recall from Chapter 1 that the nursing process is a problem-solving method that involves decision making. **Critical thinking is an essential part of problem solving and decision making.** Therefore, it is essential to most aspects of the nursing process. However, even though critical thinking and the nursing process are closely related, they are not identical. **People use critical thinking in many situations outside the nursing process and in many situations in which there is no problem to solve.** For example, you think critically about what television commercials ask you to believe, and about the claims made by politicians. Figure 2–1 illustrates the relationship between critical thinking and the nursing process.

The Problem-Solving Process

Problem solving is the process of identifying a problem and then planning and taking steps to resolve it. The nursing process is one example of a problem-solving method; other methods include trial-and-error, intuition, and the scientific method.

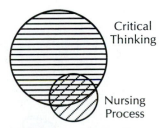

Critical Thinking

Nursing Process

Figure 2–1. Relationship of Critical Thinking to the Nursing Process

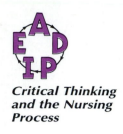

Critical Thinking and the Nursing Process

Using the **trial-and-error** method, you would try a number of solutions until you found one that worked. This is not a systematic approach, and you would probably not know why one solution worked and another did not. It is not recommended for nurses because it is inefficient and sometimes dangerous.

Intuition is the "direct apprehension of a situation based upon a background of similar and dissimilar situations and embodied intelligence or skill" (Benner and Tanner, 1984, p. 295). Schraeder and Fischer (1987) call it "immediate knowing of something without the conscious use of reason" (p. 46). Using the intuitive method, you would rely on an inner sense to provide the solution to the problem. Experienced nurses sometimes describe instances in which they somehow sensed something was wrong, and even though they could not say what prompted the feeling, they took quick action. Intuitive problem solving is neither systematic nor data-based. As a beginning practitioner, you should be cautious about flashes of intuition and discuss them with colleagues before acting upon them.

The **scientific method** is a systematic, logical approach to problem solving, based on data and hypothesis testing. You may recall from Chapter 1 that the nursing process is similar to the scientific method. Formal, deliberative problem solving is used primarily in the diagnosis and planning steps. The implementation step parallels hypothesis testing in the scientific method: in this step the nursing orders (hypotheses) are actually put into action (tested) to see if they achieve the client goals (if the hypothesis is valid).

Decision making is an important aspect of problem solving and critical thinking. Nurses make decisions in each step of the nursing process, and all problem solving requires some decisions; however, decision making is used in *other* than problem-solving situations. Nurses make value decisions (e.g., to keep client information confidential), time-management decisions (e.g., to take clean linens to the client's room at the same time as the medication in order to save steps), and scheduling decisions (e.g., to bathe the patient before visiting hours). They make decisions about which interventions are most urgent, about delegating care to others, and about whether and when to notify a physician about a client's status.

Some kinds of problem-solving may not require critical thinking. For example, in many math problems you can simply plug numbers into a formula. But the quality of a solution, especially when a problem is complex, depends heavily upon the quality of the thinking that produces it. Because nursing decisions involve many variables, nurses must think critically in order to use the nursing process effectively.

Relationship to Each Step of the Nursing Process

From the preceding sections of this chapter, you have an idea of the nature of critical thinking. Now consider some examples of how critical thinking is used in the steps of the nursing process. Table 2–1 provides an overview.

The Assessment Step

The ability to make reliable observations and to *distinguish relevant from irrelevant information* is a fundamental skill of critical thinking upon which the other critical thinking skills, such as validating, categorizing, and organizing data, are built. In the assessment phase of the nursing process, the nurse uses critical thinking skills to gather data about the patient and to validate what the patient says with what she observes. She discards information that is irrelevant or unimportant; a **relevant** fact pertains to the topic; an **irrelevant** fact does not.

Example: Martin Fry is assessing Mr. Wiley's skin. He notes that it is dry and thin and has poor turgor. This is relevant information that Martin will use in diagnosing High Risk for Impaired Skin Integrity. In this assessment, Martin also notices that Mr. Wiley has a 4-inch, white, contracted scar on his lower abdomen. This is obviously an old scar and is now irrelevant to Martin's diagnosis.

Nurses must also *distinguish between important and unimportant data.* Data can be accurate, perhaps even relevant, yet unimportant. The following example, itself relevant but unimportant, illustrates this point.

Example: Suppose you counted all the hairs on a patient's head and found that he had 350 hairs. This would be accurate if the count were confirmed, perhaps by another counter. It would be relevant if you were trying to establish that he is nearly bald. However, the actual hair count is not very important, even to establish baldness—and certainly not to his overall well-being.

During the assessment phase, the nurse *organizes and categorizes* the relevant, important data in some useful manner, usually according to a theory-based nursing framework. This, too, requires critical thinking.

The Diagnosis Step
Finding patterns and relationships and making sound inferences is an important critical thinking skill; it is the main skill used in making nursing diagnoses.

Table 2–1. Overview of Critical Thinking Throughout the Nursing Process	
The Nursing Process	**Critical-Thinking Skills**
ASSESSMENT	Observing Distinguishing relevant from irrelevant data Distinguishing important from unimportant data Validating data Organizing data Categorizing data
DIAGNOSIS	Finding patterns and relationships Making inferences Stating the problem Suspending judgment
PLANNING	Generalizing Transferring knowledge from one situation to another Developing evaluative criteria Hypothesizing
IMPLEMENTATION	Applying knowledge Testing hypotheses
EVALUATION	Deciding whether hypotheses are correct Making criterion-based evaluations

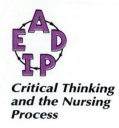

Critical Thinking and the Nursing Process

You form concepts by generalizing from personal experience, impressions, theories, and other knowledge. When you see patterns in a set of particular examples, such as dog, cat, bear, and elephant, you generalize to form the concept *animal*. A **generalization** is the relationship between two or more concepts, such as the qualities dogs, cats, bears, and elephants have in common, that makes them fit the concept *animal*.

You make **inferences** when you tentatively assign meaning to data that you see or hear. You may not know for sure what the data means, but you may believe you do, perhaps on the basis of past experience.

Example: You see your dog standing outside the door. You know she is there because you can see her—you have clear evidence. But suppose you are inside your house and you hear a scratching noise at the front door. You might again believe your dog is standing at the door, but this time the evidence is different. You don't actually see the dog, but the sound you hear makes you **infer** that she is at the door.

Obviously, some inferences are supported by more or better evidence than others. If you hear your dog's chain rattling and hear her barking as well as scratching at the door, you could be pretty sure she is outside the door (Wilbraham et al., 1990).

"Generalizing inferences can be defined as conclusions that summarize a series of observations to suggest a pattern, on which explanations and predictions can be based" (Eggen and Kauchak, 1988, p. 28). When diagnosing, nurses draw inferences from cues provided by client data. It is important for their inferences to be correct.

A critical thinker suspends judgment when evidence is lacking. This is what nurses do when they identify a possible rather than an actual or potential patient problem. Nurses must weigh the evidence and decide if their conclusions are warranted on the basis of the data they have.

Nurses use both inductive and deductive reasoning in the diagnosis step when they look for patterns and relationships among the various pieces of client data they have collected. **Inductive** reasoning begins with specific details and facts and uses them to arrive at conclusions and generalizations. When reasoning inductively, you assume that what is true of a sufficient number of individual cases is true of all cases or that certain pieces of data, when they occur together, suggest a particular interpretation.

Example: If you observe in a large number of cases that ice melts when warmed to 32° F, you will reason that all ice melts at 32° F.

Example: A nurse who observes that a client has oral pain, a coated tongue, dry mouth, decreased salivation, and halitosis (bad breath), will conclude that the client has "Altered Oral Mucous Membrane" (a nursing diagnosis).

The validity of an inductive conclusion depends upon the number of observations made, and upon the quality of those observations. Think about the difference in the certainty of the conclusions drawn in the two examples above. When scientific induction leads to conclusions that are almost invariably true (e.g., ice melts at 32° F), those conclusions can be used as the major premises for deductive reasoning.

Deductive reasoning begins with a major theory, generalization, fact, or *major premise* that generates the specific details and predictions. You reason from the universal to the particular—what is true of a class of things is true of each member of that class.

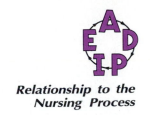

Relationship to the Nursing Process

Example:

Fact (major premise)	All ice melts at 32° F.
Fact (premise)	It is warmer than 32° F in this room.
Conclusion	The ice in the patient's water pitcher will melt.

Example:

Premise	In a nursing diagnosis, *fear* is defined as a feeling of dread related to an identifiable source that the person validates. The defining characteristic is the ability to identify the object of fear.
Fact	Billy Adams says he is scared of shots. He screams and tries to run away when the nurses come to his room to give him an injection or draw blood. His pupils dilate and his pulse rate increases.
Conclusion	Billy Adams is experiencing Fear (a nursing diagnosis).

In deductive reasoning, if the facts in the premises are true, then the conclusion must be true. However, we sometimes assume that generalizations are true when they may not be. The following is an example of wrongly assuming that a major premise (the first statement) is always true.

Premise	All infections cause fever.
Fact	Mr. Annas's temperature is 102° F.
Incorrect conclusion	Mr. Annas has an infection.

First of all, not all infections produce fever, although most do. Secondly, something other than an infection can produce fever (e.g., heat prostration). An error in reasoning may also be made if the *minor premise* (the second statement, or the patient data) is incorrect. For example, if Mr. Annas had a hot drink before his temperature was taken, the 102° reading would be incorrect. You might again conclude incorrectly that he has an infection.

The Planning Step

A nurse involved in setting client goals uses her knowledge and critical thinking skills to "form valid generalizations, explanations, [and] predictions" (Eggen and Kauchak, 1988, p. 34). *Developing and applying evaluative criteria* are also critical thinking skills; nurses use the goals written in this phase as criteria for evaluating the effectiveness of their care.

When planning nursing interventions and giving the rationale for them, the nurse "*makes interdisciplinary connections and uses insights from one subject to illuminate and correct other subjects*" (Paul, 1988a, p. 1. My italics). Critical

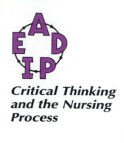

Critical Thinking and the Nursing Process

thinking also involves *making reasonable hypotheses* (Norris, 1985). After making the nursing diagnoses, the nurse hypothesizes that particular interventions will relieve the problem and help the client achieve her health goals. Generating nursing interventions is similar to generating hypotheses in the scientific method.

The Implementation Step

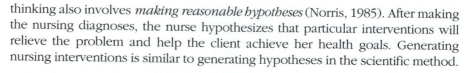

In this phase the nurse *applies her knowledge* and principles from nursing and related courses to each specific patient-care situation. As mentioned before, the ability to apply, not simply memorize, principles is a mark of critical thinking.

Example: A nursing student has learned the principles *Heat is lost through evaporation* and *The normal newborn is at risk for cold stress.* Although she has never bathed a newborn and has not memorized the procedure for doing so, she prevents cold stress by uncovering only the parts she is bathing, and drying the infant well.

Carrying out the nursing orders in the implementation phase can be compared to *hypothesis testing* in the scientific method. The nursing orders must be translated into action (or tested) in order to decide whether they were successful.

The Evaluation Step

In the evaluation phase, the nurse uses new observations to determine whether patient goals have been met, that is, whether the nursing orders (hypotheses) were successful (correct). *Using criterion-based evaluation* (see implementation above) is a critical-thinking skill.

Example: When bathing the newborn, the student realizes she must evaluate the results of her actions; that is, she must determine whether she has kept the infant warm enough. The most obvious criterion to use is that the infant's body temperature should be at least 98° F. Although no rule states that she should take the baby's temperature after a bath, she does so in order to evaluate whether she has achieved the goal of avoiding cold stress.

HOW CAN CRITICAL THINKING BE DEVELOPED?

Awareness is the first step in developing critical thinking. Now that you have an idea of what it means to think critically, you need to become aware of your own thinking style; you need to think about thinking. In this text you are asked to think critically about the nursing process.

It requires a great deal of practice to develop critical-thinking skills and a critical attitude. Most of the exercises in this book require you to practice critical-thinking skills, even though they don't always state which ones you are using. In addition, a special "Practice in Critical Thinking" exercise appears at the end of every chapter. Each of these discusses a different critical-thinking skill and asks you to apply it. The exercise at the end of this chapter applies to the material in Chapter 1, which had no critical-thinking exercise because the subject had not yet been presented.

Nurses need to use critical thinking in applying the nursing process and achieving the purpose of nursing. You are taking the first steps along the path to critical thinking when you believe in the importance of understanding rather than memorizing, and when you trust your own ability to make sense of evidence and principles.

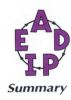

Summary

SUMMARY

Critical thinkers:
- ✓ see connections between concepts and ideas
- ✓ use logic
- ✓ recognize the difference between fact, inference, and assumption
- ✓ evaluate reasons and arguments
- ✓ consider issues before forming an opinion
- ✓ believe in their ability to think things through and make decisions

Skill-Building Activities

Discuss this exercise with your classmates. Compare your thinking with theirs.

An assumption is an idea or concept we take for granted (e.g., people used to assume the world was flat). Assumptions can be true or false (e.g, that assumption was proved false when Columbus sailed around the world instead of off the edge). You can better

Practice in Critical Thinking: Assumptions

evaluate someone's reasoning if they tell you what assumptions it is based on. You can only evaluate assumptions—yours or someone else's—if you recognize them. Make it a habit to look for hidden, unstated assumptions. **Start with this text!** To help you begin, an assumption in Chapter 1 is that nurses ought to use the nursing process.

1. Why is that statement an assumption? Could you say it is a fact instead? Why or why not?

2. What evidence does the author give you that the assumption is true?

3. How could you prove to yourself that this assumption is (or is not) true? What further evidence is needed?

4. What other assumptions can you find in Chapter 1? Write them here.

Applying the Nursing Process

(Answer Key, p. 373)

1. Your text gave reasons to justify the assertion that nurses need to be critical thinkers; these are listed below. Write the letters that match them to the correct examples.

_____ Nursing is an applied discipline.

_____ Nursing draws on knowledge from other subjects and fields.

_____ Nurses deal with change in stressful environments.

_____ Nurses make frequent, varied, and important decisions in their work.

a. Sally Sims works in an intensive-care unit. Today she performed neurological checks on her patient every hour. When her client stopped breathing she helped resuscitate him and put him on a ventilator. He has three different intravenous solutions running. She also had to attend an in-service meeting to learn how to use the new IV pump. When she returned to the unit, she learned that her client was to receive a new, experimental medication and now needed neuro checks every 15 minutes.

b. Patrick Kirk is taking a psychology course because he wants to understand his patients better. Today at work, he looked up a new medication in a pharmacology book. He also reviewed the inflammatory process in a physiology text.

c. Recalling that local lack of nutrients and oxygen results in tissue damage, Nurse Mason turns his immobile patient at least every 2 hours to prevent pressure sores.

d. Today Nurse Wiles chose to use a smaller-than-usual needle to inject a client with frail tissues and little muscle mass. She decided to let a patient's family stay past visiting hours because the patient needed their support. When another patient had symptoms of low blood sugar, she decided to give him some juice and wait to see how he responded before calling the physician.

2. Look at each of the responses to the case below. Which nurse(s) demonstrated critical thinking? Circle the correct letter(s).

Nurse: A   B   C   D

Case.   The night nurse has just reported as follows: "Mr. Stewart doesn't look very good to me. He said he felt 'sick' when I took his vital signs at 0600. Probably he just needs some orange juice." The day nurse is floating to a new unit and does not know any of her patients today. She knows from the night report that Mr. Stewart is 80 years old, he is diabetic, and his vital signs were within normal limits at 0600.

Nurse A, realizing that the regular staff probably knew the patients better than she did, followed the night nurse's advice and immediately gave Mr. Stewart some orange juice before making rounds on her other patients. After making rounds she returned to see if he was feeling better.

Nurse B, realizing that she was not an expert on diabetes, immediately called Mr. Stewart's physician and relayed the night report so that she could get orders about how to proceed.

Nurse C went to Mr. Stewart's room immediately after report, took his vital signs, listened to his heart and lungs, and asked him to describe how he was feeling. Unable to recall the symptoms of low blood sugar, he looked them up in a nursing text before giving Mr. Stewart the orange juice. His plan was to call the physician if Mr. Stewart's condition did not improve within the hour.

Nurse D gave Mr. Stewart the orange juice immediately. She then charted that Mr. Stewart had a hypoglycemic reaction (low blood sugar) and initiated a care plan for that problem, including nursing orders to give orange juice as needed and to reassess the patient within 30 minutes.

3. In the situations above, for each nurse who did not use critical thinking, explain what the nurse did wrong. In your explanations, use the information from "The Nature of Critical Thinking" in Chapter 2.

4. Which thinking does the situation demonstrate: critical, creative, associative, or directed?

   a. _____ Mr. Adams is having difficulty understanding the calorie content of different foods, so his nurse thinks of an entirely new way to present the information to him.

   b. _____ The nurse determines that a client is too weak to sit at the lavatory and assigns an aide to bathe him.

   c. _____ Prior to surgery, Ms. Morris's nurse notices that her facial expression is tense and her hands are trembling. The nurse analyzes the relationship between these cues and recognizes that the client is anxious.

   d. _____ The nurse notices that Ms. Ginsburg is left alone in the corridor to wait for surgery. She imagines how lonely the client must feel, and she is reminded of the time her mother was in the hospital. She wonders if her mother is still following her low-salt diet. She pats Ms. Ginsburg's hand as she walks by to another client's room.

5. Enter the letter for the kind of knowledge demonstrated by the following examples:

   (S) Scientific, (E) Ethical, (P) Practice wisdom

   a. ___ The nurse is having lunch with colleagues who are discussing her client's personal life. One of them says, "I heard she made all that money in real estate. Is that true?" The nurse replies, "I can't discuss personal data about her, especially where it could be overheard."

   b. ___ Mr. Castaneda is reading his wife's chart, which was accidentally left at her bedside. The nurse says, "I'm sorry, Mr. Castaneda, but I must have Ms. Castaneda's permission in order to give you information that is in the chart."

   c. ___ After reading several research reports, the head of the newborn nursery discontinued the requirement that parents must wear special gowns when holding the infants.

   d. ___ The nurses on a surgical floor urge patients to ambulate to help promote the return of peristalsis after surgery. No one can say exactly how it helps, but they all remember patients who passed flatus after ambulating (and some who didn't).

REFERENCES

Benner, P., and Tanner, C. (1984). *From Novice to Expert: Excellence and Power in Clinical Nursing Practice.* Menlo Park, CA: Addison-Wesley.

Carper, B. (1978). Fundamental patterns of knowing in nursing. *Advances in Nursing Science, 1:*(October) 13–23.

Eggen, P., and Kauchak, D. (1988). *Strategies for Teachers: Teaching Content and Thinking Skills.* 2nd ed. Englewood Cliffs, NJ: Prentice Hall.

Jameton, A. (1984). *Nursing Practice: The Ethical Issues.* Englewood Cliffs, NJ: Prentice Hall, pp. 71–79.

Kim, H. (1983). *The Nature of Theoretical Thinking in Nursing.* Norwalk, CT: Appleton-Century-Crofts.

Neuman, B. (1972). The Betty Neuman model: A total person approach to viewing patient problems. *Nursing Research, 21*(3): 264–69.

Norris, S. (1985). Synthesis of research on critical thinking. *Educational Leadership,* (May): 40–45.

Paul, R. (1988a). *The Critical Student and Person.* From The Eighth Annual and Sixth International Conference on Critical Thinking and Educational Reform. The Center for Critical Thinking and Moral Critique, Sonoma State University, Rohnert Park, CA 94928.

Paul, R. (1988b). *What, Then, Is Critical Thinking?* From The Eighth Annual and Sixth International Conference on Critical Thinking and Educational Reform. The Center for Critical Thinking and Moral Critique, Sonoma State University, Rohnert Park, CA 94928.

Roy, C. (1980). The Roy adaptation model. In Riehl, J. and Roy, C., eds., *Conceptual Models for Nursing Practice.* 2nd ed. New York: Appleton-Century-Crofts.

Schraeder, B., and Fischer, D. (1987). Using intuitive knowledge in the neonatal intensive care nursery. *Holistic Nursing Practice, 1*(3): 45–51.

Wilbraham et al. (1990). *Addison-Wesley Chemistry, Critical Thinking Worksheets.* Menlo Park, CA: Addison-Wesley.

Ziegler, S., Vaughan-Wrobel, B., and Erlen, J. (1986) *Nursing Process, Nursing Diagnosis, Nursing Knowledge: Avenues to Autonomy.* Norwalk, CT. Appleton-Century-Crofts.

CHAPTER 3

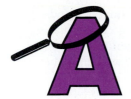

ASSESSMENT

OBJECTIVES

Upon completing this chapter, you should be able to do the following:
- Relate the assessment step to the other steps of the nursing process.
- Differentiate between subjective and objective data.
- Compare initial and ongoing assessment.
- Describe effective interview techniques.
- State the contents of the initial comprehensive nursing assessment of a client.
- Use a nursing framework to structure data collection.
- Describe nursing assessments that are pertinent to well clients.
- Explain why and how data should be validated.
- Explain the need for honesty and confidentiality when collecting data.

ASSESSMENT: THE FIRST STEP OF THE NURSING PROCESS

Assessment is the first step in the nursing process. It is the systematic gathering of relevant and important patient information for use in identifying health problems and planning and evaluating nursing care. **Data** is the set of information or facts about the patient. Some examples of data follow:

Blood-pressure reading	Amount of fluid intake
Hourly urine output	Patient's statements about his pain
Color of the urine	Results of lab tests

During the assessment step, the nurse collects, validates, records, and organizes data into predetermined categories (see Figure 3–1). The data collected during assessment must be accurate and complete because it forms the basis for the decisions made in the remaining steps of the nursing process. Incorrect or incomplete data can cause incorrect diagnoses and ineffective nursing interventions.

Standards of Practice Standard I of the American Nurses Association *Standards of Nursing Practice* identifies data collection as a nursing responsibility:

> "The collection of data about the health status of the client/patient is systematic and continuous. The data are accessible, communicated, and recorded." (American Nurses Association, 1973)

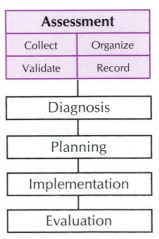

Figure 3–1. The Assessment Step

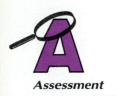

Assessment

Assessment is the systematic gathering of relevant and important patient information for use in identifying health problems and planning and evaluating nursing care.

Nursing Models and Frameworks

A **conceptual framework** is a loosely organized set of concepts and statements expressing the relationships among them. A nursing conceptual framework provides an overall structure that can be used to guide nursing practice. When a framework has been tested in practice and is well-enough organized to give clear, explicit direction to practice, education, and research, it is called a **nursing model**. Theories can be developed from models. A **theory**, like a model, is made up of concepts, but it is even more organized, detailed, and specific. A model must be tested and used extensively in practice before it is developed enough to become a theory. For the purposes of this chapter, you do not need to determine whether a theorist's ideas are a framework, a model, or a theory. Regardless of the level of development, they all present ideas about patients, health, and nurses, as well as what nursing is and does. Any level of organized concepts (framework, model, or theory) can be used to guide data collection.

Models and frameworks guide data collection by indicating the significant data. A nursing model will produce data useful in planning nursing care; a medical model will result in data useful for medical diagnoses and treatments. Just as they define the scope of nursing (Chapter 1), nursing models also describe the nature and causes of health problems, as well as the ways in which people respond to health problems. Gordon's framework, for example, directs nurses to collect data about common patterns of behavior that contribute to health, quality of life, and achievement of human potential (Gordon, 1987, p. 92). The Roy Adaptation model (1976) directs the nurse to collect data about stimuli affecting the client's adaptation in the physiologic, self-concept, role-function, and interdependence modes. Particular nursing models are discussed in more detail under "Organizing the Data" later in this chapter.

Critical Thinking in Assessment

Assessment is more than simply writing information on an assessment form; good judgment is needed to make good assessments. You will need critical thinking skills and a good knowledge base to decide which assessments to make, how much information you need, where and how to get that information, and which data is meaningful. When performing assessments, you will use your experience and knowledge from nursing and other courses to apply principles and theories about basic human needs, anatomy and physiology, disease processes, human growth and development, human behavior, socioeconomic patterns and trends, and various cultures and religions. Recall from Table 2–1 that the following critical-thinking skills are used in the assessment phase:

Observing	Validating data
Distinguishing relevant from irrelevant data	Organizing data
Distinguishing important from unimportant data	Categorizing data

These skills can be developed through knowledge and practice, as discussed in Chapter 2. The "Practice in Critical Thinking" exercise at the end of each chapter, and the other exercises in this text provide some of the practice you need to develop critical-thinking skills.

The Purpose of Nursing Assessment

The purpose of nursing assessment is to provide data about the patient's patterns of health and illness, deviations from normal, strengths, coping abilities, and risk factors for health problems. The nursing assessment focuses on patient responses to health problems—unlike the medical assessment, which focuses on disease processes and pathology. A nursing assessment may produce information about a medical diagnosis, but this is not the focus of the assessment. For example, when admitting a patient to the hospital for surgery, the nurse is interested in his disease symptoms and the nature of the surgery, but her primary interest is in how the symptoms affect his ability to care for himself, what he expects to result from the surgery, how his recovery period will affect his life, and what his main concerns are at this time.

Relationship to Other Steps of the Nursing Process

Recall from Chapter 1 that even though the steps of the nursing process are discussed separately for ease in understanding them, they are actually interrelated and overlapping. This is especially true of the assessment step because complete, accurate data provides the foundation for the other steps. The usefulness and validity of the nursing diagnoses depend greatly upon the quality of the data collected in the assessment phase. When planning goals and nursing orders, the nurse uses patient data to decide which goals are realistic and which nursing orders will be most effective.

Assessment overlaps with diagnosis in the sense that the nurse may begin to formulate a tentative problem in her mind while she is still collecting data. Assessment overlaps with the implementation and evaluation steps in that the nurse continues to collect patient data as she is carrying out these steps. For instance, as the nurse is bathing a patient (implementation), she is observing his skin condition and joint mobility. After the nursing orders have been carried out, during the evaluation phase, the nurse collects data to determine patient progress toward goal achievement (e.g., she observes the skin to see if turning and positioning the patient have prevented pressure sores).

COLLECTING THE DATA

Data collection is an important part of the assessment step. Nurses collect data of various types, from a number of sources, and at different times during the patient's illness. This section will help you develop your data-collection skills.

Types of Data

Data is classified as subjective and objective. Subjective data is sometimes called **covert data** or *symptoms*; objective data is sometimes called **overt data** or *signs*. Both types of data are needed for a thorough assessment.

Subjective data can be verified only by personal experience. Such data is not measurable or observable; it can be obtained only from what the client tells you. Subjective data includes the client's thoughts, beliefs, feelings, sensations, and perceptions of self and health (e.g., pain, dizziness, nausea, sadness, and happiness).

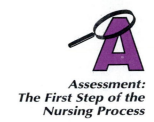

Assessment: The First Step of the Nursing Process

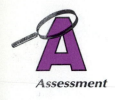

Assessment

You may not always be able to obtain subjective data. Some clients, such as infants, unconscious people, or the cognitively impaired, may not be able to provide subjective data, or their data may be unreliable. Although you will usually obtain subjective data from the client, data from significant others and other health professionals may also be subjective if it consists of opinion and perception rather than fact.

> **Example:** Subjective Data: The client's wife says, "He doesn't seem so sad today."
>
> Objective Data: The nursing assistant reports that she has taken the patient's pulse and it is 98.

Objective data can be detected by someone other than the client. You will usually obtain it by observing and examining the client. Examples of objective data include the following:

Pulse rate	Skin color
Urine output	Skin turgor
Results of diagnostic tests or X rays	Posture

When used in the nursing process, the terms *subjective* and *objective* have the special meanings described above. *Subjective* does not suggest biased information or personal interpretation of meaning, as it does in common use, and *objective* does not necessarily carry the common meaning of *impartial*.

Sources of Data

The nurse may gather data from a variety of sources, which fall into two broad categories: primary and secondary. You should use the most reliable source of data, whether it is the client or a significant other, and you should indicate the source on the client's record.

Primary Sources

The client is the **primary** data source; all other data sources are **secondary.** Primary source data can be subjective or objective; that is, it can be obtained from what the client tells you or by observation and examination.

> **Examples:** Laboratory data (WBC = 15,000).
> Temperature 100°F.
> The client states that he has a headache.
> The client's skin is pale and damp.

Secondary Sources

Secondary data is obtained from sources other than the client (e.g., other people, client records). It can be subjective or objective. *Significant others*, such as family or friends, can supplement and validate data obtained from the client. They are especially valuable sources when the client is a child or has difficulty communicating. When possible, you should get the client's consent before collecting data from significant others.

Other health-care providers, such as the physician, social worker, dietitian, respiratory therapist, and other nurses, can provide information about the areas of client functioning with which they are involved. Sharing information among

---

Equivalents

Subjective data	Objective data
Covert data	Overt data
Symptoms	Signs

disciplines is especially important when the client is being transferred from one institution to another (e.g., from a nursing home to a hospital) or discharged from the institution for follow-up care at home.

The client's written record from present and past hospitalizations can be used to help plan the initial nursing assessment and to confirm the other data. Reading the records, or **chart**, before you see the client can help you to formulate goals for the interview and prevent you from covering topics already assessed by someone else. Be aware, however, that it can also give you predetermined ideas about the client. Failure to approach the client with an open mind can cause you to miss some data. Whatever your choice, the client's record should be reviewed early in the data-collection process.

Information from nursing and other literature may be important to the assessment process, especially for students and beginning practitioners. For example, if you have never cared for a client with trigeminal neuralgia, it would be important to read the textbook picture of the disease in order to know what signs and symptoms to look for when assessing the client. The literature also provides helpful information about developmental norms, cultural differences, and spiritual practices to use as a guide during data collection.

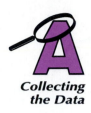

Collecting the Data

Initial Versus Ongoing Assessment

Assessment begins with the nurse's first contact with the client and continues throughout all subsequent nurse-client encounters. Although initial and ongoing assessment both involve data collection, they differ in purpose and, usually, in scope.

Initial Assessment

The **initial assessment** is made during the first nurse-client encounter. Except in emergency situations, the initial assessment is comprehensive, consisting of all subjective and objective data pertinent to the client's present health status. When the assessment is performed upon admission of the client to a health-care agency, it is called the **admission assessment.**

The Nursing Data Base The end product of the initial comprehensive assessment is the **nursing data base**; in fact the initial assessment is also called **data base assessment.** Figure 3–2 illustrates the place of the data base in the overall scheme of the assessment step. The complete data base consists of the nursing history and physical examination, as well as data from the patient's records, consultations, and a review of the literature. Figure 3–3 is an example of a nursing data base. You may wish to ask your instructor to share examples of other data bases with you.

The **nursing history** is obtained by interviewing the patient. It contains subjective data about the effects of the illness on the patient's daily functioning and ability to cope. It considers the whole person, including data about all the patient's basic needs, not just the biological ones. The specific content of a nursing history varies in different settings (e.g., a long-term care facility would require different information than a walk-in clinic) and with different nursing models. Regardless of setting or model, a nursing history usually includes the following general content areas:

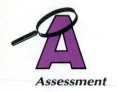

Assessment

Biographical information (e.g., age, sex and marital status)

Past health status (e.g., previous hospitalizations, childhood diseases)

Family, psychosocial, and environmental history (e.g., number of people living at home, job setting, exposure to toxic materials)

Usual habits and patterns of daily living (e.g., bedtime rituals)

Client's expectations of caregivers (i.e., what he thinks will be done for him; what he wants the nurse to do to help)

Client's perceptions of health status and illness (e.g., does he realize the implications of his illness? For example, does he think his arthritis will be cured?)

History of the present illness and information about the current state of health

Review of symptoms and their effect on the client's functioning

Coping abilities, strengths, and supports

Client's main concerns (e.g., instead of worrying about the anesthetic and surgical complications, the client's main concern may be about what the scar will look like)

Spiritual well-being (e.g., the client's source of strength or hope)

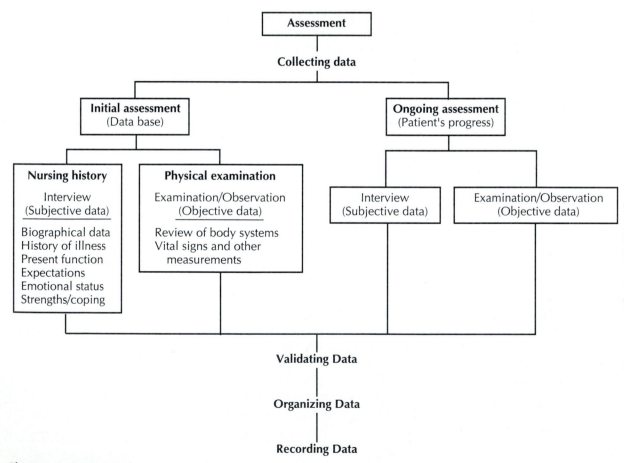

Figure 3–2. Overview of Assessment

GYNECOLOGIC ASSESSMENT TOOL

Name _NIKKI WINTERS_   Age _37_   Sex _F_
Address _110 South Cain, Liberal, KS_   Telephone _631-1098_
Significant other _John A. Winters, husband_   Telephone _Same_
Date of admission _4-6-91_   Medical diagnoses _Endometriosis, dysmenorrhea_
Allergies _Penicillin_

COMMUNICATING ▪ A pattern involving sending messages
(Read, write, understand English)(circle) _____   Other languages _Ø_
Intubated _Ø_   Speech impaired _Ø_
Alternate form of communication _Ø_

VALUING ▪ A pattern involving the assigning of relative worth
Religious preference _none_   Important religious practices _none_
Cultural orientation _Born and raised in Midwest_   Cultural practices _"Nothing in particular"_

RELATING ▪ A pattern involving establishing bonds
Role
Marital status _Married 16 years_   Age & health of significant other _36. Good health._
    Patient's description of marriage _"We're a pretty good team." "I'm lucky to have him."_
    Quality of relationship with partner _Good_
Sexual relationships (satisfactory/(unsatisfactory))
    Physical difficulties/effects of illness on relationship _↓ frequency of intercourse because of pain. "Won't be problem after surgery"_
    Changes in sexual behavior _(See above)_
    Abnormal lesions/discharges in sexual partner _Ø_
    Fear of intercourse _Ø_   **Mistrust of men** _Ø_
Role in home _Wife, mother. Makes decisions with husband_
Number of children _3_   Ages _15, 13, 12_   **Quality of Relationship with children** _Good_
Occupation _Works 3 days a week as bank teller_   Financial support _Her salary and husband's_
    Job satisfaction/concerns _Nice people. "It brings in extra money"_ Physical/mental energy expenditures _"Normal, I guess"_

Socialization
Quality of relationships with others _Friends at work; neighbors_ Patient's description _"Good." "I talk to my mom a lot."_
    Significant others' descriptions _Oldest child says, "Gets along with everybody."_
    Staff observations _Quiet, but not withdrawn_
    Verbalizes feelings of being alone _No._   Attributed to _Ø_

KNOWING ▪ A pattern involving the meaning associated with information
Current health problems _Admitted for TAH and BSO. States heavy bleeding, constant spotting, abd. cramps – past 6 mo._
Current medications _Tylenol, Ibuprofen, "iron pills"_
Previous illnesses/hospitalizations/surgeries _Childbirth: 1975, 1977, 1978. Appendectomy: 1969_

History of the following:	Patient	Family member
Anemia/blood dyscrasias	_Anemia (current)_	_Ø_
Cancer	_Ø_	_Ø_
Diabetes	_Ø_	_Ø_
Heart disease	_Ø_	_Father died from M. I._
Hypertension	_Ø_	_Ø_
Hysterectomy	_Ø_	_Ø_
Sickle cell disease	_Ø_	_Ø_
Smoking	_1/2 Pack per day for 16 years._	_Ø_
Stroke	_Ø_	_Ø_
Thyroid disease	_Ø_	_Ø_

Vaginal infection _Occasional "yeast"_
Venereal disease _Ø_
Maternal diethylstilbestrol use _No_
Other _Ø_
Menstrual/menopause history
    Age of onset _11_   Length of cycle _Normally 28 days_
    Amount/type of flow _Last 6 mo: Heavy for 10-14 days; spotting between_

Figure 3–3. A Nursing Data Base: Human Response Patterns. Adapted from Guzzetta et al. (1989). *Clinical Assessment Tools For Use With Nursing Diagnoses.* (St. Louis: C. V. Mosby, pp. 149-54.) Reprinted by permission.

Type of contraception used _Tubal Ligation_   Complications of contraception ___none___

Last menstrual period _"spotting" at present_   Associated symptoms _Abd. cramps, backache_

Number & outcome of each pregnancy _3. All normal vaginal deliveries. Labors 8-12 hours._

Complications of pregnancy, delivery, or abortions _none_

History of sexual assault: yes/(no)   **Time/place** _____

   Brief description of events _____

   Authorities notified: yes/no

Perceptions/knowledge of illness/tests/surgery _"Medicine didn't help the pain or irregular periods - so I'm having my uterus removed"_

Expectations of therapy _Will not have menses. Will cure pain, anemia_

Misconceptions _None_

Readiness to learn _Attentive, interested_

   Request information concerning _Return to work; "will I need help when I go home."_

   Educational level _High School_   Learning impeded by _–_

Orientation

Level of alertness _Fully alert_

   Orientation: Person ____✓____   Place ____✓____ Time ____✓____

   Appropriate behavior/communication _yes_

Memory

Memory intact: (yes)/no   Recent ____✓____ Remote ____✓____

FEELING ▪ A pattern involving the subjective awareness of information

Comfort

   Pain/discomfort: (yes)/no   Onset _6 mo. ago_   Duration _Intermittent; Several X a week_

     Location _Abd, back_   Quality _"cramps"_   Radiation _____

     Associated factors _Heavy bleeding c̄ period; "Spotting" between_

     Aggravating factors _Intercourse_   Alleviating factors _Heating pad, Ibuprofen_

Emotional Integrity /States

   Recent stressful life events _Ø_

   Verbalizes feelings of _"Worry" that husband will think she is less "womanly" after surgery._

     Source _____

   Evidence of posttrauma response: Anger _Ø_

     Phobias/nightmares _Ø_   Self-blame/shame _Ø_

     Depression/guilt _Ø_   Denial/emotional shock _Ø_

     Expressions of numbness _Ø_

   Physical manifestations: Crying _Ø_   Silence _Ø_   Trembling hands _Ø_

     Avoids interactions with others _Ø_   Hysterical _Ø_   Other _Ø_

MOVING ▪ A pattern involving activity

Activity

   History of physical disability _Ø_   Use of device (cane, walker, artificial limb) _Ø_

     Limitations in daily activities _Ø_

   Verbal report of fatigue or weakness _Last 2 months - "tire easily"_   Exercise habits _None - only housework_

Rest

   Hours slept/night _8_   Feels rested: (yes)/no

   Sleep aids (pillows, meds, food) _None_   Difficulty falling/remaining asleep _No_

Recreation

   Leisure activities _Read, sew, watch T.V._

   Social activities _Play cards with other couples. "Kids' activities"_

Environmental Maintenance

   Home maintenance management

   Size arrangement of home (stairs, bathroom) _Split-level_   Safety needs _None_

   Home responsibilities (patient) _Cook, clean, laundry_

   Home responsibilities (partner and/or children) _"They do the yard and car."_

Health Maintenance

   Health insurance _Husband's employer_   Regular physical checkups _No_

Self-Care

   Ability to perform ADLs: Independent ____✓____   Dependent _____

   Specific deficits _Will need help with housework after discharge_

   Discharge planning needs _Her mother will come to help out._

Figure 3–3. (continued)

Oxygenation

Complaints of dyspnea _____*0*_____ Precipitated by _____*0*_____ Orthopnea _____*0*_____

Rate *16* Rhythm *Reg* Depth *normal*

Labored/unlabored (circle) Breath sounds *clear* Cough; productive/nonproductive _____*0*_____

Sputum: Color _____*0*_____ Amount _____*0*_____ Consistency _____*0*_____

Physical Regulation

Immune Lymph nodes enlarged _____*0*_____ Location _____*0*_____ WBC count *9800*

   Differential _____–_____ PT _____ PTT _____–_____ Platelets _____–_____

Body temperature Temperature *98°* Route *Oral* Intervention _____–_____

Nutrition

Eating patterns

   Number of meals per day *2. Snacks a lot*

   Special diet *No*

   Food preferences/intolerances *Eats fried foods. Lots of chips and cola.*

   Food allergies *0*

   Fluid intake *Doesn't drink much water or other fluids*

   Diet history: sample diet *Breakfast: bacon, eggs, toast, coffee. Snacks: chips, cheese, cola. Dinner: meat, potatoes, corn, dessert.*

   Appetite changes *none*

   Difficult swallowing _____–_____ History of ulcers _____–_____ Heartburn _____–_____

   Presence of anorexia/nausea/vomiting _____

Condition of mouth/throat *Mucous membranes pink, moist. No lesions*

Weight *128* Height *5'2"* Ideal body weight *120*

Current therapy

   NPO *for OR* NG suction _____*0*_____

   Enteral nutrition _____*0*_____

   IV fluids *1000 cc Lact. Ringers before O.R. @ 125 cc/hr*

   TPN _____*0*_____

Labs

   Hemoglobin *92 g/dl* Hematocrit *32%* RBC _____*0*_____

   Na⁺ _____–_____ K⁺ _____–_____ Cl⁻ _____–_____ Glucose *124*

   Cholesterol *160* Triglycerides _____–_____ Fasting _____–_____

   Thyroid function test _____–_____

Elimination

Gastrointestinal/bowel

   Usual bowel habits *Once a day, usually; Sometimes q̄2-3 days*

   Alterations from normal *Constipated sometimes*

   Remedies used *None*

   Abdominal examination *Soft. Tender to deep palpation*

      Bowel sounds *Active, all 4 quadrants*

PERCEIVING ▪ A pattern involving the reception of information

Self-Concept

Presenting appearance *Neat; no make-up*

Patient's description of self *"Nothing special; sort of plain, I guess"*

Effects of illness/surgery on self-concept *I'm afraid my husband won't find me very attractive - it might change how he feels.*

Verbalizes positive feeling about being female *I'm glad I could have babies - men can't do that.*

Meaningfulness

Verbalizes hopelessness *No* Perceives/verbalizes loss of control *No*

Sensory/Perception

History of restrictive environment *No* Vision impaired *No* Glasses/Contacts *Myopia*

Auditory impaired _____*0*_____ Hearing aid _____*0*_____

Kinesthetic impaired _____*0*_____ Gustatory impaired _____*0*_____

Tactile impaired _____*0*_____ Olfactory impaired _____*0*_____

Reflexes: Biceps   R _____ L _____ Triceps   R   L _____ _____

      Brachioradialis R _____ L _____ *(Deferred)* Knee   R   L _____ _____

      Ankle   R _____ L _____ Plantar   R   L _____ _____

      Ankle clonus _____ Nuchal rigidity _____

      Other _____

Figure 3–3. (continued)

EXCHANGING ▪ A pattern involving mutual giving and receiving
Circulation

Cerebral

Neurologic changes/symptoms *Ø*

Pupils: Left 2 ③ 4 5 6 mm   Right 2 ③ 4 5 6 mm

    Reaction: Brisk _____ ✓ _____ Sluggish _____ Nonreactive _____

Verbal response *Appropriate*

Motor response *Appropriate*

Cardiac

Apical rate & rhythm *88 reg.*

Heart sound/murmurs *S₁ S₂ - No murmurs*

Dysrhythmias *Ø*

BP: R *130/88*   L *132/86*   Position *Sitting*

Peripheral

Jugular venous distension: yes/(no)   R _____ L _____

Pulses; *Strong, regular*

Skin temp *Warm*   Color *Good*   Turgor *Good*

Capillary refill *< 2 sec*   Edema *Ø*

Physical Integrity

Tissue Integrity: Rashes *Ø*   Lesions *Ø*

Petechiae *Ø*   Bruises *Ø*

Ecchymosis *Ø*

Abrasions *Ø*   Lacerations *Ø*

Surgical (incisions)/dressings *RLQ abd. (old appendectomy)*

Renal/urinary

Usual urine pattern *Voids q2-3 hrs.*

Alterations from normal *None*

Urine: Color *yellow*   Odor *"Normal"*   Catheter *Ø*

Urine output: 24 hour *"Don't know"*   Average hourly *"Don't know"*

Bladder distention *None*

Genitalia

Breast examination *Deferred. Doesn't do self-exam.*   External genitalia examination *Not done*

Vaginal discharge *Red-brown*   Odor *None*

Unusual vaginal discharge *"Heavy periods – spotting between"*

HCG _____ LH _____ FSH _____

CHOOSING ▪ A pattern involving the selection of alternatives
Coping

Patient's usual problem-solving methods *Consider all consequences. Do what's best for everybody.*

Family's usual problem-solving methods *Discuss. Husband usually makes final decision if can't agree.*

Patient's method of dealing with stress *"Be alone a while"*

Family's method of dealing with stress *"Try not to get on each other's nerves"*

Patient's affect *Congruent with verbalization*   Physical manifestations *Normal facial mobility*

Support systems available *Mother. Friends. Husband. Children. "I hate to ask them, though."*

Participation

Compliance with past/current health regimens *"Took all the pills – didn't help." Taking Fe⁺⁺ now.*

Willingness to comply with future health care regimen *"Oh, sure. I want to get well. I can stay home from work a while."*

Judgment

Decision-making ability

Patient's perspective *"It's ok. I guess."*

Others' perspective *Not available*

Prioritized nursing diagnosis/problem list

1. *Abd. and back pain r/t endometriosis (r/t incision, post-op)*
2. *High risk for constipation r/t effects of anesthesia, analgesics, ↓ mobility and ↓ fluid and fiber.*
3. *Possible self-concept disturbance r/t loss of uterus*
4. *Altered health maintenance r/t possible lack of understanding of cardiac risk factors.*

Signature *Sheryl Ibarra, RNC*   Date *4-6-91*

Figure 3–3. (concluded)

48

The **nursing physical examination** is a systematic assessment of all body systems, using observation and examination skills (to be discussed later in this chapter). It is concerned with identifying strengths and deficits in the client's functional abilities rather than with identifying pathology. The physical examination produces objective data.

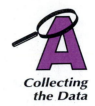

Ongoing Assessment

Ongoing assessment consists of data gathered after the data base is completed—ideally, during every nurse-patient interaction. The data is used to identify new problems and to evaluate the status of problems that have already been identified. See Table 3–1 for a summary comparison of initial and ongoing assessment.

Comprehensive Versus Focus Assessment

A **comprehensive assessment** provides an overall picture of the client's health status. The nurse obtains data about all the client's body systems and functional abilities, without necessarily having a particular health problem in mind. The initial assessment of a client is usually comprehensive.

A **focus assessment** may be used in both initial and ongoing assessments. In a focus assessment, the nurse gathers data about an actual, high-risk, or possible problem that has been identified (Alfaro, 1990; Carpenito, 1989). The assessment focuses on a specific topic or particular area of the body instead of the client's overall health status. Data from focus assessments is used to evaluate the status of existing problems and to identify new problems.

Example: *Evaluation of an existing problem.* The care plan for Hassim Asad included the problem of Fluid Volume Deficit. When performing ongoing assessment during Mr. Asad's bath, the nurse noted that his oral mucous membranes were moist and that he had good skin turgor—signs that his fluid-volume problem was resolving.

Example: *Identification of a new problem.* After his bath, Mr. Asad mentioned that his head was beginning to hurt. He had not mentioned headaches before. The nurse took his blood pressure, and questioned him about the nature and onset of the pain. Mr. Asad's blood pressure was elevated, and he was having blurred vision. The nurse elevated the head of the bed, relieving his pain somewhat, and notified the physician of this new development.

Table 3–1. Initial Versus Ongoing Assessment	
Initial Assessment	**Ongoing Assessment**
Admission assessment	Focus assessment
Data base assessment	Focuses on specific problems
Comprehensive assessment	Focuses on identified problems (can also be used to identify new problems)
Can include focus assessment	
Used to make initial problem list	Data is used to evaluate goal achievement and problem resolution.

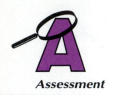

A focus assessment is not limited to ongoing data collection; it can also be used in the initial assessment when the client reports a symptom or other unusual findings. Any symptom or difficulty the client reports should be expanded on by asking further questions about it (e.g., When did it begin? What makes it worse? What relieves it?). When a client needs repeated in-depth assessment of a particular problem area, most agencies have special assessment forms for recording the ongoing focus assessment (e.g., a flow sheet for hourly neurological assessments).

Data-Collection Methods

Three methods of collecting data are used in both comprehensive and focus nursing assessments: observation, physical examination, and interview.

Observation

Observation is the conscious, deliberate use of the physical senses to gather data from the patient and his environment. Train yourself to begin observing as you first enter the patient's room. What is he doing? Does he show signs of distress, such as restlessness or pallor? What is in the environment? Are the side rails up? Are there any safety hazards? Is all the equipment working? Is the intravenous solution running? Who are the people in the room and how do they interact with the patient? Closer observations will disclose data such as skin temperature, breath sounds, and drainage odors.

> **Example:** The nurse sees that there is pink, serous drainage on Akiro Takata's cast. She sees that his toes are pink, and they are warm to her touch. She does not smell any unusual odor from the cast. She hears that Mr. Takata's breathing is quiet and not labored.

Physical Examination

A complete data base requires both subjective and objective data. **Physical examination** provides objective data that can be used to validate the subjective data obtained in the interview or clarify the effect of the patient's disease on her ability to function. The data from the initial physical examination serves as a baseline for comparing the client's later responses to nursing and medical interventions.

> **Example:** *Physical examination* might include the following activities:
>
> | | |
> |---|---|
> | Taking the client's vital signs | Auscultating bowel sounds |
> | Weighing the client | Listening to heart sounds |
> | Measuring head circumference | Palpating an infant's fontanels |

In a complete physical examination, the nurse assesses all body parts in an orderly, systematic manner. One approach is to proceed from *head to toe*. In this case, the head and neck would be examined first, and then the shoulders, chest (including heart and lungs), and back. Another approach is to examine each of the *body systems* in a predetermined order, for example, respiratory, neurological, cardiovascular, musculoskeletal, and so on. Whatever approach you choose, the examination should follow the same order each time to prevent omission of data.

In an admission assessment, the nurse usually conducts a complete physical examination, but this can vary depending upon the severity of the illness and the kind of information needed. During ongoing assessment, the nurse examines specific body areas, systems, or functions, instead of the entire body. These examinations are made to obtain data related to the patient's complaints, previously identified problems, and responses to nursing and medical interventions.

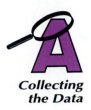

Example: A client who is taking an antibiotic complains, "I itch all over." The nurse examines his skin for rash or discoloration.

You will use the techniques of inspection, auscultation, palpation, and percussion when performing a physical examination. Like the nursing process, these require practice. Refer to a text on the fundamentals of nursing or physical assessment for in-depth discussion of these techniques and other aspects of the physical exam.

Inspection is done visually, either with the naked eye or with instruments such as an otoscope, which is used in examining the ears. Abdominal distention and skin pallor are examples of data found on inspection. Inspection is an active process in that the nurse must know what to look for. It is also a systematic process, more thorough and detailed than observation.

Auscultation uses the nurse's hearing. Using *direct* auscultation with the unaided ear the nurse can hear sounds such as the client's coughing. A stethoscope is used for *indirect* auscultation to amplify the sounds made within the client's body, such as crackles and wheezes in the lungs.

Percussion is the striking of a body surface, usually with the tip of the finger, to elicit sound or vibration. Different sounds are produced, depending upon whether the finger strikes over a solid, fluid-filled, or air-filled area. It is useful, for instance, in determining whether a patient's abdomen is distended with air or fluid.

Palpation uses the sense of touch. The finger pads are usually used because they are the most sensitive to tactile stimulation. The nurse uses palpation, for example, to check for bladder distention and to obtain the patient's pulse rate and strength.

Interview

A **nursing interview** is a planned, structured communication in which the nurse questions a patient to obtain subjective data. An interview may be informal, or formal and planned, as in an admission interview. During ongoing assessment, interviews may be brief, narrowly focused interactions between nurse and patient, but they are still purposeful, structured communication.

Purpose During the initial assessment, the main purpose of the interview is to obtain subjective data for the nursing history. At the same time, the nurse usually orients the patient to her surroundings and gives her some information about her stay (e.g., how to call for help, where to put her belongings). In addition to asking questions, the nurse should provide enough teaching and counseling to relieve some of the patient's anxieties. For both nurse and patient, impressions gained in the initial interview form the basis for the beginning of the nurse-patient relationship.

Preparing for the Interview As a rule, you should begin by reviewing the chart, so you will know who the patient is and what you want to accomplish; but be careful not to form preconceived ideas. After forming some goals for the interview, think of some initial leading questions. Schedule a time when you will be free from interruptions—not too close to mealtime, treatment time, or visiting hours. Provide privacy, wait until visitors are gone, or ask them to leave the room.

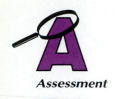

Be sure the patient is comfortable: ask if he is thirsty or needs to use the bathroom. Consider the patient's emotional state, as well. If he is very anxious or frightened, you may need to relieve his anxiety before proceeding with the interview.

Types   There are two basic types of interview: directive and nondirective. A **directive interview** is highly structured. The nurse controls the subject matter and asks questions in order to obtain specific information. This is an efficient way to obtain factual, easily categorized information, such as age, sex, and analysis of symptoms. A directive interview uses mainly **closed questions**, which call for brief, specific responses. Closed questions are especially effective in emergency situations or when the patient is very anxious. Remember, however, that a directive interview and closed questions are not very effective in helping a patient to express emotion, nor in getting information about personal or emotionally charged matters.

A **nondirective interview** allows the patient to talk about whatever she wishes, in the order and at the pace she chooses. The nurse clarifies, summarizes, and uses open-ended questions and comments to encourage communication. An **open-ended question** may specify the topic of discussion, but it is broad and requires elaboration from the patient. Such questions are good for eliciting feelings, attitudes, and beliefs. Nondirective interviewing is time-consuming and can result in a great deal of irrelevant data; however, it is useful in helping a patient to express feelings and in promoting communication. Table 3–2 gives examples of open-ended and closed questions.

The nursing interview requires a combination of directive and nondirective techniques. Use directive questioning to obtain the more specific information on the nursing history (e.g., biographical information, previous surgeries, childhood diseases). Then use broad statements to guide the patient to talk about other topics, such as sleep patterns, pain, and usual routines; finally, follow up or clarify those responses with specific, directive questions.

Example:

Nurse:	(Closed question) How many times have you been pregnant?
Patient:	Four.
Nurse:	(Closed question) Were there any problems with your other deliveries?
Patient:	Yes, with my last one.
Nurse:	(Open-ended question, directing topic) What happened?

Table 3–2. Open-Ended and Closed Questions

Closed	Open-Ended
When was the accident?	Tell me about your accident.
Are you in pain?	Describe the pain to me.
Was this a planned pregnancy?	What were your thoughts when you found out you were pregnant?

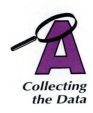
Patient: I was in labor a long time, and then something happened to the baby's heart rate. They did an emergency Caesarean section.

Nurse: (Open-ended question) What plans have you made for this delivery?

The last, broad question elicits information about a topic of the nurse's choice. A more directive, closed question along the same lines would be, "Do you plan to have a C-section again this time?" If the nurse wanted to explore the patient's feelings, she might have said, "What are your concerns for *this* delivery?"

Common Interviewing Problems   *The interviewer's own discomfort* may interfere with data collection. Students, especially, may feel they are imposing upon the patient by asking so many questions. This is true, in part, because they may not have a clear idea of how the information is to be used. To cope with this, be sure you understand the purpose of your interview and explain it to the patient during the introduction phase.

Students and nurses alike may be uncomfortable asking personal questions of a complete stranger. It helps to remind yourself that nurses are concerned with the whole person and that the data is needed in order to give comprehensive care. Also, when beginning the interview, you should encourage the patient to respond only if he feels comfortable. Remember that he can choose which information he wishes to give you, thereby preserving his privacy. You will usually find that the patient is at ease if you are at ease. In fact, it may be that the patient has felt the need to talk about a certain subject, but was not comfortable with introducing it himself.

Family and visitors may be a good source of data, but they may also inhibit the patient's response. It can be embarrassing for the patient to discuss personal information in front of others. For example, if you are interviewing a woman with her husband in the room, she will not feel free to tell you she uses oral contraceptives if she is doing it secretly against his wishes.

Spouses often answer the questions you address to the patient, making it difficult to get accurate subjective data. Unless the visitor is an important source of information (e.g., when the patient is a child), postpone the interview, or ask the visitor to step out for a few minutes.

The *interviewer's curiosity* may become a problem. There is a fine line between interest and curiosity. Do not become overly enmeshed in the details of the patient's story; focus on getting the information you need for planning care. Patients appreciate interest, but they resent curiosity. A patient who perceives you as too curious will be less inclined to give information.

The *patient's responses* can create a barrier. Because patients may respond to some questions with tears or anger, interviewers are sometimes afraid to ask questions that might upset them. It may be hard to accept another's expression of feelings, but it is important that you learn to do so. Avoiding all potentially upsetting topics can leave large gaps in the data base. It may help you to know that the patient usually feels better after expressing emotions—even though you may be uncomfortable.

Failure to adapt techniques to the patient's special needs can cause her unnecessary stress and result in incomplete or incorrect data. Some patients (e.g., the elderly, children, or those with sensory deficits) require special

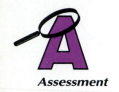

Assessment

interviewing techniques. You may need to speak more slowly, position yourself so the patient can read your lips, or modify your terminology. Be sensitive, also, to cues that the patient is becoming too tired or ill to continue with the interview.

VALIDATING THE DATA

Validation is the act of verifying data to be sure it is correct and factual. Failure to validate data may cause you to jump to faulty conclusions or misperceive what the client has said. Errors, biases and misperceptions in the data can result in inappropriate or ineffective nursing care. One way to help prevent this is to make it a habit to compare your interview and physical examination data. Most data-

---

Box 3–1. Guide for Interviewing

1. Plan ahead.
Read the chart. Think of some initial, leading questions.
Provide for privacy. Ask visitors to leave, pull the bed curtain.
Schedule enough time for the interview.
Reduce distractions. Turn off the television.
Be sure the client is comfortable.

2. Introduce yourself and set the time limit at the beginning of the interview.

3. Use the patient's name.

4. Sit down. Make eye contact. Listen.

5. Start with nonthreatening subjects and symptoms that caused the client to seek help. Beginning with the client's present complaints assures him that the questions are important.

6. Follow client leads for expanding on a subject or introducing a new topic. Don't just start at the top of the form and work mechanically down the page.

7. Refer to yourself as *I*, not *we*, as in "*We* need some information from you," or "*We* need to fill out this form." These statements indicate lack of personal involvement on the part of the nurse, and they create psychological distance between nurse and client.

8. Use language the patient can understand (many patients do not know the meaning of *void*, or *vital signs*), but don't talk down to the patient ("Let me check your tummy"). If you are not sure he understands, ask him to explain what the words mean (e.g., "Explain what happens when you have diarrhea").

9. Use neutral statements and reflection to get information. Don't phrase everything as a question. You can obtain information from a statement like, "Tell me about your job" rather than "Where do you work?" Too many questions may make you seem curious instead of concerned.

10. Use open-ended questions to encourage the client to talk. Avoid closed questions that require only a one-word or yes/no answer.

11. Avoid "why" questions when possible (e.g., "Why were you unable to stop smoking?") For many people, *why* connotes disapproval and may provoke a defensive response.

12. Provide encouragement to continue, by nodding or saying, "Um-hmm," or "Yes. . . ."

13. If the patient is rambling, allow him to finish a sentence before interrupting to redirect the conversation. Then try, "You hadn't finished telling me about. . . ."

collection forms are set up to facilitate this. In ongoing assessments, as well as in the admission assessment, always remember to *compare subjective and objective data* to see if they are in agreement. Data should be verified when the subjective and objective data do not agree—that is, when what the patient tells you is different from what you observe.

Example: The patient states she has never had high blood pressure. However, the nurse obtains a reading of 190/100. (This data should be validated.)

As a rule, you need to *validate data when there is a discrepancy in the patient's statements*—that is, when she tells you different things at different times in the interview.

Example: Early in the interview, the labor patient stated this was her first pregnancy. Later, when asked about prior hospitalizations, she said, "Once, in 1986, to have my appendix removed; and in 1988 when I had a miscarriage." (The nurse needs to ask more questions to verify exactly how many pregnancies the patient has had. The patient may not have understood that a miscarriage is counted as a pregnancy; or she may simply have forgotten to count it.)

You can *validate data as you collect it, or you can wait until the end of the assessment* to check out incongruities and inconsistencies. Data can be validated by asking more questions or by observing or examining the client further. You can also validate data by rechecking your own measurements or asking a colleague to verify them for you. In the example of a B/P reading of 190/100, the nurse would probably repeat the blood pressure measurement, perhaps in the patient's other arm. If she had difficulty hearing the blood pressure, she might ask another nurse to check it for her.

It is important to validate some, but not all, data. It would be impossible to validate the enormous amount of data collected by most nurses, and it is not necessary. As you gain experience, you will be able to tell more easily which data you need to validate. Until then, consult with a more experienced nurse or an instructor if you have questions about validating information.

ORGANIZING THE DATA

ANA Standard I requires that data collection be systematic. This means that in addition to collecting and validating the data, the nurse organizes related cues into predetermined categories. Grouping related data helps the nurse to find the patterns necessary for identifying client strengths, health problems, and risk factors. Most health-care agencies and schools of nursing have printed forms for the nursing data base. These forms organize the nursing history and the physical examination according to the framework or nursing theory the agency prefers. Using these forms enables you to organize the data at the same time you collect and record it, making the assessment more efficient. For ongoing assessments, you will not always have a data-collection form, so you will need to organize the data after you collect it. Frameworks are used to organize both initial and ongoing assessment data.

A **framework** is, very simply, a way of looking at something. Suppose a patient is trembling. A nurse using only a psychological framework might conclude the patient is frightened; a nurse using only a biological framework

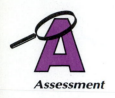

Assessment

might conclude that the patient is cold. A variety of frameworks are useful in collecting and organizing patient data: some focus on human needs, some on adaptive responses, others on self-care abilities, and so on. No matter which model you use, it is important to use it consistently in order to become familiar with it. Even if you do not use a form to collect data, you will still classify related cues according to your chosen framework when you are finished. Using a framework gives you a special way to view the patient, helps you to make thorough, systematic assessments, and makes the data more meaningful.

Maslow's Hierarchy of Needs

A popular non-nursing framework for data collection is Maslow's Hierarchy of Needs. According to Abraham Maslow's theory (1970), all people have the same basic human needs. Starting with the most basic, these are physiological, safety and security, love and belonging, self-esteem, and self-actualization. In general, the more basic needs must be met before the individual can meet the other, higher, needs. For example, someone who is homeless and has nothing to eat has little energy for thinking about self-esteem or expanding his mind. Using this framework, the nurse focuses on the extent to which the client's needs are being met. Data is collected and related cues are grouped according to each of the basic needs. Table 3–3 is an example of how data might be organized using Maslow's Hierarchy of Needs.

Roy's Adaptation Theory

Sister Callista Roy's Adaptation Theory of Nursing (1976) is frequently used as a framework for data collection. See Appendix B for a nursing data base adapted from Roy's theory. Roy views patients as biopsychosocial beings, constantly adapting to external and internal environmental demands. She theorizes that the patient needs nursing care when she cannot adapt along one of four modes: physiological, self-concept, social, and interdependence. Using this framework, the nurse would collect data about the patient's ability to adapt in those categories and about the types of environmental stimuli that affect her adaptation:

Physiological	Balance must be maintained in the areas of exercise and rest, nutrition, elimination, fluid and electrolytes, oxygen and circulation, temperature regulation, sensory regulation, and the endocrine system.
Self-concept	Developing a positive self-concept, including the physical self, moral-ethical self, and self-ideal. Includes self-esteem and psychological integrity.
Social role	Ability to function in various roles, such as parent, spouse, worker, and so on.
Interdependence	Achieving balance between dependence and independence.

Gordon's Functional Health Patterns

Marjory Gordon's framework (1987) groups data into 11 Functional Health Patterns, applicable to all clients. Gordon proposes that all human beings have "certain functional patterns that contribute to their health, quality of life, and achievement of human potential" (p. 92). These patterns are the focus of nursing assessment. The nurse uses assessment data to determine whether the client's functioning is positive, altered, or at risk for being altered in each of the patterns. Refer to Table 3–4 for a typology (description) of Gordon's Functional Health Patterns. See Appendix C for an example of an assessment form organized according to Gordon's model.

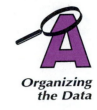

NANDA—Unitary Person Framework

The Unitary Person Framework, created by theorists from The North American Nursing Diagnosis Association (NANDA, 1989), considers a person to be an open system in continuous interaction with the environment. People are thought to be developing continuously toward increasing complexity and diversity, a process that is observed throughout a person's life stages and from generation to generation. A person is healthy, in this framework, if his pattern of energy exchange with the environment enhances his integrity and moves him toward his life's potential.

Table 3–3. Using Maslow's Hierarchy of Needs to Organize Data

Basic Needs	Examples of Data Categories
I. Physiological Survival needs	Oxygen Nutrition Fluids Body temperature, warmth Elimination Shelter Sex
II. Safety and Security Need to be safe and comfortable	Physical safety: infection, falls, drug side effects Psychological security: Knowledge of procedures, bedtime rituals, usual routines, fear of isolation, dependence needs Pain avoidance
III. Love and Belonging Need for love and affection	Information about significant others, social supports
IV. Esteem and Self-Esteem Need to feel good about self	Changes in body image (e.g., puberty, surgery) Changes in self-concept (e.g., ability to perform usual role in family) Pride in capabilities
V. Self-Actualization Need to achieve maximum potential Need for growth and change	Extent to which potential is being achieved Autonomy Motivation Problem-solving abilities Ability to accept help Ability to give help Feelings about accomplishments, roles

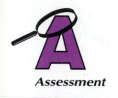

Assessment

Each person, in interaction with his environment, is characterized by a unique pattern and organization, manifested by the nine Human Response Patterns. The patterns reflect the whole person, including the person's health. NANDA uses these Human Response Patterns as a framework for classifying nursing diagnoses; however, they can also be used to organize assessment data. Table 3–5

Table 3–4. Typology of Eleven Functional Health Patterns

Health-perception/ health-management pattern	Describes client's perceived pattern of health and well-being and how health is managed. Examples: adherence to health-promotion and illness-prevention measures, compliance with medication regimen, follow-up visits to the physician.
Nutritional-metabolic pattern	Describes pattern of food and fluid consumption relative to metabolic need and pattern indicators of local nutrient supply. Includes condition of skin, teeth, hair, nails, mucous membranes, height, and weight.
Elimination pattern	Describes patterns of excretory function (bowel, bladder, and skin). Includes client's perception of "normal" function, changes in function, any devices used.
Activity-exercise pattern	Describes pattern of exercise, activity, leisure, and recreation. [Note: May include cardiovascular and respiratory status, and assessment of mobility and activities of daily living.]
Cognitive-perceptual pattern	Describes sensory-perceptual and cognitive pattern. Includes vision, hearing, taste, touch, smell, pain perception, and pain management. Includes cognitive functions such as language, memory, and decision making.
Sleep-rest pattern	Describes patterns of sleep, rest, and relaxation. Includes client's perception of quality and quantity of sleep and energy. Includes sleep aids and routines the client uses.
Self-perception/ self-concept pattern	Describes self-concept pattern and perceptions of self (e.g., body comfort, body image, feeling state). Includes attitudes about self, perception of abilities, and general sense of worth. Note pattern of body posture, eye contact, voice, and speech.
Role-relationship pattern	Describes pattern of role-engagements and relationships. Includes client's perception of current major roles and responsibilities, and satisfaction with family, work, or social relationships.
Sexuality-reproductive pattern	Describes client's patterns of satisfaction and dissatisfaction with sexuality pattern; describes reproductive patterns.
Coping/stress-tolerance pattern	Describes general coping pattern and effectiveness of the pattern in terms of stress tolerance. Includes modes of handling stress, reserves for coping, support systems, and perceived ability to control or manage situations.
Value-belief pattern	Describes patterns of values, beliefs (including spiritual), or goals that guide choices or decisions. Includes what is perceived as important in life and any value-belief conflicts related to health.

Adapted with permission from M. Gordon (1987), *Nursing Diagnosis: Process and Application*, 2nd ed. St. Louis: C. V. Mosby, p. 93.

lists the Human Response Patterns and their descriptions, along with some examples of assessments to make for each pattern. Notice the similarity between the Exchanging pattern and Maslow's physiological needs. Figure 3–3 is a data base organized according to the NANDA system.

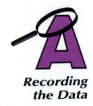

Recording the Data

RECORDING THE DATA

ANA Standard I requires that assessment data be accessible, communicated, and *recorded*. An additional consideration is that the nursing data base becomes a part of the client's permanent record. Therefore, you should record the assessment in ink on the form provided by the agency, on the same day the client is admitted. Write neatly and legibly, using only the abbreviations

Table 3–5. NANDA Human Response Patterns	
Pattern and Description	**Examples of Assessments**
1. *Exchanging*—Involves mutual giving and receiving	Nutritional status, temperature, elimination, oxygenation, circulation, fluid balance, condition of skin and mucous membranes, risk factors for injury/accidents, body systems.
2. *Communicating*—Involves sending messages	Ability to express thoughts verbally; orientation, physical impairments to speech; language barrier.
3. *Relating*—Involves establishing bonds	Type of social interactions; relationships with significant others; support system; ability to perform roles, including parenting; sexual functioning; family functioning; financial support.
4. *Valuing*—Involves the assigning of relative worth	Religious preference; relationship with deity; perception of suffering; acceptance of illness; religious practices; cultural orientation and practices.
5. *Choosing*—Involves the selection of alternatives	Ability to accept help; adjustment to health status; desire for dependence/independence; denial of problem; adherence to therapies; ability to make decisions.
6. *Moving*—Involves activity	Tolerance to activity; ability to care for self; sleep patterns; diversional activities; history of disability; home environment; safety needs; breastfeeding.
7. *Perceiving*—Involves the reception of information	Body image; self-esteem; ability to see, hear, feel, smell, taste; amount of hopefulness; perceived ability to control current situation.
8. *Knowing*—Involves the meaning associated with information	Amount of knowledge about current illness or therapies; previous illnesses; risk factors; expectations of therapy; cognitive abilities; readiness to learn; orientation; memory.
9. *Feeling*—Involves the subjective awareness of information	Pain; grieving; capacity or risk for violence; level of anxiety; emotional integrity.

Adapted by permission from the North American Nursing Diagnosis Association, *Classification of Nursing Diagnoses,* Proceedings of the Sixth Conference (St. Louis: C. V. Mosby, 1986).

59

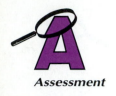

Assessment

approved by the agency. Do not try to write everything the client says word for word, as this is likely to interfere with the communication between you and the client.

Most comprehensive assessment forms provide for recording subjective and objective data separately. For clarity, you should also do that when recording data elsewhere, for instance, in a focus assessment in the nursing progress notes. Record subjective data in the client's own words when possible, using quotation marks. You may paraphrase or summarize what the client says, but do not use quotation marks in that case. Remember that *subjective data is what the client says*, not your interpretation of what she says.

> **Example:** *Exact quote*—Client states, "I feel sad and depressed today." (Correct)

> **Example:** *Paraphrasing*— Client states she feels sad and depressed today. (Correct)

> **Example:** *Interpretation*—Client is depressed. (Incorrect)

Use concrete, specific terms to describe data. Avoid vague generalities such as *good, normal, adequate,* or *tolerated well.* These words mean different things to different people. Look at the statement "Vision adequate." Does this mean the client can read newsprint without eyeglasses? Or that she can read newsprint when she is wearing glasses? Or that she can recognize a face from across the room? Or that she can see well enough to ambulate without assistance? It would be better to record "Able to read newsprint at 24 inches while wearing glasses."

Be sure to record the data, not what you think it means. The data collection form is not the place to record judgments, opinions, or conclusions. Record **cues** (what the client tells you and what you see, hear, feel, smell, and measure); not **inferences** (your judgment or interpretation of what the cues mean). Table 3–6 compares subjective and objective data (cues) with conclusions (inferences).

Table 3–6. Comparison of Data and Conclusions

Subjective Data (Cues)	Objective Data (Cues)	Conclusions (Inferences)
"My back really hurts." (Paraphrase: Patient states his back hurts.)	Lying rigidly in bed. Facial grimacing.	Patient is in pain.
"My armband is too tight, and my arm is really sore."	Left arm is hot, red, and swollen in a 4" x 4" area around the IV insertion site.	Left arm is infected at IV site.
"I'm not sure I should have this surgery. It might not even help, and it is so dangerous. I'm scared, I guess."	Tearful. Facial muscles tense. Pulse 100. Hands trembling.	Patient is frightened of surgery.

WELLNESS ASSESSMENT

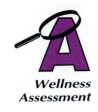

Wellness Assessment

Nurses frequently work with clients who are not ill. Nursing activities for well clients aim at promoting health and preventing illness. Therefore, data is collected in order to identify the individual's level of wellness and the presence of factors that might increase either his well-being or his risk for certain illnesses. The following are examples of activities that contribute to health and well-being:

Regularly sleeping 7 to 8 hours per night
Eating breakfast regularly
Eating regular meals with little or no snacking
Maintaining optimal weight
Frequent exercise
Moderate alcohol consumption
Avoiding smoking

Several other factors interrelate with these health habits to contribute to a person's level of wellness. A wellness assessment includes information about the following: degree of fitness, level of nutrition, sensitivity to the environment, level of life-stress, life-style and health habits, and risk factors for disease (Pinnell and de Meneses, 1986). Table 3–7 provides examples of data relevant to these factors.

Pender (1987) adds an assessment of the client's health-care beliefs, especially the client's perception of his ability to control his own health status. Persons who believe they have major control over their own health status are more likely to take the initiative in health promotion and disease prevention (e.g., breast self-

---

Table 3–7. Using a Wellness Framework to Organize Data

Degree of fitness	Exercise pattern, general appearance, muscle strength, muscle and joint flexibility, body proportions, percent of body fat.
Level of nutrition	Twenty-four-hour recall of food intake, knowledge of nutrition, effect of sociocultural beliefs on diet, analyze intake for inclusion of food from the basic four food groups and/or the Recommended Daily Allowances of essential nutrients.
Sensitivity to environment	Awareness of personal environment, including sensory stimuli and potential hazards.
Risk appraisal	Identification of client's risk factors for threats to health.
Level of life-stress	Sources of stress to the client (e.g., home, work, life events, life changes that have occurred in the past two years); client's perception of stress as positive or negative; length of exposure to stress; past coping patterns.
Life-style and personal health habits	Personal habits such as amount of sleep, weight, exercise, alcohol and tobacco use, dental care, safety and health-care practices (e.g., last Pap smear, last chest X ray). (Refer to Figure 3–4 for a self-test of healthy life-style.)

For further information, see Pinnell and de Meneses, *The Nursing Process: Theory, Application, and Related Processes* (Norwalk, CT: Appleton-Lange, 1986), pp. 89–90.

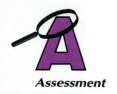
exam). Those who believe that health is the result of luck, or that "knowledgeable others" are responsible for their health may need more help in making behavior changes (Edelman and Mandle, 1986, p. 53).

Various other frameworks, including the ones discussed in this chapter under "Organizing the Data," could be used to classify wellness data. Figure 3–4 is an example of a tool that might be used to collect data about the client's life-style and health habits.

ETHICAL CONSIDERATIONS

As in all aspects of care, the nurse must be aware of her ethical responsibilities when assessing clients. According to the ANA "Code for Nurses" (1985),

> the nurse provides services with respect for human dignity and the uniqueness of the client. . . . The nurse safeguards the client's right to privacy by judiciously protecting information of a confidential nature.

Honesty and confidentiality are the issues most frequently encountered during this step of the nursing process. These issues involve the moral principles of veracity and autonomy.

Honesty

The moral principle of **veracity** holds that we should tell the truth and not lie. In assessing patients, this means that you should be honest about how you will use the data: to plan the patient's care, for research, for a student paper, and so forth. Remember when you introduce yourself to the patient to tell him what to expect from the interview and how the information will be used.

Truthfulness also affects the patient's autonomy. The moral principle of **autonomy** holds that a person has the right to be independent and to determine for himself what is to happen to him. If the patient does not know how the data will be used, he cannot make a truly informed choice about whether to participate in the interview and thereby loses some of his autonomy.

Confidentiality

Treat assessment data as confidential. Failure to do so robs the patient of his autonomy, since it removes his control over how data is used and shared. Among other things, confidentiality means that assessment notes should be kept in the patient's chart, not lying about where anyone else can read them. It also means that you should not talk about patient data at the desk, in the halls, or in the lunchroom, where casual observers might overhear.

A client may tell you something in confidence that you feel you must tell in order to protect her; for example, a client might tell you of her plans for suicide. If you believe you cannot keep the information confidential, then you are obligated (by the principle of veracity) to tell the client that, in her best interest, you must share the information with other caregivers. A similar situation arises when a client tells you something that you feel you must reveal in order to protect someone else. There is no rule about when to tell and when not to tell. You will, each time, have to balance the need to preserve autonomy against the need to protect the client or others.

healthstyle: a self-test

All of us want good health. But many of us do not know how to be as healthy as possible. Health experts now describe lifestyle as one of the most important factors affecting health. In fact, it is estimated that as many as seven of the ten leading causes of death could be reduced through common-sense changes in lifestyle. That's what this brief test, developed by the Public Health Service, is all about. Its purpose is simply to tell you how well you are doing to stay healthy. The behavior is covered in the test are recommended for most Americans. Some of them may not apply to persons with certain chronic diseases or handicaps, or to pregnant women. Such persons may require special instructions from their physicians.

Cigarette Smoking

If you never smoke, enter a score of 10 for this section and go to the next section on *Alcohol and Drugs*.

	Almost Always	Sometimes	Almost Never
1. I avoid smoking cigarettes.	2	1	0
2. I smoke only low tar and nicotine cigarettes *or* I smoke a pipe or cigars.	2	1	0

Smoking Score: _____

Alcohol and Drugs

	Almost Always	Sometimes	Almost Never
1. I avoid drinking alcoholic beverages or I drink no more than 1 or 2 drinks a day.	4	1	0
2. I avoid using alcohol or other drugs (especially illegal drugs) as a way of handling stressful situations or the problems in my life.	2	1	0
3. I am careful not to drink alcohol when taking certain medicines (for example, medicine for sleeping, pain, colds, and allergies), or when pregnant.	2	1	0
4. I read and follow the label directions when using prescribed and over-the-counter drugs.	2	1	0

Alcohol and Drugs Score: _____

Eating Habits

	Almost Always	Sometimes	Almost Never
1. I eat a variety of foods each day, such as fruits and vegetables, whole grain breads and cereals, lean meats, dairy products, dry peas and beans, and nuts and seeds.	4	1	0
2. I limit the amount of fat, saturated fat, and cholesterol I eat (including fat on meats, eggs, butter, cream, shortenings, and organ meats such as liver).	2	1	0
3. I limit the amount of salt I eat by cooking with only small amounts, not adding salt at the table, and avoiding salty snacks.	2	1	0
4. I avoid eating too much sugar (especially frequent snacks of sticky candy or soft drinks).	2	1	0

Eating Habits Score: _____

Exercise/Fitness

	Almost Always	Sometimes	Almost Never
1. I maintain a desired weight, avoiding overweight and underweight.	3	1	0
2. I do vigorous exercises for 15–30 minutes at least 3 times a week (examples include running, swimming, brisk walking).	3	1	0
3. I do exercises that enhance my muscle tone for 15–30 minutes at least 3 times a week (examples include yoga and calisthenics).	2	1	0
4. I use part of leisure time participating in individual, family, or team activities that increase my level of fitness (such as gardening, bowling, golf, and baseball).	2	1	0

Exercise/Fitness Score: _____

Stress Control

	Almost Always	Sometimes	Almost Never
1. I have a job or do other work that I enjoy.	2	1	0
2. I find it easy to relax and express my feelings freely.	2	1	0
3. I recognize early, and prepare for, events or situations likely to be stressful for me.	2	1	0
4. I have close friends, relatives, or others whom I can talk to about personal matters and call on for help when needed.	2	1	0
5. I participate in group activities (such as church and community organizations or hobbies that I enjoy.	2	1	0

Stress Control Score: _____

Safety

	Almost Always	Sometimes	Almost Never
1. I wear a seat belt while riding in a car.	2	1	0
2. I avoid driving while under the influence of alcohol and other drugs.	2	1	0
3. I obey traffic rules and the speed limit when driving.	2	1	0
4. I am careful when using potentially harmful products or substances (such as household cleaners, poisons, and electrical devices).	2	1	0
5. I avoid smoking in bed.	2	1	0

Safety Score: _____

Figure 3–4. Healthstyle: A Self Test. Courtesy of National Health Information Clearinghouse, Washington, D.C.

What Your Scores Mean to YOU

Scores of 9 and 10

Excellent! Your answers show that you are aware of the importance of this area to your health. More important, you are putting your knowledge to work for you by practicing good health habits. As long as you continue to do so, this area should not pose a serious health risk. It's likely that you are setting an example for your family and friends to follow. Since you got a very high test score on this part of the test, you may want to consider other areas where your scores indicate room for improvement.

Scores of 6 to 8

Your health practices in this area are good, but there is room for improvement. Look again at the items you answered with "Sometimes" or "Almost Never." What changes can you make to improve your score? Even a small change can often help you achieve better health.

Scores of 3 to 5

Your health risks are showing! Would you like more information about the risks you are facing and about why it is important for you to change these behaviors. Perhaps you need help in deciding how to successfully make the changes you desire. In either case, help is available.

Scores of 0 to 2

Obviously, you were concerned enough about your health to take the test, but your answers show that you may be taking serious and unnecessary risks with your health. Perhaps you are not aware of the risks and what to do about them You can easily get the information and help you need to improve, if you wish. The next step is up to you.

YOU Can Start Right Now!

In the test you just completed were numerous suggestions to help you reduce your risk of disease and premature death. Here are some of the most significant:

• *Avoid cigarettes.* Cigarette smoking is the single most important preventable cause of illness and early death. It is especially risky for pregnant women and their unborn babies. Persons who stop smoking reduce their risk of getting heart disease and cancer. So if you're a cigarette smoker, think twice about lighting that next cigarette. If you choose to continue smoking, try decreasing the number of cigarettes you smoke and switching to a low tar and nicotine brand.

• *Follow sensible drinking habits.* Alcohol produces changes in mood and behavior. Most people who drink are able to control their intake of alcohol and to avoid undesired, and often harmful, effects, Heavy, regular use of alcohol can lead to cirrhosis of the liver, a leading cause of death. Also, statistics clearly show that mixing drinking and driving is often the cause of fatal or crippling accidents. So if you drink, do it wisely and in moderation. *Use care in taking drugs.* Today's greater use of drugs—both legal and illegal—is one of our most serious health risks. Even some drugs prescribed by your doctor can be dangerous if taken when drinking alcohol or before driving. Excessive or continued use of tranquilizers (or "pep pills") can cause physical and mental problems. Using or experimenting with illicit drugs such as marijuana, heroin, cocaine, and PCP may lead to a number of damaging effects or even death.

• *Eat sensibly.* Overweight individuals are at greater risk for diabetes, gall bladder disease, and high blood pressure. So it makes good sense to maintain proper weight. But good eating habits also mean holding down the amount of fat (especially saturated fat), cholesterol, sugar and salt in your diet. If you must snack, try nibbling on fresh fruits and vegetables. You'll feel better—and look better, too.

• *Exercise regularly.* Almost everyone can benefit form exercise—and there's some form of exercise almost everyone can do. (If you have any doubt, check first with your doctor.) Usually, as little as 15–30 minutes of vigorous exercise three times a week will help you have a healthier heart, eliminate excess weight, tone up sagging muscles, and sleep better. Think how much difference all these improvements could make in the way you feel!

• *Learn to handle stress.* Stress is a normal part of living; everyone faces it to some degree. The causes of stress can be good or bad, desirable or undesirable (such as a promotion on the job or the loss of a spouse). Properly handled, stress need not be a problem. But unhealthy responses to stress—such a driving too fast or erratically, drinking too much, or prolonged anger or grief—can cause a variety of physical and mental problems. Even on a very busy day, find a few minutes to slow down and relax. Talking over a problem with someone you trust can often help you find a satisfactory solution. Learn to distinguish between things that are "worth fighting about" and things that are less important.

• *Be safety conscious.* Think "safety first" at home, at work , at school, at play, and on the highway. Buckle seat belts and obey traffic rules. Keep poisons and weapons out of the reach of children, and keep emergency numbers by your telephone. When the unexpected happens, you'll be prepared.

Figure 3–4. (continued)

In both instances, it is better from an ethical standpoint to stop the client from telling you something you cannot keep confidential. Of course this is not always possible, but often you can pick up clues from the client that she is about to disclose this kind of information. If you do, you might say something like, "This sounds like something I may not be able to keep confidential. Are you *sure* you want to go on with it?"

BOX 3–2. Guide to the Assessment Step

1. Collect data
    Interview
    Observation
    Physical examination
2. Validate data with client and significant others
    Compare subjective and objective data
    Validate conflicting data
3. Organize and record data
    Initial assessment: Use printed form (admission data base)
    Ongoing assessment: Use nursing model to organize; record on care
    plan or nursing progress notes.

SUMMARY

Assessment
✓ is the collection, validation, organization, and recording of data using interview, observation, and examination.
✓ requires critical-thinking skills, good knowledge, and an awareness of ethical issues such as confidentiality and honesty.
✓ uses directive and nondirective interviewing techniques, adapting to the special needs of the client.
✓ may involve various conceptual models to collect and organize data such as Maslow's Hierarchy of Needs, Roy's Adaptation Theory, Gordon's Functional Health Patterns, the Unitary Person Framework, or a wellness framework.
✓ includes consideration of the moral principles of veracity and autonomy.

Skill-Building Activities

When a state studies its transportation problems, the planners classify the various means of transportation in a few categories such as cars, trucks, buses, planes, and trains. This is done so that the large bulk of information about how each kind of vehicle fits into the state's transportation picture can be summarized. Generalities about each class of vehicle are more valuable in planning than the mass of unorganized data about each kind of vehicle. Also, such classification can produce new information by identifying common features of the vehicles in each category.

Similarly, when collecting patient data, nurses classify it according to their chosen theoretical framework (e.g., Maslow, Gordon, NANDA). Unclassified data about a patient might look something like this:

Harold Sims is a 35-year-old carpenter. He is married and has three children. There is a 2-inch scar on his forearm. He states he has been "short of breath" on exertion and is coughing frequently. Scattered wheezes are auscultated throughout his lungs. He is able to read newsprint without glasses. Active bowel sounds are auscultated in all four quadrants of his abdomen.

Now look at the data again, listed with the related cues in bold print:

Age 35
Works as a carpenter
2-inch scar on forearm
States he has been "**short of breath**" on exertion.
States having frequent **cough**
Scattered wheezes auscultated throughout lungs
Able to read newsprint without glasses
Married; has 3 children
Active bowel sounds auscultated in all 4 quadrants

This is only a small part of the total data collected on a patient. Notice how difficult it is to find the related items, even when they are in bold print. With a framework for data collection, related items are classified together naturally, making the data more meaningful and the patterns more obvious. A framework also helps prevent omission of data, since categories with scant or no data will be obvious when you have finished your assessment.

Learning the Skill of Classification

Let's start with an example in your community. You will classify the various jobs in your community into the following categories: agricultural, technical, medical, clerical, and other. List some local jobs that fit each classification.

Agricultural

Technical

Medical

Clerical

Other

Compare your answers with those of your classmates and discuss any differences you may have in your classifications. Explain why each job fits in its category.

Applying the Skill

Classify the following patient data using two different frameworks: Gordon's and NANDA's. Review the discussion in Chapter 3 about these frameworks and refer to Tables 3–4 and 3–5 as needed.

Discuss your answers with your classmates individually or in class. There is no answer key for this exercise because the emphasis is not on whether your answers are *correct*, but on the thinking process you used to arrive at the answers—that is, the skill of *classifying*. The only way to evaluate your thinking process is to discuss it with others and get feedback from them.

Patient Data

Age 37
States having continual vaginal bleeding for the past 6 months
States has never been pregnant
Skin warm and dry
Hears normal speech at 10 feet
Takes iron pills
Weighs 130 lb.
States "light social drinker"
States she has asthma
States she is not concerned about effect of hysterectomy on her sexuality
Works as a hairdresser
"I sleep a lot" when under stress
Blood sugar—124
Chest X ray normal
Manages all activities of daily living independently
Takes a bulk-forming laxative daily
Blood pressure 120/80

Oriented to time, place, and person
Wants to see hospital chaplain before surgery
States vision is 20/20 with glasses
Good skin turgor
Full range of motion of neck
Hemoglobin 9.5
5 feet, 5 inches tall
Has smoked 1/2 pack per day for 16 years
Lungs clear to auscultation
Allergic to penicillin
States eats 3 meals a day, but snacks often
States mother had cervical cancer
Has frequent headaches. Takes aspirin to relieve.
Unmarried
Urinates 5–6 times per day. "No difficulty"
Temperature 100°
Drinks "lots of water"
Hospitalized in 1980 for appendectomy
One formed stool per day; occasional constipation

1. **Classify the data, using Gordon's framework.** (A few items have been classified for you. Notice that some of the data appears in more than one pattern.)

Patterns	Data
Health-perception/ health-management	Takes iron pills
Nutritional-metabolic	Takes iron pills
Elimination	
Activity-exercise	States she has asthma
Cognitive-perceptual	
Sleep-rest	
Self-perception/ Self-concept	
Role-relationship	
Sexuality-reproductive	
Coping/ stress-tolerance	
Value-belief	
Other	Age 37

2. **Classify the data, using NANDA Human Response Patterns** (A few items have been classified for you. Notice that some of the data appears in more than one pattern.)

Human Response Pattern	Data
Exchanging	Skin warm and dry
Communicating	
Relating	States not concerned about effect of hysterectomy on sexuality.
Valuing	
Choosing	States not concerned about effect of hysterectomy on sexuality.
Moving	
Perceiving	
Knowing	
Feeling	
Other	

Notice that in some categories (or patterns) you may have entered no data. If you have classified the data correctly, this would indicate to you, as a practicing nurse, that your data collection is incomplete.

Adapted from *Critical Thinking Worksheets,* a Supplement of *Addison-Wesley Chemistry,* by Wilbraham et al. (Menlo Park, CA: Addison-Wesley Publishing Company, 1990).

(Answer Key, p. 374)

1. Listed below are data-collection practices observed on various nursing units. You are the quality-control nurse. Place a check mark beside the practices that meet ANA Standard I.

   a. ___ Admission data is recorded on a printed form in predetermined categories.

   b. ___ There is an admission assessment in the chart. The nursing progress notes on two different days list care given to the patient, but no assessment data about the patient.

   c. ___ The nurses record the comprehensive assessment in paragraph form on the nursing progress notes; they do not all record the data in the same order.

   d. ___ Each patient's chart contains a nursing history and physical examination. A divider with a tab makes these easy to locate.

2. Place a *C* beside the cues. Place an *I* beside the inferences.

   a. ___ The client's blood pressure is 140/80.

   b. ___ The client states he is in pain.

   c. ___ The client is afraid.

   d. ___ The client is depressed.

   e. ___ The client's wife says he forgets to take his pills.

   f. ___ The incision is draining pink fluid.

   g. ___ The incision is infected.

3. Classify the data on the next page by placing the letters in the appropriate columns. Note that most letters will be placed in *two* columns (subjective/objective and primary/secondary). The first one is done for you.

Subjective Data	Objective Data	Primary Source	Secondary Source
	a		a

a. You read in the chart that the client's blood pressure is 140/80.

b. Client's wife says he doesn't sleep well.

c. You observe that the client is pale.

d. The aide tells you the client is pale.

e. You palpate the client's pulse. It is 84 bpm.

f. Mrs. Jones says, "I can't sleep."

g. The nursing progress notes say, "Client is breathing rapidly."

h. The night nurse reports the client's temperature is 98.6°.

i. The client is coughing.

j. Client states he is cold.

k. The client is walking with a limp.

l. Urine output measured at 100 cc.

m. You feel the dressing. It is dry.

n. Client says she cannot void.

o. You auscultate wheezes in the patient's lungs.

p. Anesthetist tells you the pulse is weak and thready.

q. You palpate a weak, thready pulse.

r. Patient tells you his leg hurts.

4. Suppose your instructor gives you the following patient assignment for the next day.

> You are to perform the admission assessment, including interview and physical examination, on Melissa Bourque, who is being admitted for cosmetic surgery. Patient is a 45-year-old female. Her preoperative lab work has been done and will be on the chart, along with her medical records from the physician's office.

Will you read Ms. Bourque's chart before doing the nursing interview? Why or why not?

5. Indicate whether the *nurse* (you) obtained the data by interview (*I*), observation (*O*), or physical examination (*E*).

a. ___ You read in the chart that the client's blood pressure is 140/80.

b. ___ Client's wife says he doesn't sleep well.

c. ___ You see that the client is pale.

d. ___ You feel the dressing. It is dry.

e. ___ You count the client's pulse at 84 bpm.

f. ___ You hear the client cough.

g. ___ Client states he is cold.

h. ___ Urine output is measured at 100 cc.

i. ___ Client says she cannot void.

j. ___ You auscultate wheezes in the client's lungs.

k. ___ Anesthetist tells you the pulse is weak and thready.

6. Which of these questions would you ask *earliest* in the interview? Why?

  a. What birth control measures do you use?

  b. Do you have any allergies?

7. Identify the type of question: *C* = Closed, *O* = Open-ended.

  a. ___ Would you like a backrub?

  b. ___ Where would you like me to begin?

  c. ___ Did you sleep well?

  d. ___ How did you sleep?

  e. ___ What do you think kept you from sleeping well?

  f. ___ Are you hearing voices?

  g. ___ Tell me about the voices.

  h. ___ Are you worried about the operation?

  i. ___ How do you feel now?

  j. ___ Tell me about the delivery.

8. The client says, "I have this pain in my stomach." Write examples of questions the nurse could ask to find out more about it.

  a. A closed question:

  b. An open-ended question:

9. You need to perform the data base assessment for Stella Contini. You have read her chart and know that she is 50 years old, unmarried, and has no children. She has severe arthritis in several joints and is being admitted for a total knee replacement. Her mother and sister are at the bedside. Ms. Contini has a roommate in the adjoining bed.

  a. To *prepare* for the interview, what do you need to do?

b. There is a section on the assessment form labeled "Reason for Hospitalization." What would you say to Ms. Contini to elicit this information?

c. There is a section on the form labeled "Usual sexual functioning" and another labeled "Changes in sexual functioning since illness." Would you ask these questions? Why or why not?

10. Place a check mark beside the data that should be validated.

   a. ___ The patient tells you he is not anxious about the barium enema. He is lying quietly in bed with no obvious muscle tension. His hands are still. His skin is warm and dry.

   b. ___ The patient says, "On a scale of 1 to 10, the pain is a 10. Worst I can imagine." Less than five minutes ago, you observed the patient talking on the telephone in a normal tone of voice.

   c. ___ The patient says he smokes two packs of cigarettes a day. You observe that his teeth and fingers are brown-stained.

   d. ___ The client tells you on admission that she lives alone. In a later conversation, she refers to her roommate.

   e. ___ The data was obtained early in the interview, and then the client became confused and began to ramble incoherently.

   f. ___ The mother says her little boy "eats like a horse." You observe that the child is thin and small for his age.

11. Some of the following nursing progress notes consist of data. Others are judgments about the data or conclusions drawn by the nurse. Draw a line through each of the judgments/conclusions.

   a. Patient stated, "I feel sick."

   b. Vomited 100 cc green-tinged fluid.

   c. Patient is nauseated.

   d. Patient was tearful during the interview.

   e. Client is disoriented.

f. Tolerated clear liquids well.

g. Ambulated to bathroom with no dizziness.

h. Ms. Benitez is extremely fearful of this surgery.

i. Abdomen is distended.

j. Client states he is confused about the medication schedule.

k. Respirations normal.

l. Vision is poor.

m. Drinking adequate amount of fluids.

12. Write the correct word in the blank: Is the situation a question of *veracity, confidentiality,* or *neither?*

   a. _____ The nurse asks the patient whether he prefers a bedbath or a whirlpool bath.

   b. _____ Before beginning the interview, the nurse tells the patient she needs the information to help plan his care.

   c. _____ Nora Morenz is collecting data about pain relief measures for a research project. Because it does not change the patients' care and because they are not mentioned by name, she decides not to tell them she is collecting data for research.

   d. _____ A patient's wife overhears the staff discussing information about her husband in the lunchroom.

   e. _____ The client tells the nurse she has a knife hidden in the room and that "Someone is going to be sorry." The nurse looks for the knife, but cannot find it. She tells the client, "I am afraid for you and for the other patients. I'm sorry, but I will have to share what you've told me with the rest of the staff."

13. Under which of Gordon's functional health patterns should the following data be placed?

   a. _____ "My kids are home alone. I'm worried about them."

   b. _____ Skin pale and damp.

   c. _____ Client is blind.

   d. _____ Client states she sleeps 4 hours a night.

   e. _____ "I probably brought this illness on myself. I never got my Pap smears when I was supposed to. I guess I deserve this."

f. _____ Client has annual physical examination.

g. _____ "My doctor says I have high blood pressure. I'm supposed to stop eating salt, but I just can't do it."

REFERENCES

Alfaro, R. (1990). _Applying Nursing Diagnosis and Nursing Process: A Step-by-Step Guide._ Philadelphia: J. B. Lippincott.

American Nurses Association. (1973). _Standards of Nursing Practice._ Kansas City, MO.

American Nurses Association. (1985). _Code for Nurses with Interpretative Statements._ Kansas City, MO.

Carpenito, L. (1989). _Nursing Diagnosis: Application to Clinical Practice._ 3rd ed. Philadelphia: J. B. Lippincott.

Edelman, C., and Mandle, C. (1986). _Health Promotion Throughout the Life Span._ St. Louis, MO: C. V. Mosby.

Gordon, M. (1987). _Nursing Diagnosis: Process and Application._ 2nd ed. New York: McGraw-Hill.

Maslow, A. (1970). _Motivation and Personality._ 2nd ed. New York: Harper & Row.

North American Nursing Diagnosis Association. (1986). _Classification of Nursing Diagnoses: Proceedings of the Sixth Conference._ St. Louis: C. V. Mosby.

North American Nursing Diagnosis Association. (1989). _Classification of Nursing Diagnoses: Proceedings of the Eighth Conference._ Philadelphia: J. B. Lippincott.

Pender, N. (1987). _Health Promotion in Nursing Practice._ 2nd ed. Norwalk, CT: Appleton & Lange.

Pinnell, N., and de Meneses, M. (1986). _The Nursing Process: Theory, Application, and Related Processes._ Norwalk, CT: Appleton-Century-Crofts.

Roy, Sr. C. (1976). _Introduction to Nursing: An Adaptation Model._ Englewood Cliffs, NJ: Prentice Hall.

CHAPTER 4

DIAGNOSTIC REASONING

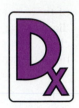

OBJECTIVES

Upon completing this chapter you should be able to do the following:
- Explain how diagnosis is related to the other steps of the nursing process.
- Differentiate between the various uses of the term *diagnosis*.
- Describe the process of diagnostic reasoning.
- Explain what is meant by a *client problem*.
- Given a client problem, correctly identify its type and status.
- Describe common diagnostic errors and explain how they can be prevented.
- Explain why and how you should verify your nursing diagnoses.

INTRODUCTION

This chapter will (1) discuss diagnosis as a step of the nursing process; (2) define *patient problem* and help you begin to differentiate between a problem and other phenomena, such as symptoms and medical diagnoses; and (3) explain the diagnostic reasoning process. In this chapter you will learn to identify three kinds of health problems:

1. Problems nurses can treat independently *(nursing diagnoses)*
2. Problems nurses treat in collaboration with other health professionals *(collaborative problems)*
3. Problems for which nurses give delegated care prescribed by others *(medical problems)*

It is essential to fully understand the concept of *patient problems* before attempting to write nursing diagnoses, because a nursing diagnosis is usually a statement of a health problem. Beginning diagnosticians often have difficulty in understanding exactly what the client's problem *is;* they are not sure if it is a symptom, a complaint, a situation, a disease, or a pathophysiology. Therefore, this chapter is intended to help you form the concept of *problem* before you attempt to work with special types of problems (e.g., nursing diagnoses).

Nursing diagnoses provide the basis for giving individualized care, but nursing care is not limited to interventions based on nursing diagnoses. Nurses use the *diagnostic reasoning process,* to draw conclusions about the client's health status and decide whether nursing intervention is needed. This means that nurses diagnose both nursing diagnoses and collaborative problems; and although they do not actually diagnose medical conditions, they must be aware

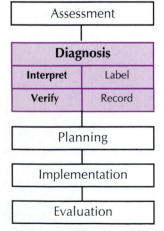

Figure 4–1. Diagnosis

of their existence and of the client's need for medical interventions. The same diagnostic reasoning process is used, regardless of problem type. Therefore, this chapter focuses on the *diagnostic process* as it applies to the identification of *all* health problems, not just to nursing diagnoses.

The diagnostic process is more than simply choosing some likely looking labels to put on a client's care plan; these labels must reflect the client's health problems accurately. This chapter will help you to identify problems correctly and accurately. Because clients have health problems *other* than nursing diagnoses, the standardized lists of nursing diagnosis labels (such as the NANDA lists found on the inside covers of your text) cannot describe all of a client's problems. This chapter deals with the broader concept of *problems,* not just nursing diagnoses; therefore it does not always use NANDA terminology. Nursing diagnoses and standardized language are presented in depth in Chapter 5.

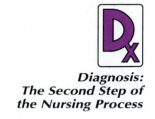

DIAGNOSIS: THE SECOND STEP OF THE NURSING PROCESS

During diagnosis, the second step of the nursing process, nurses use critical thinking skills such as making inferences, analysis, and synthesis to interpret patient data. Data is interpreted in order to identify patient health status (i.e., strengths, problems, and causes of the problems). Strengths and problems are verified with the patient, formally labeled, and recorded on the patient's care plan. The nursing activities that are a part of the diagnosis step are shown in Figure 4–1.

Relationship to Other Nursing Process Steps

Recall from Chapter 1 that the steps of the nursing process are interdependent and overlapping. Diagnosis is a pivotal step in the nursing process. All activities preceding this step are directed toward formulating the nursing diagnoses. All the care-planning activities following this step are based on the nursing diagnoses (see Figure 4–2).

Diagnosis depends on the assessment phase because the quality of the data acquired during assessment affects the accuracy of the nursing diagnoses. The following example illustrates how the two stages overlap. Like most nurses, the nurse in the example begins to think of possible meanings for some of the data (diagnosis) as she is collecting it (assessment).

Example: During the assessment interview, Nurse Adkins notices that the patient is speaking hesitantly and softly, giving brief answers, and refusing to make eye contact. She wonders if the patient is shy, withdrawn, anxious, or perhaps having difficulty with his self-concept. She continues to gather data to confirm or deny these possibilities. In the diagnosis step, she will critically examine all the patient data she has gathered and draw a firmer conclusion about its meaning.

Diagnosis also affects the planning, implementation and evaluation steps. The problems and strengths identified during diagnosis provide a focus for planning the patient's care (planning phase). When specifically and accurately stated, they guide the nurse in developing appropriate goals and nursing orders for the care plan.

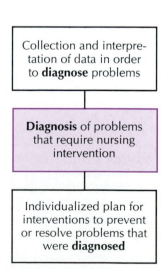

Figure 4–2. Diagnosis: A Pivotal Step

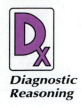

**Diagnostic
Reasoning**

The diagnosis and implementation steps sometimes occur almost simultaneously. For example, in an emergency situation a nurse may take action (implementation) as soon as the urgent problem is recognized—before she consciously makes a plan or identifies the rest of the problems, or even before completely analyzing the data. Diagnosis also overlaps with the evaluation phase. During evaluation, the nurse determines whether the patient's problems have changed status or been resolved. If not, they are reexamined to be sure they were diagnosed correctly and completely.

Terminology

Diagnosis is a key step in the nursing process. It is also the step that creates the most confusion for students and practicing nurses alike. One of the difficulties is that diagnosis is both a process and a product. That is, a nurse uses a reasoning process called *nursing diagnosis* to produce a statement of health status that is also called a *nursing diagnosis*. In order to write the statement, the nurse refers to a standardized list of terms that are sometimes called *nursing diagnoses.* You will see *diagnosis* given all these meanings in the literature. To minimize confusion, this text uses the terms adapted from Carpenito (1989) and shown in Figure 4–3.

This chapter presents *diagnosis* both as a step of the nursing process and as a nursing activity. It will also introduce *nursing diagnosis* (the problem statement). Chapter 5 discusses nursing diagnosis in more depth and explains how to use the NANDA *diagnostic labels* to write problem statements.

DIAGNOSIS: A NURSING ACTIVITY

Recall that diagnosis is a nursing activity as well as a step of the nursing process. This section includes a detailed discussion of diagnostic reasoning. First it explores the meaning of *human response* and explains how to recognize a *patient problem*. It then differentiates between actual, potential (high-risk), and possible problems and between three types of health problems: nursing diagnoses, collaborative problems, and medical conditions. Finally, it describes, step-by-step, the process of interpreting data.

Definition of Diagnosis as an Activity

Diagnosis is an intellectual activity in which critical thinking skills are used to identify patterns and draw conclusions. It is the reasoning process any expert group uses to draw conclusions about the nature and cause of their phenomena of concern. Speech therapists diagnose speaking problems, teachers diagnose learning problems, physicians diagnose diseases, and automobile mechanics diagnose engine problems. Each profession diagnoses its own particular phenomena of concern.

Recall from Chapter 1 that the phenomena of concern for nurses are human responses. In nursing, therefore, **diagnosis** is an intellectual activity that uses critical thinking skills to identify patterns and make judgments about human responses to actual or potential health problems.

Diagnosis is an intellectual activity in which nurses use critical thinking skills to identify patterns and make judgments about human responses to actual or potential health problems.

History of Diagnosis

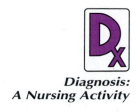

Diagnosis:
A Nursing Activity

The term *diagnosis* began to appear in the nursing literature in the 1950s. McManus (1951) used the term *nursing diagnosis* in describing the functions of a professional nurse. Fry (1953) stated that nursing diagnosis was based on the client's needs for nursing care rather than medical therapies. Until that time nursing had been conceptualized as a set of tasks, and nursing care was planned around those tasks. Nurses assisted physicians in treating diseases. They gathered data about patients, but primarily for the purpose of ensuring that doctors could make medical diagnoses, not for the purpose of planning nursing care.

In the 1960s, as the term became more common, there was some question as to whether diagnosing by nurses was encroaching on medical territory. Diagnosis was becoming an important part of the nursing process, but it was still necessary to differentiate between nursing diagnosis and medical diagnosis—to establish that the purpose and the phenomena of concern were different and that diagnosis was a cognitive process that nurses could and should use.

The ANA, in its *Standards of Nursing Practice* (1973), included nursing diagnosis as an important part of the nursing process. This legitimized it as a function of professional nurses, and several states began to use the term in their nurse practice acts. In that same year the first national nursing diagnosis task force, now the North American Nursing Diagnosis Association (NANDA), met to begin working on standardizing the terminology for nursing diagnoses (Gebbie and Lavin, 1975; Gebbie, 1976). The group continues to meet biannually to refine the diagnostic labels and the system for classifying them.

Standard II: Nursing diagnoses are derived from health status data (ANA, 1973).

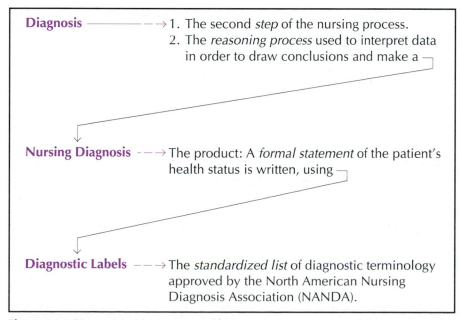

Diagnosis — — — → 1. The second *step* of the nursing process.
2. The *reasoning process* used to interpret data in order to draw conclusions and make a

Nursing Diagnosis - — → The product: A *formal statement* of the patient's health status is written, using

Diagnostic Labels - — → The *standardized list* of diagnostic terminology approved by the North American Nursing Diagnosis Association (NANDA).

Figure 4–3. *Diagnosis* in Nursing Terminology

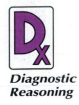

Diagnostic Reasoning

During the 1970s and 1980s, the term *nursing diagnosis* was incorporated into virtually all state nurse practice acts, making diagnosis a nursing obligation as well as a legal right. Diagnosis is now taught in most schools of nursing, commonly referred to in the literature, and frequently used by nurses to describe problem identification in their practice.

The Importance of Diagnosing

There remains little controversy over diagnosis as a nursing activity. Diagnosing is now a standard by which professional care is measured. The ANA Standard II states that "nursing diagnoses are derived from health status data." Standards III and IV further state that goals and nursing interventions should be derived from the nursing diagnoses (ANA 1973). The acceptance of diagnosing as a nursing function and as a step of the nursing process has been beneficial to clients and to the profession.

Facilitates Individualized Care Perhaps the most important benefit is that nursing diagnosis enables nurses to give individualized patient care. Even though patients with identical medical conditions may need similar "routine" nursing interventions, the priorities of care may differ for each. A prioritized list of nursing diagnoses enables the nurse to concentrate on the care most important for each individual. For example, a nurse is caring for Mary Chinn and Donald Schulz, who have had myocardial infarctions (heart attack). For these and all M.I. patients, the nurse would follow the agency standards for monitoring vital signs and observing for complications such as arrhythmias and congestive heart failure. However, a prioritized list of nursing diagnoses for each of these two patients clearly shows that each requires individualized care aside from the "routine." Nursing diagnosis helps to assure that their special needs are identified.

Makes Care Planning Easier Nurses who use nursing diagnosis find it easier to plan and give nursing care. The diagnostic labels help them to manage the large quantity and variety of patient information by organizing it into fewer, larger chunks, or concepts. A diagnostic label, such as Altered Oral Mucous Membrane, is a concept. Recall from Chapter 2 that a concept is a mental image of reality that has been generalized from many particular instances.

Example: Suppose you have collected the following data (only a small part of the complete data base for a patient): Patient states his mouth is painful. His tongue is coated. Patient has very little saliva; mucous membranes are dry. Several vesicles and ulcerations are observed in patient's oral cavity. Patient is breathing through his mouth; strong odor noted. Patient is receiving head and neck radiation therapy.

As a concept, the following nursing diagnosis gives you the same picture as that entire set of data:

Altered Oral Mucous Membrane related to mouth breathing, insufficient fluid intake, and radiation therapy.

Once you have grasped the concept *Altered Oral Mucous Membrane,* the term will suggest to you the presence of those cues. When you observe one cue, you will be alert for related cues that might lead you to diagnose Altered Oral Mucous Membrane. For example, when you notice that a patient is mouth breathing, you will check to see if his mucous membranes are dry and check his fluid intake. The reverse is also true. If a colleague tells you, "Mr. Anzio has Altered Oral Mucous Membrane related to mouth breathing and insufficient fluid intake," you will have a picture in your mind of the condition of his mouth: his tongue is probably coated, and his mouth is probably dry and sore.

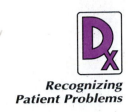

Defines the Domain of Nursing   "A profession must have a language that communicates its uniqueness and at the same time is understood by peers, other professionals, and consumers/clients" (Warren and Hoskins, 1990, p. 162). Nursing diagnoses are an important vehicle for describing nursing's unique contributions to health care—for defining the domain of nursing. Diagnostic language makes it clear that nurses do far more than simply carry out physicians' orders for treating disease. It enables nurses to communicate to administrators, legislators, consumers, and insurance providers the specific nature of the health conditions they treat. In addition to promoting interdisciplinary communication, nursing diagnoses are used for measuring nursing work loads and for staffing and budgeting purposes.

Improves Communication Within the Profession   Communication among nurses also improves when nurses in education, research, and practice all use a standard language to describe the patient's health status. When a physician says a patient has diabetes, other physicians all have a similar mental image of the patient's health status. The same is true when nurses discuss, for example, Altered Oral Mucous Membrane.

Increases Nursing Autonomy and Accountability   Because nursing diagnoses help to delineate independent nursing functions (those performed without a physician's order), they increase nursing autonomy and accountability. As independent nursing interventions have become more visible, nurses have needed to accept more responsibility for their actions.

Facilitates Computerized Care Planning   Nursing diagnoses provide a system for storing and retrieving patient information as well as for care planning. As health-care institutions begin to fully utilize computer technology, patient records and care plans are being computer-generated and stored. When the nurse makes a nursing diagnosis for a patient, the computer can generate a comprehensive list of nursing orders that have been stored for that diagnosis. The nurse simply selects the appropriate orders and individualizes them to fit any special needs of the patient.

RECOGNIZING PATIENT PROBLEMS

Since diagnosing involves problem identification, you must know what a problem is. You must be able to differentiate a problem from other phenomena, such as symptoms or treatments. A **health problem** is recognized by the following characteristics:

- It is a human response to a life process, event or stressor.
- It is a health-related condition that both the client and the nurse wish to change.
- It requires intervention in order to prevent or resolve illness, or to facilitate coping.

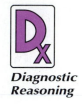

- It results in ineffective coping/adaptation or daily living that is unsatisfying to the client.
- It is an undesirable state.

How you define and recognize *patient problems* depends to a degree upon the nursing framework you use. For example, in the Roy model (1984), you would recognize a problem as a failure of adaptation. In the Gordon (1987) model, a health problem occurs when a health pattern is dysfunctional; that is, when it does not meet expected norms.

Human Responses

When learning to differentiate between patient problems and other phenomena, remember that the focus for nursing diagnosis and care is in the area of human responses. Recall from Chapter 1 that **human responses** are human reactions to an event or a stressor.

Examples of Human Responses	
Changes in:	
Body appearance:	Posture, skin color
Body function:	Inability to move a joint; difficulty in swallowing
Symptoms:	Fever, elevated white-blood-cell count
Knowledge:	Knowledge of foods low in salt
Skills:	Ability to change own dressing
Emotions:	Anger, sadness

In most frameworks, a stressor is anything that causes a change in the body's equilibrium, or steady state. Illness, the environment, resource limitations, loss of supports, and reduced coping ability can all be sources of stressors; indeed, almost anything can cause a human response.

Human responses occur in several *dimensions*. They can be biological (physical), psychological, interpersonal/social, or spiritual.

Example: Consider the following possible responses to the stressor of having a myocardial infarction (heart attack).

Physical response:	Pain
Psychological response:	Fear
Interpersonal/social response:	Returning to work before he is well
Spiritual response:	Praying

Human responses occur at different *levels:* cellular, systemic, organic, or whole-person (organismic). A single stressor can cause multilevel responses. A cellular response occurs at the level of individual cells; for example, the ability of a cell to use glucose may change. Systemic responses occur in body systems, such as the circulatory or respiratory system (e.g., peripheral vasodilation or an increased respiratory rate). Localized skeletal muscle fatigue—in a runner's calves, for instance—is an example of organic response. Nursing occurs at and affects all levels, but nursing diagnosis is usually at the whole-person or possibly the systemic level.

Example: A person who is severely burned loses large amounts of body fluids. If the fluids are not replaced, she responds at the cellular level by losing water from the cells into the bloodstream (cellular dehydration). At the systemic level, the sympathetic nervous system responds to the trauma by decreasing the activity of the gastrointestinal system. At the whole-person level, the person may respond by perceiving pain or, later, by social isolation.

Responses to stressors can be helpful or harmful. Remember, not all human responses are problems. A human response becomes a health problem when it results in ineffective coping or daily living that is unsatisfying to the client. Human responses may be adaptive, helping to restore health, or they may be maladaptive and damaging to health. In fact, a response can be helpful at one time and harmful at another.

Example: Ms. Mason has a "chest cold" and a severe cough. She feels very ill. Her psychological response is *fear* (that she may have pneumonia). The fear motivates her to see her physician for treatment—an adaptive response.

Example: Later Ms. Mason has an episode of postmenopausal bleeding. Her psychological response is again *fear* (that she may have cancer). This time she is overwhelmed by her fear. She avoids seeing a physician because she is afraid he will tell her she has cancer, thereby making it real. This time the fear was a maladaptive response because it immobilized her instead of motivating her to act.

Refer to Table 4–1 for additional examples of stressors and various types and levels of human responses. Notice that a response can become a stressor that produces still *another* response (e.g., Ms. Mason's fear produced avoidance).

Common Errors in Problem Identification

While learning, students sometimes confuse problems with various phenomena that are related but not the same. It may help to have some examples of things that are *not* problems so that you can avoid these errors. The examples on the following pages describe situations that may be incorrectly identified as problems.

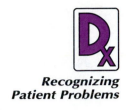

Recognizing Patient Problems

Table 4–1. Various Levels of Stressors and Human Responses

Stressor	Human Response	Type	Level	Effect
Blocked coronary artery, causing decreased O_2 to heart muscle	Damage to heart muscle (ischemia)	Physical	Cellular and organic	Maladaptive
	Pain	Psychological & physical	Whole-person (organismic)	Adaptive, if causes decreased activity, conserving O_2; maladaptive, if causes fight-or-flight response, increasing demand for O_2
	Fear of death	Psychological	Whole-person	Can be adaptive or maladaptive (see above)
Fear of death from heart attack	Increased heart rate	Physical	Systemic	Usually maladaptive
	Praying	Spiritual	Whole-person	Probably adaptive

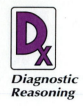

Diagnostic Reasoning

A medical diagnosis while it is a patient problem, should not be used in a nursing diagnosis. Although nurses do provide disease-related care, that is not their primary responsibility. More holistically, *nursing is concerned with the effect of the disease upon the person* and his ability to function. A patient with a medical diagnosis of diabetes mellitus might respond with one or more problems such as lack of motivation to follow diabetic diet, hopelessness because of the incurable nature of the disease, or fear of injecting his own insulin. The following are examples of problem responses that may be associated with medical diagnoses. You can see that the disease and the problem are not identical.

Medical Diagnosis	*Patient Problem (Responses)*
Diabetes mellitus	Increased risk of infection
	Inadequate knowledge of diabetic diet
	Fear of injections
	Altered self-concept
	Feelings of hopelessness
Emphysema	Inability to perform usual work role; loss of job
	Fatigue
	Inability to cook, clean, and care for self
	Fear and anxiety because of difficulty breathing

Pathology and pathophysiology are not patient problems. Of course you must understand the pathophysiology of the patient's illness in order to make nursing diagnoses and plan care. However, *nurses focus on the effects of pathology on the person's functioning.* The pathophysiology of asthma is a narrowing of the bronchial airways. Physicians are concerned with determining the best medication to produce bronchial dilation. Nurses focus on the problems that result from airway constriction, such as inability to give self-care, loss of appetite, and anxiety—all of which are related to difficult breathing and lack of oxygen. Following is an example of pathophysiology and some associated problems.

Pathophysiology	*Problems (Responses)*
Loss of elasticity of lungs; loss of alveolar integrity	Inability to perform usual work role; loss of job
	Fatigue, inability to cook, clean, and care for self
	Fear and anxiety because of difficulty in breathing

Although pathophysiology should not be considered a problem, it may sometimes be the etiology (cause) of a problem, as discussed later in this chapter (see "Diagnostic Reasoning Process").

A nursing problem or nursing goal is not a patient problem. The problem should be viewed from the patient's perspective, not the nurse's. "Foley catheter not draining properly" is a problem for the nurse; the patient's problem is that she is at risk for bladder distention or bladder infection because of the improper drainage. *The patient's problem is the response* (1) that will occur if the nurse's problem is not corrected or (2) that is causing the nurse's problem. Note the following examples.

Nursing Problems or Goals	*Patient Problems*
Patient is noisy; disturbs other patients	Anxiety
	Confusion or disorientation
	Fear of abandonment
Prevent infection	High risk for infection

In the first example, the patient's noisy behavior is a human response, but it is not a problem *to the patient*. It is a symptom of her problem—perhaps that she is anxious, disoriented, or afraid. In the last example, preventing infection is not the *patient's* problem. The patient's problem is that she may acquire an infection if the nurse does not intervene.

A nursing action or routine is not a patient problem. Notice that the following nursing actions/routines are statements of activities that the *nurse* is to perform—the focus is on the nurse. Problems are statements of client health status—the focus is on the client.

Nursing Action or Routine	*Client Problems*
Give emotional support	Anxiety (or possibly fear or grief)
Keep Foley catheter patent	High risk for urinary tract infection
Teach about Basic Four Food Groups	Lack of knowledge about nutritional needs

Diagnostic tests or treatments are not patient problems. The *problem is the patient's response* to the tests and treatments: anxiety, adjustments in daily living, changes in relationships, and so on. Listing the patient's tests and treatments does not provide enough direction for nursing interventions, and fails to individualize the diagnosis. In the following examples you can see that patients may respond in different ways to the same treatment.

Test or Treatment	*Problems (Responses)*
Has a new colostomy	Lack of knowledge and skill in caring for appliance
	Fear of social contact, embarrassment
	Impaired skin integrity around stoma
Must stay on salt-free diet	Lack of motivation to change eating habits
	Lack of knowledge of high-sodium foods

The patient's equipment is not a problem. *The problem is the effect of the equipment on the patient, or the patient's response to it.* Different patients have different responses to the same equipment.

Equipment	*Problem*
Patient has a cast on her leg	Decreased mobility
	Itching
Patient has dentures	Change in body image
	Speech distortion

A patient need is not the same as a patient problem. An unmet need may be the *cause* of a problem, but it is not the same as a problem. The following examples should clarify the difference.

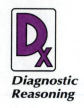

Need	Problem
Need	*Problem*
Needs more sleep	Fatigue; sleep-pattern disturbance
Unmet nutritional needs	Altered nutrition: less than body requirements
Needs emotional support	Grief; altered self-concept; anxiety

Types of Problems

Recall from the "Introduction" section that nurses analyze data to identify three kinds of problems: (1) nursing diagnoses, (2) collaborative problems, and (3) other (usually medical) problems. As a nurse, you will be involved in giving care for all three problem types, and you must be able to distinguish between them. Although nursing responsibility is different for each type, one is not more important than the other. Be careful not to force nursing diagnosis labels onto collaborative problems. Be equally careful not to overlook nursing diagnoses and attempt to fit all the patient's care under "Potential complications of . . . "

Recognizing Nursing Diagnoses

Recall that the phenomena of concern for nursing practice are human responses. It follows that nursing diagnosis should be applied to human responses. At its ninth national conference, NANDA (1990) adopted an official definition of **nursing diagnosis:**

> A nursing diagnosis is a clinical judgement about individual, family, or community responses to actual or potential health problems/life processes. Nursing diagnoses provide the basis for selection of nursing interventions to achieve outcomes for which the nurse is accountable. (p. 114)

A **nursing diagnosis** is a statement of an actual or potential (high-risk) health problem that nurses can legally identify and for which they can prescribe the primary interventions for treatment and prevention. The key term here is *primary.* Nurses may not prescribe *all* the care for a nursing diagnosis (for instance, most patients with a nursing diagnosis of Pain have medical orders for analgesics), but if it is a nursing diagnosis, the nurse can prescribe *most* of the interventions needed to prevent or resolve the problem. Usually the nurse does not need to confer with a physician about treatments for nursing diagnoses.

Because human responses vary, you cannot predict with certainty which nursing diagnoses will occur with a particular disease or treatment. As you can see from the preceding examples, any number of nursing diagnoses may or may not occur with a medical diagnosis. You cannot assume, for example, that someone with diabetes will have Fear of Injections or Lack of Knowledge about a diabetic diet.

For a well client, a nursing diagnosis is a statement reflecting the client's healthy responses, or strengths, in areas where the nurse can intervene independently to promote growth or maintenance of the healthy response; for example: Maintenance of Positive Self-Concept or Potential for Enhanced Self-Concept. Wellness diagnoses are discussed in more detail in Chapter 5. NANDA (1990) defines a **wellness diagnosis** as follows:

> A wellness nursing diagnosis is a clinical judgment about an individual, family, or community in transition from a specific level of wellness to a higher level of wellness. (p. 117)

Nursing diagnosis:

A statement of an actual or high-risk health problem that nurses can

○ Legally identify and treat

○ Prevent or resolve primarily by independent nursing actions

---

Examples of Nursing Diagnoses

Impaired Skin Integrity (excoriation) related to incontinence

High Risk for Infection (of abdominal incision) related to poor nutritional status

Dysfunctional Grieving related to unresolved guilt feelings

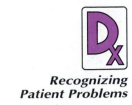

Recognizing Collaborative Problems

Carpenito (1991) states that **collaborative problems** are "certain physiological complications that nurses monitor, to detect their onset or changes in status. Nurses manage collaborative problems by utilizing both physician-prescribed and nursing-prescribed interventions to minimize the complications of the events" (p. 5). Independent nursing interventions for collaborative problems focus mainly on monitoring the patient's condition and preventing the development of the complication. Definitive treatment of the condition requires both medical and nursing interventions.

Because there are a limited number of physiological complications for a given disease, collaborative problems tend to be present any time a particular disease or treatment is present; that is, each disease or treatment has particular complications that are always associated with it. Nursing diagnoses, on the other hand, involve human responses, which vary greatly from one person to the next. Therefore, the same set of nursing diagnoses cannot be expected to occur with a particular disease or condition; and a single nursing diagnosis may occur as a response to any number of diseases. For example, all postpartum patients have similar collaborative problems (potential complications), such as postpartum hemorrhage and thrombophlebitis. But not all new mothers have the same nursing diagnoses. Some might experience Alteration in Parenting (delayed bonding), but most will not. Some might have a Knowledge Deficit problem; others will not.

Appendix D is a list of collaborative problems that are commonly associated with the different body systems (Carpenito, 1989). Table 4–2 lists examples of collaborative problems associated with various tests and treatments.

Recognizing Medical Diagnoses

Medical diagnoses are a type of patient problem. Although medical diagnoses and nursing diagnoses are both reached by the use of the diagnostic reasoning process, they are quite different. A **medical diagnosis** identifies a disease process or pathology and is made for the purpose of treating the pathology. It does not necessarily consider the human responses to the pathology.

Example: The physician diagnoses hypertension and prescribes antihypertensive medications and a low-salt diet. The nurse will diagnose and treat the patient's and family's responses to the medical diagnosis. Is the patient motivated to change his diet? What changes will the family need to make to incorporate the diet change into their menu plan? Does the patient understand the importance of taking his medications, even though they may have unpleasant side effects? If the patient is hospitalized, the nurse will give the medications prescribed by the physician.

As long as the disease process is present, the medical diagnosis does not change. Nursing diagnoses, on the other hand, change as the client's responses change. In the preceding example, the nursing diagnosis might initially be "High risk for Noncompliance with Medication Regimen related to lack of understanding of therapeutic effects and side effects of the drug." However, as the patient gains knowledge of the drug and takes it as ordered, this diagnosis would no longer apply. If the patient found the side effects unpleasant and continued to

Collaborative problems:

○ Usually physiological complications of a disease or treatment.

○ Nurses collaborate with other health-care professionals to treat and prevent.

○ Independent nursing actions focus on prevention and monitoring for onset of problem.

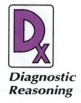

Diagnostic Reasoning

skip doses of the drug, the diagnosis might change to actual "Noncompliance with Medication Regimen. . ." Remember that clients who have the same medical diagnosis may have very different nursing diagnoses. Consider the previous example of Mary Chinn and Donald Schulz, who both have a medical diagnosis of myocardial infarction (heart attack), but have very different nursing diagnoses.

Nurses make observations pertinent to patients' medical diagnoses and perform treatments delegated by the physician. Although nurses do not diagnose or prescribe treatments for medical problems, nursing judgment is required. They

Table 4–2. Examples of Collaborative Problems Associated with Tests and Treatments

Test or Treatment	Collaborative Problem (Potential Complications)	
Arteriogram	Allergic reaction Renal failure Hemorrhage; hematoma	Thrombosis at site Paresthesia Embolism
Bronchoscopy	Airway obstruction (bronchoconstriction)	Hemorrhage
Cardiac catheterization	Site-hemorrhage or hematoma Cardiac arrhythmias, infarction, perforation Paresthesia	Embolism Hypervolemia Hypovolemia
Casts and traction	Misalignment of bones Bleeding Edema	Impaired circulation Neurological compromise
Chest tubes	Bleeding → hemothorax Blockage or displacement → pneumothorax	Septicemia
Foley catheter	Urinary tract infection	Bladder distention
Hemodialysis	Bleeding Air embolism Fluid shifts Electrolyte imbalance	Transfusion reactions Hepatitis B Shunt clotting; fistulas
Intravenous therapy	Infiltration	Phlebitis
Medications	Side effects Toxic effects; overdose	Allergic reactions
Nasogastric suction	Electrolyte imbalance Gastric ulceration → hemorrhage	
Tracheal suctioning	Hypoxia	Bleeding
Surgery	Excessive bleeding → shock Atelectasis Paralytic ileus	Fluid imbalance Electrolyte imbalance Infection
Assisted ventilation	Airway obstruction (tube plugged or displaced) Ineffective O_2–CO_2 exchange Tracheal necrosis	Acid-base imbalance Pneumothorax Respirator dependence

must know the pathophysiology of the disease and understand why the medications or treatments are being given, as well as the client response they are expected to produce. See Table 4–3 for a summary comparison of the three types of patient health problems.

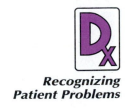

Status of Problems

Problems may be actual, potential, or possible. A care plan should include all three types. A comprehensive nursing care plan includes measures for prevention and detection of high-risk and possible problems, as well as treatment of actual problems.

Actual Problems

An **actual** problem is one that is actually present at the time you make the assessment. It is diagnosed by the presence of associated signs and symptoms. For an actual problem, nursing care is directed toward relieving or resolving the problem.

Example: A patient who has had a cholecystectomy (removal of her gallbladder) has a history of smoking, and has been reluctant to turn, cough, and deep breathe because of pain. She has begun to cough frequently and reports shortness of breath. The nurse auscultates abnormal breath sounds and notes that the client is pale and listless. These signs and symptoms indicate an *actual problem*: *Ineffective Airway Clearance*.

Table 4–3. Comparison of Nursing Diagnoses with Collaborative Problems and Medical Diagnoses

Nursing Diagnoses	Collaborative Problems	Medical Diagnoses
Describe human responses of all kinds.	Involve human responses—mainly physiological complications of disease, tests, or treatments.	Do not consider human responses other than disease and pathology.
Nurses can diagnose.	Nurses can diagnose.	Physician must diagnose.
Nurse orders most interventions to prevent or treat.	Nurse collaborates with physician to prevent and treat (need medical orders).	Physician orders primary interventions to prevent or treat.
Nursing focus: treatment and prevention.	Nursing focus: prevent and monitor for onset or status of condition.	Nursing focus: monitor and implement physician's orders for treatment.
Independent nursing actions.	Some independent actions, but mostly for monitoring and preventing.	Dependent nursing actions.
Can change frequently.	Can change frequently; present when disease or situation is present.	Remains the same while disease is present.

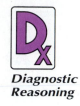

Diagnostic Reasoning

Potential (High-Risk) Problems

A **potential** (or **high-risk**) problem is one that is likely to develop if the nurse does not intervene. Potential problems are diagnosed by the presence of risk factors that predispose a patient to developing a problem. Nursing care is directed toward preventing the problem by reducing the risk factors; or toward early detection of the problem to lessen its consequences.

A potential problem can be either a nursing diagnosis or a collaborative problem. If the problem is a nursing diagnosis, it is labeled *High Risk*. If the problem is collaborative, it is labeled *Potential*.

Example: A patient has just had a cholecystectomy. She has a long history of heavy smoking and respiratory infections. She is reluctant to cough and deep breathe, and moves about in bed only with much encouragement. She is taking morphine (which can depress respirations) for pain control. This patient does not have any symptoms of a respiratory problem. However, given her history and present risk factors, she will probably develop one unless the nurse is aggressive in persuading her to be more mobile and to breathe deeply. The risk factors (her history, pain, narcotics, and immobility) indicate a *potential nursing diagnosis: High Risk for Ineffective Airway Clearance.*

A potential (high-risk) nursing diagnosis should be used only for those patients who have a higher-than-normal risk for developing a problem—those who have more risk factors than the general group to which they belong. NANDA guidelines from the 1990 Conference include the following definition:

> A high-risk nursing diagnosis is a clinical judgment that an individual, family, or community is more vulnerable to develop the problem than others in the same or similar situation. (p. 116)

For those who have the same risk as the general population, a *collaborative problem (potential complication)* should be used. For example, *all* patients having a general anesthetic are at risk for respiratory problems. However, for those who have no risk factors in addition to the surgery, routine postoperative "turn-cough-deep breathe" treatment is adequate; their care plan could be based on the collaborative problem, "Potential Complications of Surgery (respiratory)." On the other hand, if a patient is a smoker and is having general anesthesia for a cholecystectomy (a high abdominal incision), his respiratory status merits special attention. He is at higher risk than the general population of cholecystectomy patients, so a nursing diagnosis of "High Risk for Altered Respiratory Function related to high abdominal incision and splinting" should be written.

As a further example, any new parent could develop Altered Parenting (delayed bonding). However, not every new parent requires nursing intervention to keep this problem from developing. Therefore, you would not use the nursing diagnosis "High Risk for Altered Parenting" for every new mother. You would use it for those who have more risk factors than other new parents.

Possible Problems

A **possible** problem, similar to a physician's rule-out diagnosis, is one that you tentatively believe to exist; you have enough data to suspect a problem, but not enough to be sure. Nursing care is then directed toward gathering focus data to confirm or eliminate the diagnosis. Using possible problems can help keep you from: (1) omitting an important diagnosis and (2) making an incorrect diagnosis because of insufficient data.

Cues

Actual Problems
- Problem present
- Signs and symptoms present

Potential (High-risk) Problems
- Problem may develop
- Risk factors present

Possible Problems
- Unsure if problem is present
- Some signs/symptoms present, but not definitive
- Data incomplete

Example: Still another patient who has had a cholecystectomy has *no* history of smoking and has been adhering to the schedule of turning, coughing, and deep breathing every two hours. She is slightly pale, and reports that she feels "a little short of breath." There are no other signs of respiratory distress, but the nurse wants to be sure the situation is carefully evaluated by other shifts. So she diagnoses a *possible problem: Possible Ineffective Airway Clearance.*

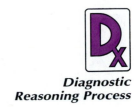

Diagnostic Reasoning Process

DIAGNOSTIC REASONING PROCESS

Now that you can recognize a patient problem and differentiate between nursing diagnoses, collaborative problems, and medical diagnoses, let us look at the intellectual process that enables you to take a patient's data base and identify the problems that apply to that individual. It cannot be overemphasized that diagnosing is more than simply choosing a label from a list. In addition to your basic knowledge (e.g., anatomy, physiology, psychology), you must master the skills of diagnostic reasoning so that your clinical judgments will be accurate. The care you deliver is the end result of the diagnoses you make; correct diagnosis lays the groundwork for efficient, effective, individualized care.

Interpreting Data

After you have organized and recorded your assessment data, it must be interpreted. This is the step in the process in which you determine what the data means.

Critical Thinking

Data interpretation includes the cognitive processes of analysis and synthesis. You will use **analysis** when "taking apart" the data base to examine and interpret each piece of data, identify deviations from normal, and identify patterns and relationships in the data. **Synthesis** means combining parts or elements into a single new entity. You will use synthesis when comparing the cue patterns to various theories, concepts, and norms in order to identify strengths and generate explanations for symptoms.

You may use both inductive and deductive reasoning to interpret data. **Inductive reasoning** begins with a set of particular facts and uses them to draw a conclusion. Induction is used to find possible patterns in information and extend them to *predict* new information.

Example:
Particular facts: Nikki Winters (Chapter 3, Figure 3–3) states that she includes very little fiber in her diet, that she doesn't drink much fluid, and that she sometimes has a bowel movement only every 2 or 3 days. She has just had a general anesthetic and is taking narcotic analgesics for pain control.

Conclusion: The nurse concludes that Ms. Winters has High Risk for Colonic Constipation. The nurse's conclusion is a *prediction* that Ms. Winters will probably become constipated if nothing is done to prevent it.

Deductive reasoning begins with a principle, generalization, or major idea and proceeds to discover or predict specific facts based on that general idea.

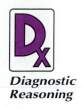

Diagnostic Reasoning

Example: Kathy Cole is a nurse in a long-term care facility, and she knows the effects of poor nutrition and immobility upon skin integrity (principles and generalizations). Based on this knowledge and her clinical experience, she maintains a turning schedule for Mr. Randall, who is paralyzed, and she observes for redness and other signs of impaired skin integrity (the specific facts predicted by the principles).

Use of Frameworks

Recall from Chapter 3 that it is important to use a framework for organizing and interpreting data. The framework's concepts (such as Maslow's concept of *hierarchy*) will help you to establish relationships between isolated pieces of data. Concepts allow clusters to stand out for your attention; for instance, the concept of *constipation* in the Nikki Winters example helped the nurse to notice that fluid, fiber, anesthesia, and narcotics were somehow related. This chapter uses the NANDA Human Response Patterns as a framework for data analysis.

Steps in Data Interpretation

This section presents data interpretation as a series of steps in order to help you understand the process. In reality, it is a complex process, not a rigid set of linear steps to be accomplished one at a time. Some steps, of course, must be taken before others, but you should use these steps as guidelines, realizing that you will do some of them simultaneously, move back and forth between them, and perhaps even intuit portions of them, especially as you gain clinical experience.

Data interpretation occurs at three levels. In the first level, you organize the data, look for inconsistencies and missing data, and compare the data to established norms. In the second level, you look for patterns and relationships in the data and hypothesize explanations (problems) for the patterns. In the final level of interpretation you determine the probable cause of the problems.

Step 1: Organize the Data. The first step in data analysis is to organize the data. If you have made an initial, comprehensive assessment, most of your data will already be grouped according to the framework of your data-collection form. That form is a part of the patient's permanent record, so you cannot mark on it. For that reason, especially while you are learning, you should rewrite the data base cues in a concise format according to your preferred framework. Summarizing information in this manner makes data gaps and inconsistencies more obvious, and makes it easier to see relationships between the cues. Nikki Winters's admission assessment form (Figure 3–3 in Chapter 3) was based on the NANDA Human Response Patterns. Box 4–1 contains Ms. Winters's admission data, listed in a more concise format (still using the NANDA framework).

Step 2: Identify Data Gaps and Inconsistencies. Ideally, your data will be complete, and you will have identified and validated incongruent data during the assessment step. However, the need for certain data may not become apparent until you cluster and begin to look for meaning in the data. After listing Ms. Winters's data, you can see that more information is needed regarding her husband's feelings about her surgery, the amount of physical and emotional support he can be counted on to give postoperatively, and her feelings about herself.

To identify inconsistencies, check to see if information given under one pattern contradicts that given under another pattern or if your objective findings conflict with what the client has said. Has the client given you the same information (concerns, strengths, etc.) as other team members? An inconsistency for Ms. Winters is that she understands the procedure and postoperative care for a hysterectomy, yet she believes the surgery may make her less attractive and diminish her sexuality.

Step 3: Compare Individual Cues to Standards and Norms. In this first level of data interpretation you use your knowledge of anatomy, physiology, psychology, developmental theory, and so on, to evaluate whether or not the cues are normal. You will compare them to such standards as norms for height and weight, lab values and nutritional requirements, social functioning, coping skills, and usual health status. Following are some examples of various kinds of significant cues:

Deviation from population norms (e.g., height 5'2", weight 240 lb).
Developmental delays (e.g., 2-year-old does not walk yet).
Changes in the patient's usual health status (e.g., loss of appetite).
Dysfunctional behavior (e.g., drug usage, withdrawal from social contact).
Changes in the patient's usual behavior (e.g., poor hygiene, grooming).

It may help you to circle or highlight the significant or abnormal data, as was done for Ms. Winters's data in Box 4–1.

Step 4: Establish Patterns (Cue Clusters) and Relationships in the Data. In the second level of data interpretation, each cue is interpreted in the context of the other cues. As you compare data across the categories of your framework, some apparently normal data may take on new significance. In Box 4–1, under the Relating pattern, Ms. Winters's comment about her husband ("I'm lucky to have him") at first sounds positive. However, after noting her comments in the Feeling and Perceiving categories, it seems the Relating comment may be significant. That is why it is circled in Box 4–1, even though it seems normal when considered by itself.

Begin this step by looking for *cues that are repeated* in more than one category (in the NANDA framework a category is called a *pattern*). For example, Ms. Winters expressed concern about her sexual relationship in response to questions asked in the Knowing, Feeling, and Perceiving patterns, and she reported a history of sexual dissatisfaction in the Relating pattern. Because she mentioned this repeatedly, you may conclude that it is an important area for her.

Next, examine data across categories and begin to *group together (cluster) the cues that seem related*. Try to determine the relationship between facts. Does Ms. Winters's failure to have regular physical exams (Health-Maintenance pattern) have anything to do with her lack of exercise (Activity and Recreation pattern), or with her smoking (Knowing)? Has her self-concept (Perceiving) been affected by her unsatisfactory sexual relationship (Relating)? Does a hemoglobin of 9.2 g/dl (Exchanging) have anything to do with her statement that she is too tired to do housework (Moving: activity)?

While you are learning, it is a good idea to make a second written list to cluster your cues. This one will be much shorter than the first one because you will omit the healthy responses and list only significant data. The way you form your cue clusters and make your new list will depend on whether you reason deductively or inductively.

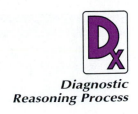

***Diagnostic
Reasoning Process***

93

Box 4–1. Nikki Winters's Data Organized by Human Response Patterns

Communicating

Reads, writes, understands English.

Valuing

Born and raised in Midwest.
No religious practices.
No unusual cultural practices.

Relating

Married 16 yrs. Husband 36, good health.
Children 15, 13, 12.
States of marriage, "We're a pretty good team."
"I'm lucky to have him."
Says relationship "good."

Sexual relationship unsatisfactory. Infrequent intercourse past 6 months because of pain.
"That won't be a problem after surgery."
States role as wife, mother.
Relationship with children good.
Occupation: Bank teller, part-time; likes the people and extra money. Live on husband's salary + hers.

Socialization: Has friends at work, neighbors.
"I talk to my mom a lot."
Oldest child says "Gets along with everybody."
Is quiet, but not withdrawn.

Knowing

TAH & BSO tomorrow.
Dysmenorrhea for past 6 months.
Medications: Tylenol, Ibuprofen, "iron pills."
Previous illnesses; Hospitalized only for appendectomy, childbirth.
History of illness & health habits: No major illnesses except present. Anemic.
Occasional vaginal infection ("yeast").
Smokes 1/2 pack/day X 16 years.
Family history: Father died of M.I.

Knowing (continued)

Menstrual history:
Age of onset: 11; normal cycle 28 days (before illness).
Has had tubal ligation.
Presently having scant vaginal flow, reddish brown.
Past 6 mo. abd. cramps & backache with menses.
History: 3 normal pregnancies with vag. delivery.
Understands need for surgery.
Understands removing uterus will stop menses; expects it will cure pain and anemia.
Attentive, interested. High school education.
Requested information about amount of help needed on discharge; when to return to work.
Alert and oriented X 3. Memory intact.

Feeling

Abd. cramping and lower back pain intermittent past 6 mo.
Vaginal bleeding associated with cramping.
Somewhat relieved by heating pad, Ibuprofen.
Pain aggravated by intercourse.
No recent stressful life events.
Feels "worry" that husband will find her "less a woman" after surgery.

Moving

No disabilities or assistive devices.
Last 2 months tires easily.
No exercise; just housework.
Sleeps 8 hrs. Feels rested.
Recreation: Reads, sews, watches TV. Plays cards with other couples; children's activities.
Has sole responsibility for cooking and housework.

(continued)

Moving (continued)

Husband and children do yard and car.

Health Maintenance: Has insurance.
No regular physical checkups.
Independent ADLs pre-op.
Mother will come to help out after
surgery.

Perceiving

Neat. No make-up.
Describes self as "nothing special—sort of
plain."
Afraid husband won't find her attractive
after surgery; "it might change how he
feels."
Feelings about being female: "I'm glad I
could have babies; men can't do that."
No verbal or nonverbal cues of hopelessness or loss of control.
Wears glasses for myopia.

Choosing

Problem solving: Considers all conse-
quences; does "what's best for every-
body."
Family problem solving: Discuss.
Husband usually makes final decision if
can't agree.
Dealing with stress: Be alone a while; "Try
not to get on each other's nerves."
Minimal facial mobility.
Support systems: Mother. Friends. Hus-
band. Children.
"I hate to ask them" (for help).
Has complied with therapies in past.
Taking Fe^{++} now.
Agrees to comply with post-op routines.
States decision-making abilities "OK, I guess."

Exchanging

No neurologic changes. Pupils equal and
reactive.
Appropriate verbal & motor response.
AP 88, regular. S$_1$, S$_2$, no murmurs; EKG
normal.

Exchanging (continued)

BP 130/88(R), 132/86(L), sitting.
Peripheral pulses strong, regular.
Capillary refill < 2 seconds; no clubbing.
Skin warm; color good; good turgor.
Skin intact, no lesions.
Old appendectomy scar RLQ abdomen.
No c/o dyspnea.
Resp 16, regular; normal depth; unlabored
breathing.
Breath sounds clear bilaterally.
No lymph node enlargement.
WBC 9,800.
Temp 98.6 orally.

Nutrition: 2 meals/day with snacks (a lot).
No special diet. Eats a lot of chips and
colas.
Drinks very little fluid.
Sample diet low in fiber.
No appetite changes.
Mucous membranes moist, pink; no
lesions
5'2", 128 lb.

NPO for surgery after midnight.
IV 1000 cc Lactated Ringers @ 125cc/hr
in A.M.
Hgb 9.2 G/DL, Hct 32%.
Cholesterol 160, Glucose 124.

Elimination: BM x 1/day;
sometimes every 2–3 days.
Sometimes constipated; uses no laxatives.
Abd. soft, tender to deep palpation.
Bowel sounds active in all 4 quadrants.
Voids every 2–3 hrs; yellow, normal odor,
no odor.
Couldn't estimate quantity.

Genitalia: Does not do breast self-exam.
Cannot pinpoint LMP. Constant spotting or
heavy bleeding past 6 months.
Scant, red-brown vaginal discharge now;
no odor.

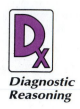

Diagnostic Reasoning

Recall that **deductive reasoning** begins with a major theory or generalization that generates the specific details and predictions. Therefore, if you use a deductive approach to group the abnormal data, you would begin by listing all the abnormal data (circled in Box 4–1) under the appropriate categories of your framework. For example, the abnormal cues from two of the categories would be listed in the following manner:

Exchanging (Elimination)
Sometimes has bowel movement
   only every 2–3 days.
States sometimes constipated.

Exchanging (Nutrition)
Diet not well balanced.
Inadequate fluid and fiber.
Hemoglobin 9.2 g/dl, Hct 32%.
NPO for surgery.

The **inductive approach,** shown in Table 4–4, will be used in the remaining steps of data interpretation in this chapter. Recall that inductive reasoning begins with specific details and uses them to arrive at a conclusion or generalization. Using an inductive approach in Step 4, you would make your new list of cue clusters by grouping together all significant cues (the circled cues in Box 4-1) that seem to be related, regardless of the pattern in which they were collected on your initial assessment tool.

Referring to Table 4–4, notice that the same cue may appear in several groupings. When you find a fact that seems significant, look for all the other facts that may be related. Remember that some cues that seem normal at first may take on different meaning when grouped with other cues. Taken by itself, the fact that Ms. Winters gets no regular exercise seems unremarkable. But taken with the other cues in Cluster 3, it may indicate a problem of Health Maintenance in the Moving pattern.

Next, decide which framework pattern is represented by each cue cluster. Identifying the general area (pattern) in which the problem occurs helps to narrow your search for the specific problem. A cue cluster may involve more than one pattern. If so, list them all; it may be that the cue cluster represents more than one problem. For example, Cluster 1 involves both the Relating and Feeling patterns—there are two problems in this cue cluster.

Another possibility is that only one pattern is involved, but it is not yet possible to be sure which one. In that event, you may be better able to identify the pattern after you begin to define the specific problems. For example, Cluster 3 seems to be associated with both Moving and Knowing. Only as you begin to decide cause and effect does it becomes clear that the *problem* occurs in the Moving pattern.

Step 5: Draw Conclusions About Each of the Groups of Cues (Identify Problems). In this part of the reasoning process you make the final judgments about the meaning of the cue clusters. The following discussion continues to use the inductive process; it would vary slightly if you were using a deductive approach.

First, *think of as many possible explanations (hypotheses) as you can for each cue cluster.* This helps keep you from drawing premature conclusions about the meaning of the data. You may rule out some hypotheses because of insufficient data and confirm others based upon your knowledge and

Table 4–4. Related Cues Suggesting Unhealthy Responses: Inductive Method

Related "Unhealthy" Cues (Clusters)	NANDA Pattern	Informal Problem Statement
Cluster 1 Sexual relationship unsatisfactory: infrequent intercourse past 6 months because of pain. States, "That won't be a problem after surgery." Dysmenorrhea past 6 months. Scant vaginal flow, reddish brown. No odor. Past 6 months, abd. cramps and backache with menses. Abd. cramping and lower back pain intermittent, past 6 months Vaginal bleeding associated with cramping. Pain aggravated by intercourse. Can't pinpoint LMP. Constant spotting or heavy bleeding, past 6 months.	Relating: role Feeling: comfort	(Symptoms of her medical problem: endometriosis) (Medical/collaborative problem) Actual Pain Pre-op: secondary to endometriosis
Cluster 2 Anemic. Takes "iron pills." Constant spotting or heavy bleeding past six months. Last 2 months, tires easily. No exercise except housework. Recreation is sedentary: TV, reading . . . Hgb 9.2, Hct 32%	Moving: activity or ~~Exchanging: nutrition~~	(Medical problem) Anemia secondary to uterine bleeding
Cluster 3 Smokes 1/2 pack/day × 16 years Father died of M.I. No regular physical checkups. No exercise except housework. 2 meals/day with a lot of snacks. Does not eat a balanced diet. Does not do breast self-exam.	Moving: health maintenance or ~~Knowing~~	(Nursing diagnosis) Actual Increased Risk of Heart Attack—plus other unhealthy life-style habits
Cluster 4 Worried that husband will feel she's "less a woman" after surgery. Afraid husband won't find her attractive after surgery; "it might change how he feels." States, "I'm lucky to have him." Unsatisfactory sexual relationship past 6 months. Husband makes final decisions when they can't agree. Describes self as "nothing special; sort of plain."	~~Feeling: emotional~~ or Perceiving: self-concept	(Nursing diagnosis) Possible Low Self-Esteem
Cluster 5 States occasional constipation. BM every 1–3 days. Sample diet includes very little fiber, few fluids.	Exchanging: elimination	(Nursing diagnosis) High Risk for Constipation

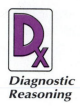

experience. In your own words, write the hypotheses that express the possibilities most accurately. For Cluster 1 in Table 4–4, some possible explanations follow:

1. Mr. and Ms. Winters presently have an unsatisfactory sexual relationship because of Ms. Winters's disease symptoms. The data directly supports this explanation. However, this cue cluster is the result of a medical problem that will most likely be resolved by the surgery. Removal of Ms. Winters's uterus should stop her pain and bleeding and allow her to resume satisfactory sexual intercourse. No nursing intervention is needed in this pattern, so the problem should not be included in the care plan.

2. Mr. and Ms. Winters may have a problem resuming a satisfactory sexual relationship, possibly because of her ideas about the effects of hysterectomy upon her sexuality.

3. Ms. Winters has a physical comfort problem: chronic pain caused by her endometriosis. Tomorrow there will be pain as a result of the surgery, but for simplicity we will not consider it in this data analysis.

4. Ms. Winters does not have enough information about her surgery. You can probably reject this explanation because there are several examples of knowledge on her data base. The exception is that she believes the hysterectomy may have a negative effect on her sexuality.

Next, *for each of your explanations, make one of the following judgments*:

• There is no problem.

• There is an actual problem. Client data indicates a need for assistance in making a change.

• There is a potential (high-risk) problem. There are no signs and symptoms of an actual problem, but risk factors exist. A problem may occur if you do not intervene.

• There is a possible problem. You have reason to suspect a problem, but not enough data to confirm it.

Table 4–4 includes the judgments (informal problem statements) made about all five cue clusters. For the explanations identified above for Cluster 1, you would probably make the following judgments:

1. There is an actual problem with sexual functioning that is caused by a disease process. However, the surgery will cure Ms. Winters's pain and bleeding, so the problem should be resolved after surgery. No problem need be written on the care plan.

2. There is no problem. There is not enough data to support high risk for difficulty in resuming the sexual relationship.

3. There is an actual problem of pain.

4. There is no knowledge problem. There *are* two cues that indicate misunderstanding about the effects of hysterectomy, but they will be addressed with Cluster 4. Other data shows that, overall, Ms. Winters's knowledge is adequate.

Step 6: Determine the Probable Etiology of the Problems.   This step begins the third and final level of the diagnostic reasoning process. In this step you determine the most likely causes of the problems you identified in Step 5. These are the problem **etiologies**—the physiological, psychological, sociological, spiritual, or environmental factors believed to be causing or contributing to the problem. The etiologies must be correctly identified in order for your nursing actions to be effective.

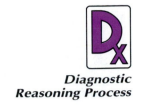

Diagnostic Reasoning Process

To identify etiologies, ask yourself, "What is *causing* this problem?" and ask the patient, "What do you think may be causing this problem?" You may find the Yura and Walsh (1988) categorization of etiologies in Box 4–2 helpful.

In the first level of data interpretation, you compared assessment data to standards and norms to see if problems existed. In the next level, you interpreted the cues in relation to other cues, identified broad problem areas, and then hypothesized more specific problems to explain the cue clusters. In this final level of data interpretation, you apply your knowledge and experience to the data in order to decide which responses are problems and which are causes. You must make inferences in this step, because you cannot actually *observe* the link between problem and cause. For example, from Table 4–4, observations for Ms. Winters (states "sometimes constipated" and "BM every 1–3 days") allow you to conclude that she has a problem: High Risk for Constipation. However, you cannot observe that her low fiber and fluid intake are the cause of this problem. You must infer this link between the problem and cause on the basis of your knowledge of normal nutrition and the physiology of elimination.

You will not necessarily find the etiology within the same pattern as the problem. In the following example from Table 4–4, a problem in the Moving pattern is caused by a stressor in the Knowing pattern:

		NANDA Pattern
Problem:	Altered Health Maintenance (increased risk of M.I. and other unhealthy life-style factors)	Moving
Etiology:	Possible lack of information about health promotion and disease prevention	Knowing

---

Box 4–2. Types of Etiologies

Personal and situational occurrences
Philosophic, ethical, and religious
Medical, dental, pharmacologic, and nursing
   therapies (commissions and omissions)
Pathophysiologic states
Psychopathologic states
Legal states and occurrences
Physiologic miscalculation and/or nonacceptance
Congenital alterations (reparable and irreparable)
Political impacts and impositions

Communication alterations
Environmental affronts/impositions
Social and economic affronts
Education, information, or knowledge deficits
Heredity and genetic impacts
Cultural imposition
Geographic and climate affronts
Functional role structure and impact

Adapted with permission from Yura and Walsh, *The Nursing Process* , 5th ed. (Norwalk, CT: Appleton & Lange, 1988), pp. 129–30.

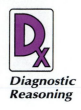

Diagnostic Reasoning

Different clients may have the same problem, but different etiologies. For example, failure to comply with the prescribed medication regimen (Noncompliance) may be caused by denial of illness in Patient A and by forgetfulness in Patient B. Furthermore, a problem can have any number of etiologies. For example, Patient C may fail to comply with the prescribed medication regimen *both* because he is denying his illness and because he is forgetful. When possible, you should focus on those contributing factors that can be influenced by independent nursing interventions.

Step 7: Determine the Problem Type: Nursing Diagnosis, Collaborative Problem, or Other. All of Ms. Winters's problems are nursing diagnoses, except two; the nurse can order definitive actions to prevent or treat all but these two problems. Clusters 1 and 2 in Table 4–4 indicate problems that are essentially medical. The pain and unsatisfactory sexual relationship in Cluster 1 are being caused by the endometriosis, and can be expected to resolve after surgery. In Cluster 2, Ms. Winters tires easily because her excessive bleeding has caused her to become anemic. The surgery and possibly the prescription for iron pills can be expected to cure this problem. You could collaborate in resolving this problem by teaching her about foods high in iron and by teaching her about her medications; but the definitive therapy is medical and surgical.

Ms. Winters does have some other collaborative problems (e.g., potential hemorrhage, potential IV infiltration/phlebitis) that are not apparent from the cue clusters in Table 4–4. They are identified from the fact that she will have surgery and intravenous therapy, and would occur for any patient having these treatments.

Step 8: Make the Final Decision About Which Pattern of Your Framework Each Problem Represents. Relating problems to framework patterns (see Table 4–4, center column) will help you to choose labels when you begin to write your diagnostic statements. You need a good understanding of your framework to select the appropriate pattern names. For instance, you must know something about the NANDA Human Response Patterns in order to know what cues and problems are associated with the patterns Exchanging and Knowing. It may help you to look back at the types of questions your assessment tool uses for each pattern. For the problems above, some helpful questions might be, "Is this problem one of

1. Relating? Does it involve establishing family and social bonds? Does it involve sexual relationships?

2. Knowing? That is, does it involve the meaning associated with information? Do these cues have something to do with the patient's lack of information?

3. Feeling? Do these cues seem to indicate a problem of physical or emotional comfort?

4. Perceiving? Do these cues involve the way in which the patient receives information, or her self-concept?"

For example, Cluster 3 at first appears to involve both the pattern of Moving and Knowing. The most reasonable explanation of the cues is that Ms. Winters's lack of knowledge (Knowing) is causing her unhealthy life-style (Moving). Her unhealthy life-style is the problem—the human response that needs to be

100

changed. In this step, you are categorizing the problem, not the etiology; so this cue cluster fits best in the Moving pattern. When you write your formal diagnoses (in a later step) you will look first in the Moving pattern to find the correct label.

Follow this same process for each group of cues until you have listed and identified the appropriate pattern for all the patient's problems. Refer to the Problem Statements in Table 4–4 for a preliminary list of Ms. Winters's problems (not yet labeled formally with NANDA terminology).

Step 9: Identify Client and Family Strengths.   The client's strengths should be integrated in the plan of care. Examine your original list of cues (see Box 4–1), and ask the client and family how they have coped successfully with past problems and what they see as their strengths. Strengths are those areas of normal, healthy functioning that will help the client to prevent or resolve problems. The following are some of Ms. Winters's strengths:

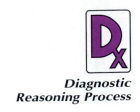

Diagnostic Reasoning Process

Communicating	Communicates adequately in dominant language
Relating	Stable family situation
	Adequate financial support (works only part time)
	Has adequate social network
Perception	No perceptual or sensory difficulties

Errors in Diagnostic Reasoning

Although you can never be certain that a diagnosis is correct, your diagnoses must be highly accurate. Keep your mind open to all possible explanations of the data clusters. The following errors keep you from noticing important cues or from thinking of certain explanations for the data. Recognizing some common diagnostic errors may help you avoid them by applying the appropriate critical thinking skills.

Premature Data Interpretation   Be sure you identify a *pattern* of behavior; do not make a judgment based on only one or two cues. In the following example, the nurse should have gathered more data before interpreting the patient's cues to mean Pain.

Example: The nurse, making a routine, hourly postoperative observation of Ms. Foley, sees that she is crying. The nurse says, "Oh, I'm sorry. I'll be right back with your pain medication," and leaves the room. On checking the medication record, the nurse discovers that Ms. Foley has already received her analgesic. She was actually crying because her physician had just told her that the surgery was not as successful as they had hoped it would be.

Critical thinkers do not usually make this error because they make it a habit to be sure they have all the evidence, and they suspend judgment when evidence is incomplete.

Personal Bias   Bias is the tendency to slant one's judgment in a particular way. A biased conclusion is based on personal theories and stereotypes more than on reason. We all have ideas about what people are like and what causes them to behave in certain ways, and even why they become ill. Many of these ideas are based on life experience and may or may not be accurate. Some people, for example, believe they will catch a cold if they get their feet wet or go outside with wet hair; other people believe that illness is punishment for wrongdoing.

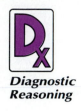

To what extent do you believe that people cause themselves to become ill, and how much is just bad luck? If you feel strongly that people are responsible for good health practices, then you may be less open-minded about a lung-cancer patient who has a 40-year smoking history or an emphysema patient who asks to be taken off the ventilator so he can have a cigarette. This personal theory may affect data interpretation for patients with AIDS or other sexually transmitted diseases.

Stereotypes are beliefs about groups of people. *Fat people are jolly, men avoid commitment,* and *women are emotional,* are examples of stereotypes. A negative stereotype (e.g., *adolescent males are violent*) is a **prejudice**. Stereotypes are expectations about a person based on beliefs about his group (physicians, elderly people, nurses, Americans, etc.). They are formed by our culture and based more on hearsay than on actual fact or experience. The nurse who relies on stereotypes instead of patient data will not recognize the uniqueness of each individual. One common example of this is referring to patients by their medical diagnosis or their room number, (e.g., "the hysterectomy patient in 220," or just "the lady in 220").

Forming Premature Conclusions Based on Context or Information About the Client   Nurses sometimes make judgments before they even meet the client, based on information about the client's medical diagnosis, the type of setting, the client's record, or what other professionals say about the client. Such information can help you to hypothesize nursing diagnoses, but be careful not to let it bias your thinking.

Example: Nurse Thomas has read about the relationship between loss of a body part and grieving. She also recognizes childbearing as an important aspect of a woman's identity. She therefore expects that her hysterectomy patients will grieve over the loss of childbearing ability. This nurse fails to see her clients as individuals and is quick to develop a Grieving diagnosis at the first sign of crying, sadness, or other emotional upset, based upon what she "knows."

Patients become upset for many reasons, and Nurse Thomas's inference of grief is highly inaccurate for some of them.

Relying Too Much on Past Experience   Basing conclusions on past experience with similar situations is a common and legitimate practice. This is different from stereotyping, since stereotypes are based on little or no experience. Generalizing from experience can help you to formulate tentative diagnoses, but it can also lead to error unless you validate your assumptions. Although many patients behave similarly in similar situations, it is an error to assume that they all will.

Example: Suppose Nurse Thomas, in the earlier example, had not read about loss of body parts, grief, or female identity. Suppose instead that she had taken care of several hysterectomy patients, all of whom *did* experience grief. In this case, Nurse Thomas's expectations of grief would be based upon her experience. She would have used the specific cases she experienced to generalize a rule about *all* cases.

Relying Too Much on Authority   Experienced nurses, teachers, the nursing literature, and textbooks are all good sources of ideas about the meaning of client data. However, you should critically examine even this information and remain open to new information and ideas. The patient problems you formulate with the help of an authority must be verified the same as other problems.

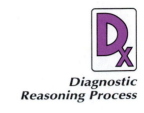

Diagnostic Reasoning Process

Empathizing/Identifying with Patient   **Empathy** is the ability to imagine intellectually what another person might be experiencing or feeling. It is achieved by placing yourself in the patient's position and imagining what your reactions would be *if you were that person*. Empathy is an important and valued aspect of therapeutic relationships because it can increase your understanding of the patient and your ability to interpret data and predict behavior. Because you know that people share certain basic human needs, behaviors, and feelings (e.g., need for food, feelings of fear and love), you can predict a patient's behavior, to some extent, on the basis of what your own would be in the same situation. The more similar you are to the patient, the more likely your predictions are to be accurate. The danger, of course, is in failing to recognize the uniqueness of individual responses—in assuming, without verifying, that the patient will feel as you would.

Example: Dina Duggan has always felt, "I can handle anything, no matter how bad, if I just know what it is. It is the unknown and the unexpected that I can't cope with." On the basis of this feeling, Dina was always careful to explain in detail what her patients could expect when sending them for diagnostic tests or treatments. Imagine her surprise when she began to teach a patient about a bone marrow aspiration and the patient stopped her, saying, "If you don't mind, I'd really rather not hear about it now. I would rather just have them tell me what to do right when it needs doing. If I start to think about things like that ahead of time I worry and get worked up into a state before it even happens."

Avoiding Errors

Except for the first two, most of these sources of error are also legitimate sources of hypotheses about the meaning of patient data; they cause problems only when you rely too heavily on them. The following suggestions may help you to avoid diagnostic errors.

Verify. To prevent error, hypothesize *possible* explanations of the data, realizing that all diagnoses are only tentative until they are verified. Begin and end the diagnostic process by talking with the client and family. When you are collecting data, ask them what their health problems are and what they believe the causes to be. At the end of the process, ask them to verify your diagnoses.

Build a good knowledge base and acquire clinical experience. You will need to apply knowledge from many different areas in order to recognize significant cues and patterns and generate hypotheses about the data. For example, nurses use principles from chemistry, anatomy, physiology, disease processes, communication, teaching, growth and development, and pharmacology—to name a few. Each subject helps you to understand patient data in a different way and improves the accuracy of your diagnoses.

Be sure you have a working knowledge of what is normal. You need to know the norms (what is normal for most people) for such things as vital signs, lab tests, motor skills and speech development, skin color, breath sounds, and so on. In addition, you must determine what is normal for a particular individual, taking into account age, physical makeup, life-style, culture, and the person's own perception of what is normal. For example, normal blood pressure for adults is in the range of 110/60–140/80. However, you may obtain a blood pressure of 90/50 that is perfectly normal for a particular individual. For another person with long-standing hypertension, 150/90 may be normal. Findings should be compared to the patient's baseline data when possible.

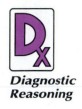

Diagnostic Reasoning

Consult resources. Whether you are a student or an experienced nurse, whenever you are in doubt about a diagnosis, you should consult appropriate resources: professional literature, agency policies, nursing colleagues, and other professionals. If you have not memorized the definitions and characteristics of the various diagnostic categories, consult a nursing diagnosis guide, such as the one in the back of your text, to be certain your patient's signs and symptoms truly fit the label you have chosen.

Base your diagnosis on patterns—that is, on behavior over time—rather than on an isolated incident. For example, you cannot diagnose Actual Low Self-Esteem for Nikki Winters on the basis of the two cues obtained in the admission interview (see Table 4-4). There is no data to show that she has ever had these thoughts before or that she will again. You will need to see if her feelings persist or if other data is found to support the cues.

Finally, *improve your critical thinking skills* by applying them to every area of your life: the music you hear, the newspapers you read, and the conversations you have with friends. Be aware of and avoid errors in thinking such as overgeneralizing or stereotyping, making unwarranted assumptions, oversimplifying, and drawing premature conclusions. Review Chapter 2 as often as you need to, and do the critical thinking activities that follow the other chapters in this text.

Verifying the Diagnosis

After tentatively diagnosing the client's problems and strengths, you should verify your conclusions. A diagnosis is your interpretation of the meaning of the data, and interpretation is not the same as fact. You can never be certain that an interpretation is correct, even after verifying it. There is always some risk that it is less accurate than it should be. Try not to think of diagnoses as right or wrong, but as being on a continuum of more or less accurate. Make your diagnoses as accurate as possible, but remain open to changing them as you get new data or insights.

Ideally, you should verify the problems and strengths with the patient to be sure her perception of the situation is the same as yours. If she is unable to participate in the decision making, you may be able to verify your diagnoses with significant others.

Example: You might say to Ms. Winters, "It seems to me that one of your problems has been the unsatisfactory sexual relationship caused by your pain and bleeding. One of your concerns might be to avoid any problems in resuming sexual intercourse after surgery. Does this seem accurate to you?"

If the patient confirms your hypothesis, you will include the problem on her care plan. If the patient does not agree with the problems you have hypothesized, you will clarify and restate them until they accurately reflect her health status. You may occasionally include a problem in a care plan even though the patient denies it; it may be a problem the patient is not aware of or one she is denying unconsciously.

Example: Ms. Winters may not perceive that she has Low Self-Esteem. Yet, because your data suggests it, you may wish to continue to assess for this problem and use nursing interventions to promote self-esteem. If you want to assure that other nurses will also do this, you must include the problem on Ms. Winters's care plan as a possible problem.

You should further validate each tentative diagnosis by comparing it to the criteria in Box 4–3. If the client verifies it and it meets the criteria, your diagnosis should be high on the accuracy continuum.

Box 4–3. Criteria for Validating Diagnoses

- The data base is complete and accurate.
- The data analysis is based on a nursing framework.
- The cue clusters demonstrate existence of a pattern.
- The cues are truly characteristic of the problems hypothesized.
- There are enough cues present to demonstrate existence of the problem.
- The tentative cause-and-effect relationship is based on scientific nursing knowledge and clinical experience.

Labeling and Recording Diagnoses

After selecting and verifying the client's problems and strengths, the next step is to state them formally. To determine the labels for the nursing diagnoses, you simply compare the cue clusters to the definitions and defining characteristics for the NANDA diagnostic labels in your Nursing Diagnosis Guide. The process of selecting labels and recording diagnostic statements for nursing diagnoses and collaborative problems is covered in detail in Chapter 5.

Box 4–4. Steps of the Diagnostic Process

Interpret the data

Level One

1. Organize entire data base in concise format, according to your chosen framework.
2. Identify and remedy any remaining data gaps or inconsistencies.
3. Identify significant cues by comparing individual cues to standards and norms. Circle these cues.

Level Two

4. Identify patterns and relationships among the significant cues. Make a new list in which you cluster the related significant cues.
5. Using your knowledge of the framework, decide which category or pattern each cue cluster represents. A cluster may involve more than one framework pattern.
6. Identify the problems. Think of as many explanations as possible for each cue cluster. Then decide which hypothesis best explains the cue cluster. (Note: You may sometimes identify both problems and etiologies in this step.)
7. Determine the status of each problem: Actual, potential (high-risk), possible, or no problem.

Level Three

8. Determine the etiologies of the problems.
9. Identify problem type: nursing diagnosis, collaborative problem, medical problem, or other.
10. Identify client strengths and supports.

Verify the data

11. Verify problems and strengths with client, family, and other professionals or references.
12. Decide in which pattern of the framework the problem occurs. (*continued*)

Label the data
13. Label the problem. Write the formal problem statements, both nursing diagnoses and collaborative problems.
14. Prioritize the problems.

Record the data
15. Record the nursing diagnoses and collaborative problems on the appropriate documents: patient care plan, chart, and so forth.

SUMMARY

The diagnostic process is summarized in Box 4–4.

Diagnosis
✓ is a pivotal step in the nursing process.
✓ focuses on human responses to disease and other stressors in the area of health.
✓ is the process of *interpreting data, verifying* hypotheses about the data (with the client or other professionals), *labeling* the problems, and *recording* the diagnoses in priority order.
✓ may identify nursing diagnoses or collaborative or other health problems.
✓ may identify actual, high risk, or possible problems.
✓ requires critical thinking, *not* making premature judgments or relying on experience or empathy.

A nursing diagnosis
✓ involves human responses to disease and other stressors.
✓ is a problem that nurses can independently treat or prevent.

Skill-Building Activities

In everyday life we make many decisions about what is true. These range from very simple things like "My dog is standing outside the door" to very complex things like "The world is built of tiny bits of matter called atoms." Have you ever stopped to think about how you know what is true?

We think some things are true because we have direct evidence. For instance, you might see your dog standing outside the door. You know that she is there because you can see her. We also believe things are true even when we do not have such clear evidence. Suppose you are in your house and you hear a scratching noise coming from the front door. Just as before, you might believe that your dog is standing at the door, but this time the evidence is different. You don't actually see your dog, but the sound you hear makes you think she is at the door. This is the best explanation you can think of for the noise. We call this process *making an inference*. An **inference** is something we believe to be true based on careful consideration of the evidence.

We cannot be totally sure of the truth of our inferences. Obviously, however, some inferences are supported by more evidence than others. In the preceding example, if you hear your dog's chain rattling and hear her barking and scratching, you can be pretty sure that she is outside the door. If, on the other hand, all you heard was some scratching you would be less sure about your inference. It could be you heard some other animal, like a raccoon.

Sometimes we get so used to making a particular inference that we do not even realize we are inferring. If every time you hear scratching at the door you go and find your dog, then you assume that the scratching always means your dog is out there because you have tested your inference many times. Many of the so-called "facts" of science are really inferences that we make so often that we do not stop to consider that we are making an inference. It is important to remember, though, that things like problems and etiologies are really inferences from evidence. In many cases they have never been observed directly.

Learning the Skill

Practice thinking about inferences by answering the following questions.

1. While sitting in a sunlit room, you notice that the direct sunlight has stopped coming through the window. List several things you might infer.

2. A few minutes after the sunlight stopped coming through the window, you observed drops of water falling from the sky. Does this provide any additional evidence for one of your inferences? Explain.

3. Can you be sure that what you have inferred is true?

Applying the Skill

In nursing diagnosis, we use the patient's signs and symptoms (cues) as evidence to support our inferences about the patient's problems and their etiologies. Some problems can be directly observed (e.g., Altered Skin Integrity), but others must be inferred (e.g., Low Self-Esteem). We can never, however, directly observe the link between the problem and the etiology; the cause of the problem is always inferred.

1. State whether the following are cues or inferences.

   _____ The nurse's interpretation of the data

   _____ Weight 250 lbs

   _____ Obesity

   _____ Temperature 100° F

   _____ Anxiety

2. In the following case, circle the cues.

Maria Gutierrez had a routine surgery and an uneventful recovery-room period. She was returned to her room at 4:00 P.M., still drowsy, but responding to her name. A Foley catheter was in place, draining clear, pale yellow urine. Her IV was patent; 1000 cc of D_5LR was running at 75 cc per hour. Her skin turgor was good. Her vital signs were B/P 124/76–130/82, pulse 72–86, and respirations 12–20 throughout the evening. At 8:00 P.M. she was helped to sit on the side of the bed for about 15 minutes. She moved slowly and complained of incisional pain, which she rated 10 on a scale of 1 to 10 (10 being the worst). She administered her own morphine by use of a PCA pump, and rated her pain as "about 5" when she was lying still. Her abdominal dressing was dry and intact throughout the night, as was her vaginal pad. At 9:00 P.M. she had sips of a carbonated drink. At 9:20 she complained of nausea.

3. In the preceding case, the nurse made several inferences. Write the cues that led the nurse to make each of the following inferences (use the cues you circled above).

   a. Ms. Gutierrez was drowsy from the anesthetic.

   b. There was no problem with Ms. Gutierrez's urinary system.

   c. Ms. Gutierrez was adequately hydrated.

   d. Ms. Gutierrez was experiencing acute incisional pain.

   e. The morphine was effective in relieving her incisional pain.

   f. Ms. Gutierrez became nauseated because her GI motility had not fully returned after her anesthesia.

4. Do all of these inferences have an equal amount of supporting evidence? Which ones do you think need more evidence?

5. Examine the explanations for each cue cluster. Circle the parts that are inferred and underline the parts that have direct evidence to support them.

a. *Cues:* Your patient has just had general anesthetic. Bowel sounds are absent to auscultation. Patient drank 100 cc of fluid and immediately vomited. Patient complains of nausea.

Explanation: Nausea and vomiting caused by decreased gastrointestinal activity secondary to general anesthetic.

b. *Cues:* Your patient has just been admitted to the hospital. He is pale and trembling. His palms are cool and damp. He speaks rapidly.

Explanation: Anxiety related to being in a strange environment.

c. *Cues:* Your patient is unable to drink anything. He is vomiting and experiencing severe diarrhea. In fact, his output for the past 12 hours has been 500 cc greater than his intake. His skin turgor is poor; his mucous membranes are dry.

Explanation: Fluid Volume Deficit caused by being unable to drink and by diarrhea and vomiting.

6. Now, for each inference in item 5, write whether you think the evidence is adequate or inadequate. If it is inadequate, what else do you need to know in order to make that inference?

*Adapted from *Critical Thinking Worksheets,* a Supplement of *Addison-Wesley Chemistry,* by Wilbraham et al. (Menlo Park, CA: Addison-Wesley Publishing Company, 1990).

Applying the Nursing Process

(Answer Key, p. 375)

1. Match the terms to the correct definitions.

   a. Diagnosis   **1.** ___ A list of specific labels/titles developed by NANDA to describe health states that nurses can legally diagnose and treat

   b. Diagnostic labels   **2.** ___ A two-part or three-part statement about a client response to a situation or health problem

   c. Nursing diagnosis   **3.** ___ The second step of the nursing process

                                       4. ___ The process by which data are interpreted and problems identified

2. (True or false) A nursing diagnosis

   a. ___ should be used to label all problems a nurse can identify.

   b. ___ is a problem that nurses are able, licensed, and legally responsible to treat.

   c. ___ is a statement of a client problem.

   d. ___ cannot be a statement of a potential (high-risk) problem.

   e. ___ is a nursing judgment.

   f. ___ describes medical conditions.

   g. ___ includes the etiology of the problem, when known.

3. You are Head Nurse on a hospital unit, and your job is to encourage the staff nurses to begin using nursing diagnoses on their care plans and in their charting. One nurse says, "I didn't learn that when I went to school, and I've done just fine without it all these years. I can't see any reason to do all that extra work." What would you say to persuade her that nursing diagnosis is important to her practice?

4. Place a check mark (✔) beside the words or phrases that are patient problems.

   a. ___ Appendicitis

   b. ___ Catheter obstruction

   c. ___ Decreased peripheral circulation

   d. ___ Asthma

   e. ___ Delayed parent-infant bonding

   f. ___ Having bowel resection surgery

   g. ___ NPO (nothing by mouth)

   h. ___ Constipation

   i. ___ Activity intolerance

   j. ___ Needs skin care

   k. ___ Low white-blood-cell count

   l. ___ Uncooperative

   m. ___ Needs constant attention

5. In the following situation, circle the stressors, and underline the responses.

   Ms. Sato developed a blood clot in her right thigh. Her thigh was swollen and warm to the touch. It was also slightly red. An intravenous catheter was inserted in her right forearm, and she was started on a Heparin drip. She was placed on complete bedrest. That evening, she rang for the nurse several times, asking to have her leg checked and requesting pain medication. She was observed reading her Bible each time the nurse entered the room. Twenty-four hours later, when her clotting time returned to normal, the Heparin was discontinued.

6. Now list Ms. Sato's *responses* (from Question 5) below. Write whether each occurred at the cellular, systemic, organic, or whole-person *level*. Also indicate whether it was in the physical, psychological, interpersonal, or spiritual *dimension*. The first one is done for you.

Response	Level	Dimension
Thigh swollen	Organic	Physical

7. Complete the following nursing diagnoses by adding etiologies to the problems given. Remember that a problem can be caused by any number of different etiologies. Use your knowledge of the medical condition to suggest appropriate etiologies.

For a client with a medical diagnosis of	Problem	r/t Etiology
Fractured femur	**a.** Acute Pain	
	b. High risk for Impaired Skin Integrity:pressure sores or excoriation	
Pneumonia	**a.** Ineffective Breathing Patterns	
	b. Activity Intolerance	

8. Match the terms to the correct statements.

N—Nursing diagnosis

C—Collaborative problem

a. ___ Deals mainly with physiological complications.

b. ___ A two-part or three-part statement about a client response to a situation or health problem.

c. ___ A physiological complication resulting from pathophysiology or disease process.

d. ___ Independent nursing interventions are mainly to monitor for symptoms and prevent condition.

e. ___ Nurse can order definitive treatment.

f. ___ Requires medical intervention.

g. ___ Can be expected to be present any time the disease or treatment is present.

h. ___ Can be a physiological, psychosocial, spiritual, or interpersonal problem.

9. Fill in the blanks with the status of each of the following problems.

A—Actual problem   **Pot**—Potential (high-risk) problem   **Pos**—Possible problem

a. ___ A client states he is experiencing stomach pain.

b. ___ A blind client is at risk for falls in an unfamiliar environment.

c. ___ The problem is likely to occur if certain preventive nursing actions are not begun.

d. ___ Risk factors are the etiology for the problem.

e. ___ Data not sufficient to confirm or rule out the diagnosis. More data needed.

f. ___ Client has a group of related signs and symptoms.

g. ___ Similar to a physician's "rule-out" diagnosis.

h. ___ Nurse prescribes interventions to prevent by reducing risk factors and/or monitoring status and onset of the problem.

i. ___ Nurse prescribes interventions to treat the problem, as well as monitor status.

j. ___ Problem is identified mainly to assure additional data collection.

k. ___ The patient has arthritis. Her knee is red and swollen. She states that it is very painful. She has a/an _____ problem of Pain.

l. ___ The patient has arthritis. Her knee is red and swollen. The status of her Pain diagnosis is _____.

m. ___ The patient has arthritis. Her knee is red and swollen. You see she is limping. The status of her Pain diagnosis is _____.

10. Place an *N* beside the problem statements that are nursing diagnoses. Some have etiologies and some do not. Circle the part (or parts) of the statements that the nurse can independently treat or prevent.

a. ___ Potential Arrhythmia r/t myocardial infarction

b. ___ Low Self-Esteem r/t perceived sexual inadequacy

c. ___ High Risk for Skin Breakdown

d. ___ Perineal Rash and Excoriation r/t urinary incontinence

e. ___ Confusion and Disorientation r/t inadequate cerebral oxygenation 2° CVA.

11. Using the NANDA framework, group the following cues *inductively* into the correct patterns of the framework. The Unitary Person patterns are Exchanging, Communicating, Relating, Valuing, Choosing, Moving, Perceiving, Knowing, and Feeling. Decide the NANDA pattern in which the *problem* occurs. (You will probably have two or three cue clusters.) Refer to chapter 3 for a review of this framework.

Cues: Ms. Petersen's blood pressure is 190/100. She says she hasn't been taking her "blood-pressure pills" because "they don't make me feel any better." She says she also has trouble remembering to take them. She is 50 pounds overweight. She says she works long hours and doesn't have time to cook—tends to eat fast food and snacks a lot. Her job is sedentary, and she does not engage in any physical exercise. For fun, she likes to "eat at a nice restaurant."

Cue Clusters	NANDA Pattern in Which Problem Occurs

12. Now look at the problems and etiologies you have identified for the cue clusters in Exercise 11. Write nursing diagnoses for the cue clusters (Problem r/t etiology). Use NANDA terminology if you wish, or simply state the problem and its etiology in your own words. You should have two nursing diagnoses.

13. In your own words, write the most likely explanation for each of the following cue clusters.

    a. An elderly client with left-side paralysis has a red, broken area of skin over his sacrum.

    b. Larry VanHuff has had severe diarrhea for two days. Today he has been vomiting each time he takes fluids by mouth. He does not yet have symptoms such as poor skin turgor or dry, sticky mucous membranes in his mouth.

14. Match the diagnostic error with the case illustrating it.

    a. ___ Mike Skarda actually hears very well; but because he is elderly, his new nurse speaks loudly when talking to him.

    b. ___ Sharon Weiss feels it is cruel to prolong life by using heroic technology. When Mr. Ivanov's family will not agree to a "Do not resuscitate" order, Sharon fails to identify their guilt feelings and need for support.

    c. ___ All the caesarean birth moms Susan Stone has cared for have been ambulatory by 24 hours post-op. Her nursing text indicates that this is the norm. When Susan asks her patient to walk to the chair so she can make her bed, the patient says, "You will need to help me." Assuming the patient is being overly anxious, Susan says, "You can do it. Just go slow." However, this particular mom cannot walk without her cane and leg braces.

    d. ___ When a young woman with long, blond hair is brought to the emergency room in critical condition, the nurse (herself a young woman) becomes immobilized, thinking "Poor thing. That could be me!"

1. Premature data interpretation

2. Personal bias

3. Stereotyping

4. Generalizing from past experience

5. Relying on authority

6. Empathy

REFERENCES

American Nurses Association. (1973). *Standards for Nursing Practice.* Kansas City, MO.

Carpenito, L. (1989). *Nursing Diagnosis: Application to Clinical Practice.* 3rd ed. Philadelphia: J. B. Lippincott.

Carpenito, L. (1991). *Nursing Care Plans and Documentation: Nursing Diagnoses and Collaborative Problems.* Philadelphia: J. B. Lippincott.

Fry, V. (1953). The creative approach to nursing. *American Journal of Nursing, 53*(3): 301–2.

Gebbie, K. (1976). Development of a taxonomy of nursing diagnosis. In Walter, J., et al., *Dynamics of Problem-Oriented Approaches: Patient Care and Documentation.* Philadelphia: J. B. Lippincott.

Gebbie, K., and Lavin, M. (1975). *Classification of Nursing Diagnoses: Proceedings of the First National Conference.* St. Louis: C. V. Mosby.

Gordon, M. (1987). *Nursing Diagnosis: Process and Application.* New York: McGraw-Hill.

McManus, L. (1951). Assumption of functions of nursing. In *Regional Planning for Nursing and Nursing Education.* New York: Teachers College Press.

North American Nursing Diagnosis Association. (1990). *Taxonomy I—Revised 1990.* St. Louis.

Roy, Sr. C. (1984). *Introduction to Nursing: An Adaptation Model.* Englewood Cliffs, N.J.: Prentice Hall.

Warren, J., and Hoskins, L. (1990). The development of NANDA's nursing diagnosis taxonomy. *Nursing Diagnosis, 1*(4): 162–68.

Yura, H., and Walsh, M. (1988). *The Nursing Process: Assessing, Planning, Implementing, Evaluating.* 5th ed. Norwalk, CT: Appleton & Lange, 129–30.

CHAPTER 5

WRITING DIAGNOSTIC STATEMENTS

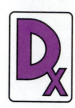

Upon completing this chapter, you should be able to do the following:
- Briefly describe the history of the North American Nursing Diagnosis Association.
- Discuss issues associated with the NANDA system of labeling and classifying nursing diagnoses.
- Use the NANDA Ninth Conference diagnostic labels to write precise, concise, and accurate nursing diagnoses.
- Write collaborative problem statements in correct format.
- List guidelines for improving the quality of diagnostic statements.
- Describe the ethical issues involved in writing diagnostic statements.
- Write diagnostic statements describing wellness states.
- Prioritize client problems using a basic needs or a preservation of life framework.

INTRODUCTION

In Chapter 4 you learned to analyze data in order to identify and verify nursing diagnoses, collaborative problems, and patient strengths. This chapter explains how to use the NANDA standardized terminology to write nursing diagnoses, describes formats for various kinds of problem statements, and presents frameworks for prioritizing a patient's problems. Figure 5–1 highlights the aspects of the diagnosis step that are emphasized in this chapter.

THE NORTH AMERICAN NURSING DIAGNOSIS ASSOCIATION

In the 1950s and 1960s the need for consistency in the profession was recognized. During this period, several studies were done to identify patient problems requiring nursing intervention. These evolved into lists of *nursing problems* (Abdellah et al., 1960) and *client needs* that might require basic nursing care (Henderson, 1964). While neither of these was actually a list of patient problems, they did demonstrate that nursing care focuses on something other than disease processes.

In 1973, the American Nurses Association published the *Standards of Nursing Practice*, which identified nursing diagnosis as an important function of the professional nurse. During that same year, nursing faculty members at St. Louis University, led by Kristine Gebbie and Mary Ann Lavin, initiated a project to

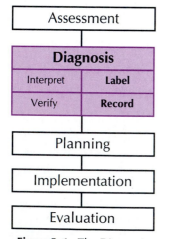

Figure 5–1. The Diagnosis Step in the Nursing Process

identify and categorize problems that should be considered *nursing diagnoses*. A national task force was formed to implement the project. One hundred nurses attended the First Conference on Nursing Diagnosis in 1973 (Gebbie, 1976a). This group continued to meet every two years and, at the Fifth Conference in 1982 (Kim et al., 1984), formally became the North American Nursing Diagnosis Association (NANDA). In 1990, there were over 1,400 members throughout the United States and Canada. NANDA membership consists of nurses from education, practice, research, and administration, as well as from all nursing specialty areas (e.g., intensive care, maternal-child, home health). This diversity assures input from a variety of perspectives.

The major function of the early groups was to generate, name, and implement diagnostic categories. At the First Conference a tentative list of diagnostic labels was formulated, but not approved. Thirty-seven of those were accepted (approved for use) at the second national conference (Gebbie, 1976b). Diagnostic titles were rapidly generated and accepted until the Fifth Conference. At the Ninth Conference, in 1990, only two new titles were accepted, bringing the total number of approved labels to 100.

By the Fifth Conference, in 1982, emphasis was shifting from generating new diagnosis labels to clarifying existing labels and developing etiologies and defining characteristics. Other important issues began to emerge: the need for a classification system (taxonomy) and the need for a theoretical framework on which to base the taxonomy. These priorities still exist, along with others, such as promoting research to validate the diagnostic labels and encouraging nurses to use standardized labeling in their practice.

At the Seventh Conference, in 1986, the group accepted the nine Human Response Patterns as the organizing framework for Taxonomy I (McLane, 1987). Taxonomy development is ongoing; Taxonomy I was revised in 1990 (see Box 5–1), and Taxonomy II will be presented at the 1992 conference. Notice in Box 5–1 that the taxonomic levels are numerically coded to aid in computer applications. The Human Response Patterns were not developed as a conceptual framework for nursing assessments and interventions; however, they may begin to serve that purpose as the relationships between the patterns are demonstrated, and as they are related to other nursing knowledge. In fact, this is already being proposed (England, 1989; Fitzpatrick, 1990; Guzzetta, 1989). You may recall that the Nikki Winters data base (Figure 3–3 in Chapter 3) is organized according to the NANDA Human Response Patterns.

NANDA continues to meet every two years to discuss and accept new diagnostic labels, hear committee reports, and offer continuing education programs. Work is carried on between conferences by a large group of members serving on many standing committees and by 23 Regional Nursing Diagnosis Association groups. The accompanying list of the standing committees will give you an idea of the scope of NANDA activities.

New and modified diagnostic labels are discussed at each biannual conference, but new diagnoses are no longer voted on at the national conference. Since the Sixth Conference (1984), they must go through the Diagnosis Review Committee before a mail vote by the membership. Changes in accepted labels undergo the same process as proposed new diagnostic labels. Any professional nurse wishing to submit a nursing diagnosis would follow the review process summarized in Box 5–2.

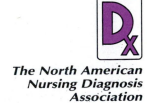

The North American Nursing Diagnosis Association

NANDA STANDING COMMITTEES

Bylaws
Diagnosis Review
Finance
International
Nominating
Public Relations/Membership
Program
Publications
Regional Affairs
Research
Taxonomy

Writing Diagnostic Statements

Box 5–1. Taxonomy I, Revised 1990

Bracketed items and blank spaces represent areas that are yet to be named, described or voted in.

1. EXCHANGING
    1.1 *Altered Nutrition*
        1.1.1
        1.1.2 [Systemic]
            1.1.2.1 More Than Body Requirements
            1.1.2.2 Less Than Body Requirements
            1.1.2.3 Potential for More Than Body Requirements
    1.2 [*Altered Physical Regulation*]
        1.2.1 [Immunologic]
            1.2.1.1 Potential for Infection
        1.2.2 [Temperature]
            1.2.2.1 Potential Altered Body Temperature
            1.2.2.2 Hypothermia
            1.2.2.3 Hyperthermia
            1.2.2.4 Ineffective Thermoregulation
        1.2.3 [Neurologic]
            1.2.3.1 Dysreflexia
    1.3 *Altered Elimination*
        1.3.1 Bowel
            1.3.1.1 Constipation
                1.3.1.1.1 Perceived
                1.3.1.1.2 Colonic
            1.3.1.2 Diarrhea
            1.3.1.3 Bowel Incontinence
        1.3.2 Urinary
            1.3.2.1 Incontinence
                1.3.2.1.1 Stress
                1.3.2.1.2 Reflex
                1.3.2.1.3 Urge
                1.3.2.1.4 Functional
                1.3.2.1.5 Total
            1.3.2.2 Retention
    1.4 [*Altered Circulation*]
        1.4.1 Vascular]
            1.4.1.1 Tissue Perfusion
                1.4.1.1.1 Renal
                1.4.1.1.2 Cerebral
                1.4.1.1.3 Cardiopulmonary
                1.4.1.1.4 Gastrointestinal
                1.4.1.1.5 Peripheral
            1.4.1.2 Fluid Volume
                1.4.1.2.1 Excess
                1.4.1.2.2 Deficit
                    1.4.1.2.2.1 Actual (1) Actual (2)
                    1.4.1.2.2.2 Potential
        1.4.2 [Cardiac]
            1.4.2.1 Decreased Cardiac Output

Box 5-1. (continued)

1.5   *[Altered Oxygenation]*
   1.5.1 [Respiration]
      1.5.1.1 Impaired Gas Exchange
      1.5.1.2 Ineffective Airway Clearance
      1.5.1.3 Ineffective Breathing Pattern
1.6   *[Altered Physical Integrity]*
   1.6.1 Potential for Injury
      1.6.1.1 Potential for Suffocation
      1.6.1.2 Potential for Poisoning
      1.6.1.3 Potential for Trauma
      1.6.1.4 Potential for Aspiration
      1.6.1.5 Potential for Disuse Syndrome
 *1.6.2 Altered Protection
      1.6.2.1 Impaired Tissue Integrity
         1.6.2.1.1. Altered Oral Mucous Membrane
            1.6.2.1.2.1 Impaired Skin Integrity
            1.6.2.1.2.2 Potential Impaired Skin Integrity

2. COMMUNICATION
2.1   *Altered Communication*
   2.1.1 Verbal
      2.1.1.1 Impaired

3. RELATING
3.1   *[Altered Socialization]*
   3.1.1 Impaired Social Interaction
   3.1.2 Social Isolation
3.2   *[Altered role]*
   3.2.1 Altered Role Performance
      3.2.1.1 Parenting
         3.2.1.1.1 Actual
         3.2.1.1.2 Potential
      3.2.1.2 Sexual
         3.2.1.2.1 Dysfunction
   3.2.2 Altered Family Processes
   3.2.3 [Role Conflict]
      3.2.3.1 Parental Role Conflict
3.3   *Altered Sexuality Patterns*

4. VALUING
4.1   *[Altered Spiritual State]*
   4.1.1 Spiritual Distress

5. CHOOSING
5.1   *Altered Coping*
   5.1.1 Individual Coping
      5.1.1.1 Ineffective
         5.1.1.1.1 Impaired Adjustment
         5.1.1.1.2 Defensive Coping
         5.1.1.1.3 Ineffective Denial
   5.1.2 Family Coping
      5.1.2.1 Ineffective
         5.1.2.1.1 Disabling
         5.1.2.1.2 Compromised
      5.1.2.2 Potential for Growth

The North American Nursing Diagnosis Association

Diagnosis is an intellectual activity in which nurses use critical thinking skills to identify patterns and make judgments about human responses to actual or potential health problems.

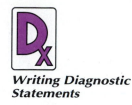

Writing Diagnostic Statements

Box 5–1. (continued)

5.2 [*Altered Participation*]
   5.2.1 [Individual]
      5.2.1.1 Noncompliance (Specify)
5.3 [*Altered Judgment*]
   5.3.1 [Individual]
      5.3.1.1 Decisional Conflict (Specify)
5.4 *Health-Seeking Behaviors* (*Specify*)

6. MOVING
6.1 [*Altered Activity*]
   6.1.1 Physical Mobility
      6.1.1.1 Impaired
      6.1.1.2 Activity Intolerance
         6.1.1.2.1 Fatigue
      6.1.1.3 Potential Activity Intolerance
6.2 [*Altered rest*]
   6.2.1 Sleep-Pattern Disturbance
6.3 [*Altered Recreation*]
   6.3.1 Diversional Activity
      6.3.1.1 Deficit
6.4 [*Altered ADL*]
   6.4.1 Home-Maintenance Management
      6.4.1.1 Impaired
   6.4.2 Health Maintenance
6.5 *Self-Care Deficit*
   6.5.1 Feeding
      6.5.1.1 Impaired Swallowing
      6.5.1.2 Impaired Breastfeeding
     *6.5.1.3 Effective Breastfeeding
   6.5.2 Bathing/Hygiene
   6.5.3 Dressing/Grooming
   6.5.4 Toileting
6.6 *Altered Growth and Development*

7. PERCEIVING
7.1 *Altered Self-Concept*
   7.1.1 Body Image Disturbance
   7.1.2 Self-Esteem Disturbance
      7.1.2.1 Chronic Low Self-Esteem
      7.1.2.2 Situational Low Self-Esteem
   7.1.3 Personal Identity Disturbance
7.2 *Altered Sensory/Perception*
   7.2.1 Visual
      7.2.1.1 Unilateral Neglect
   7.2.2 Auditory
   7.2.3 Kinesthetic
   7.2.4 Gustatory
   7.2.5 Tactile
   7.2.6 Olfactory
7.3 [*Altered Meaningfulness*]
   7.3.1 Hopelessness
   7.3.2 Powerlessness

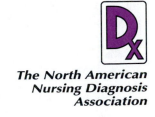

**The North American
Nursing Diagnosis
Association**

> **Box 5–1. (concluded)**
>
> **8. KNOWING**
>   8.1   *[Altered Knowing]*
>   8.1.1 Knowledge Deficit (Specify)
>   8.2   [   ]
>   8.3   *Altered Thought Processes*
> **9. FEELING**
>   9.1   *Altered Comfort*
>   9.1.1 Pain
>   9.1.1.1 Chronic Pain
>   9.2   *[Altered Emotional Integrity]*
>   9.2.1 Grieving
>   9.2.1.1 Dysfunctional
>   9.2.1.2 Anticipatory
>   9.2.2 Potential for Violence (Self or Others)
>   9.2.3 Post-Trauma Response
>   9.2.3.1 Rape-Trauma Syndrome
>   9.2.3.1.1 Compound Reaction
>   9.2.3.1.2 Silent Reaction
>   9.3   *[Altered Emotional State]*
>   9.3.1 Anxiety
>   9.3.2 Fear
>
> Adapted from *Taxonomy I–Revised, 1990* and *Taxonomy I–Revised, June 1988*, St. Louis: North American Nursing Diagnosis Association. Used by permission of North American Nursing Diagnosis Association.

NANDA distributes nursing diagnosis information by publishing the *Proceedings* of each of the conferences. This is a book made up of reports of action taken at the conference, committee reports, regional and special-interest group reports, invited papers, a section discussing new diagnostic labels, and a section containing the taxonomy and the approved diagnostic labels. In January 1990, NANDA began publishing *Nursing Diagnosis*, the official journal of the organization, which replaces the newsletter that was formerly used to communicate with members between conferences.

The Taxonomy of Nursing Diagnoses

A **taxonomy** is a system for identifying and classifying objects on the basis of their relationships. Any number of ordering principles can be used to classify things (e.g., size, weight, or color).

The first NANDA taxonomy was alphabetical and nonhierarchical (as in the list inside the front cover of this text). As mentioned previously, NANDA has since chosen Human Response Patterns as the organizing principle for its list of diagnostic labels. *Taxonomy I—Revised, 1990,* currently approved for use, is a hierarchical system in which each of the diagnostic labels is a subcategory of one of the nine Human Response Patterns (refer to Box 5–1). Each of the Human Response Patterns is a Level I concept—the most abstract. The most diagnostically useful concepts occur at Levels IV and V, which are more concrete and specific; however, a few of the approved diagnostic labels occur at levels II and III of the taxonomy (e.g., Altered Sexuality Patterns and Body Image Disturbance).

123

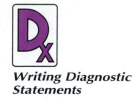

Writing Diagnostic Statements

NANDA and the ANA have worked together to adapt *Taxonomy I* for possible inclusion in the World Health Organization's 10th revision of the *International Classification of Diseases* (*ICD–10*). Some changes in terminology and numbering were made to accommodate the WHO numbering system. Inclusion of nursing diagnoses in the *ICD* would be a step toward (1) developing an international nursing data base and (2) documenting nursing care for third-party payment.

Issues Associated with the NANDA Classification System

There are various criticisms of the taxonomy and of individual diagnostic labels: too broad, too abstract, too medical, and so on. These problems will probably be corrected as the system evolves and individual diagnoses are refined. Meanwhile,

---

Box 5–2. Summary of the NANDA Review Cycle for New Diagnostic Labels

Step 1. Receipt of Diagnoses. A diagnosis is submitted to NANDA by individual nurses or a nursing group. NANDA can also initiate this step.

Step 2. Diagnoses Enter the Public Domain. NANDA reports to the membership any diagnosis submitted for review, along with the name of the person(s) submitting it.

Step 3. Diagnoses Are Reviewed by Clinical/Technical Task Forces. A panel is created to review a specific diagnosis based on individual clinical and technical expertise (they are not necessarily NANDA members). Members critique the diagnosis to be sure it meets the submission criteria.

Step 4. Diagnoses Are Reviewed by the NANDA Diagnosis Review Committee (DRC). The Committee accepts, alters, or rejects the diagnosis, and forwards its recommendations to the NANDA Board.

Step 5. Diagnoses Are Reviewed by the NANDA Board. The Board convenes to discuss the recommendations and accepts, rejects, or returns the diagnosis to the DRC for revision. Accepted diagnoses are prepared for General Assembly review.

Step 6. Diagnoses Are Reviewed by the General Assembly during the National Conference. The DRC makes any recommended changes before the diagnoses are voted on by the general membership.

Step 7. Diagnoses Are Voted Upon by the NANDA Membership. A mail ballot of proposed diagnoses is sent to all NANDA members. Approved diagnoses are published in the *Proceedings* and in the *NANDA Taxonomy* (Carroll-Johnson, 1989).

Summarized from *Taxonomy I—Revised, 1990.* Courtesy of North American Nursing Diagnosis Association.

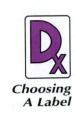
if you disagree with a diagnostic label, you do not have to use it, or you can add words to make it more specific and concrete. You should not reject the idea of standardized diagnostic terminology just because of a few unwieldy diagnoses. The system is evolving, as do all classification systems. In the medical diagnosis taxonomy, only in recent years was *toxemia of pregnancy* changed to *preeclampsia/eclampsia,* and only recently has *AIDS* become a medical diagnosis.

The more serious issues involve the whole system rather than individual diagnoses. We may be expecting too much from nursing diagnosis in terms of what it can do for the profession and for patients. Does it truly define nursing? And if so, will that make any difference in the long run? Nursing is changing rapidly and being shaped in part by events outside the profession (e.g., technology, the economy, military engagements). In our enthusiasm for this relatively new idea, we must remember that nursing diagnosis is simply an important *part* of nursing. It cannot be expected to singlehandedly remedy such problems as lack of autonomy and third-party pay; other measures will be necessary.

The nursing profession must also be cautious not to limit itself by classification or any other system. The taxonomy defines the profession as it is today, but it should not become static. Nurses must actively shape the profession (and the taxonomy) to meet tomorrow's needs, not simply reflect today's.

Some believe that choosing a diagnosis from a list of ready-made labels actually causes nurses to miss creative inferences they would otherwise make. Others believe that a step-by-step, scientific approach inhibits intuitive problem solving and prevents a holistic perspective (Kobert and Folan, 1990). Certainly we have all seen examples of the dehumanizing effects of science and technology. However, this does not have to be the case. Kritek (1985) says that "naming our phenomena of concern does not narrow our perception of clients, but broadens it. . . . When a child weeps, you work hard to discover why. You try to solve the problem. But of course, you always comfort the entire child, not just the problem. Nursing will retain its fidelity to holism if it chooses to do so" (p. 396). Using a common language and logical thinking should actually help nurses to identify and communicate unique aspects of patients that they might otherwise miss.

Even though there are still issues to resolve, "If nursing is to become a full profession, it needs to develop and accept one classification system for those functions and responsibilities that are solely those of the nurse" (Carpenito, 1989, p. 14). We do not need a perfect system in order to make progress. Nurses should use those diagnostic labels that make sense to them, and develop their own diagnoses to describe other human responses. Only through clinical use can the list be refined and expanded.

CHOOSING A LABEL

As a science emerges, a language develops to describe everyday observations. The NANDA diagnostic labels provide a common language for all nurses to use in describing health problems for any type of client and in any health-care setting. You must understand the meaning of the NANDA labels if your written statements are to accurately reflect your clinical judgments.

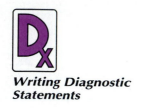

Writing Diagnostic Statements

Components of a NANDA Diagnosis

Each **diagnostic concept** has four components: label, definition, defining characteristics, and either related factors or risk factors.

Label

Also referred to as the *title* or *name*, the **label** is a concise phrase or term describing the client's health. Labels can be used as either the problem or the etiology in a diagnostic statement. Many labels include qualifying terms such as *Actual, High Risk, Ineffective, Impaired, or Increased.* NANDA has provided a list of definitions for these qualifiers (see Table 5–1).

Notice that many of the labels are very general; you cannot know what a diagnostic concept includes by looking at the label alone. For example, what do you think Activity Intolerance means? Does it mean the patient tires easily when playing football, or that he has chest pain when he walks up the stairs? What is the difference between the labels Activity Intolerance and Fatigue? The other components of a NANDA diagnostic concept help to clarify these questions.

Table 5–1. Diagnosis Qualifiers

Qualifier	Definition
Actual	Existing at the present moment; existing in reality.
Potential	Can, but has not yet, come into being; possible.
High Risk	*See* potential
Altered	A change from baseline.
Decreased	Smaller; lessened; diminished; lesser in size, amount, or degree.
Increased	Greater in size, amount, or degree; larger, enlarged.
Impaired	Made worse, weakened; damaged, reduced; deteriorated.
Depleted	Emptied wholly or partially; exhausted of.
Deficient	Inadequate in amount, quality, or degree; defective; not sufficient; incomplete.
Excessive	Characterized by an amount or quantity that is greater than is necessary, desirable, or useful.
Dysfunctional	Abnormal; impaired or incompletely functioning.
Disturbed	Agitated; interrupted, interfered with.
Ineffective	Not producing the desired effect.
Acute	Severe but of short duration.
Chronic	Lasting a long time; recurring; habitual; constant.
Intermittent	Stopping and starting again at intervals; periodic; cyclic.

From *Taxonomy I—Revised, 1990.* Reprinted by permission of the North American Nursing Diagnosis Association.

Definition

The **definition** expresses clearly and precisely the essential nature of the diagnostic label; it differentiates the label from all others. For example, the definitions for Activity Intolerance and Fatigue indicate that Fatigue is characterized by a sense of exhaustion; however, exhaustion is only a part of Activity Intolerance, in which heart changes, discomfort, and dyspnea may also be present.

Defining Characteristics

Defining characteristics are the *cues* (the subjective and objective data) that indicate the presence of the diagnostic label. For actual diagnoses, the defining characteristics are the patient's *signs and symptoms;* for high-risk diagnoses, they are *risk factors*. It is not necessary for all the defining characteristics to be present in order to use a label; usually the presence of two or three confirms a diagnosis. The defining characteristics for many labels are classified as *critical, major,* and *minor.* Newer labels specify *major* or *minor;* the earlier labels specified which characteristics were *critical.*

Critical defining characteristics are symptoms that are almost always present when the problem is present and absent when the problem is absent. If critical defining characteristics are identified for a label, they *must* be present in order to make the diagnosis.

Example: "Verbal report of fatigue or weakness" is a critical defining characteristic for Activity Intolerance. Even if the patient experiences *b, c* and *d* (below), you cannot diagnose Activity Intolerance unless *a* is present. You could, however, make the diagnosis if *only a* is present.

a. Verbal report of fatigue or weakness
b. Abnormal heart rate or blood-pressure response to activity
c. Exertional discomfort or dyspnea
d. EKG changes reflecting arrhythmias or ischemia

Major defining characteristics are those that appear to be present in all clients who have the diagnosis. NANDA defines *all* as "present in 80%–100% of those having the diagnosis" (1990). This means that as many as 20% of the clients with a diagnosis may *not* have these signs and symptoms. However, you should be skeptical about making a diagnosis if none of the major defining characteristics is present. Note that they do not *all* have to be present.

Example: You could diagnose Colonic Constipation if only one or two of the following major defining characteristics were present:

a. Decreased frequency
b. Hard, dry stool
c. Straining at stool
d. Painful defecation
e. Abdominal distention
f. Palpable mass

It is easy to see that a client with a diagnosis of Colonic Constipation might experience one or more of these symptoms in various combinations. A palpable mass is present in at least 80% of clients who have Colonic Constipation, but some clients might not have a palpable mass. Furthermore, you would probably diagnose Colonic Constipation for a client who had only symptoms *b* and *c*, but you would not make that diagnosis for a client who had only symptoms *e* and *f*.

Cues

Defining Characteristics → Actual Diagnosis

Risk Factors → High-risk Diagnosis

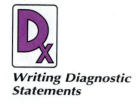
Minor defining characteristics are those that are present in many (at least half) of the clients experiencing the diagnosis. Since these signs and symptoms are not present in all clients with the diagnosis, you can make a diagnosis even if your client does not have any of the minor defining characteristics. However, the more signs and symptoms you see that fit the picture, the more sure you can be that your diagnosis is valid.

Example: If the client has the major defining characteristics, you could diagnose Colonic Constipation even if none of the following minor defining characteristics is present:

a.	Rectal pressure	**c.**	Appetite impairment
b.	Headache	**d.**	Abdominal pain

Even if *all* of these symptoms are present, though, you could not diagnose Colonic Constipation unless one of the major defining characteristics (such as straining at stool) is present. However if rectal pressure, headache, and appetite impairment are present *in addition to* one or two of the major defining characteristics, you would be even more certain that a diagnosis of Colonic Constipation is valid.

Related or Risk Factors

Related or **risk factors** are the conditions or situations that are associated with the problem in some way. They may, for instance, be conditions that precede, influence, cause, or contribute to the problem. They can be biological, psychological, social, developmental, treatment-related, situational, and so on. Each diagnostic label lists the related factors seen most often; however do not interpret this as a complete list of factors that *could* be associated with the label. Imagine, for example, the variety of situations/factors that could contribute in some way to Anxiety; it would be impossible to list them all.

Related factors are often but not always the etiologies of the diagnostic statement. A related factor may be a part of the etiology for several problems, or a single problem may have several related factors as its etiology.

Examples:

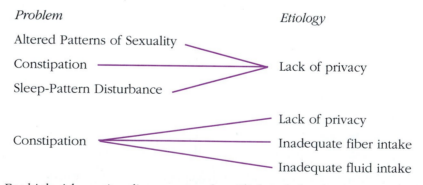

Problem	Etiology
Altered Patterns of Sexuality	
Constipation	Lack of privacy
Sleep-Pattern Disturbance	

	Lack of privacy
Constipation	Inadequate fiber intake
	Inadequate fluid intake

For high-risk nursing diagnoses, such as High Risk for Fluid Volume Deficit, risk factors are similar to defining characteristics: they are the cues that must be present in order to make the diagnosis. Some high-risk nursing diagnoses list both risk factors and related factors. Risk factors are nearly always at least a part of the etiology of the high-risk diagnostic statement.

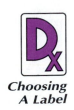

Example: Using the factors below, you might write the following diagnosis for a patient: "High Risk for Fluid Volume Deficit related to increased urinary output secondary to diuretic medications."

> *Risk factors* for the label, High Risk for Fluid Volume Deficit: Increased output, urinary frequency, thirst, altered intake

> *Related factors* for the label, High Risk for Fluid Volume Deficit: Extremes of age, excessive losses through normal routes (e.g., diarrhea), medications (e.g., diuretics)

How to Choose the Correct Label

To choose the correct label, you simply match cue clusters with the definitions and defining characteristics of one of the NANDA labels. These are found in the *Nursing Diagnosis Guide* in the back of your text. Remember, though, that there are about 100 different labels, so random searching is not practical. Actually, by the time you are ready to choose a label, you should already have narrowed the possibilities. Recall that during data interpretation you identified the most likely explanation (problem and etiology) for each cluster of cues and decided which of your framework patterns fit it best. Finding labels on the list that appear to have the same meaning as your hypothesized explanation should then be a simple matter.

Refer again to Table 4–4 in Chapter 4, the clustered abnormal cues for Nikki Winters. Cluster 5 is shown as follows:

Cluster 5	*NANDA Human Response Pattern*
States occasional constipation.	Exchanging (Elimination)
BM every 1–3 days.	
Sample diet includes very little fiber or fluids.	

(In addition, you know that Ms. Winters will have general anesthesia and morphine, both of which may cause decreased peristalisis.)

The nurse hypothesized the following explanation for Cluster 5:

> Ms. Winters's history of constipation is probably caused partly by her inadequate intake of fluids and fiber. This, together with surgery, anesthesia, and morphine, put her at more than normal risk of becoming constipated.

She concluded that this explanation represented a potential rather than an actual problem, and that the problem is a nursing diagnosis (not a collaborative or medical problem). Her informal problem statement was High Risk for Constipation.

To find the appropriate NANDA label for this problem, you could simply look at an alphabetized list (such as the one inside the front cover of this text) for labels that seem related in some way to the explanation. You would, in this case, look for labels with words like *elimination, bowel,* or *constipation.* Next, find the labels in your *Nursing Diagnosis Guide* and compare them to your cluster of cues.

It is more efficient, though, to organize your list of diagnostic labels according to a theoretical framework (the same one you used to organize your data), so that related diagnoses are listed together. Since Nikki Winters's

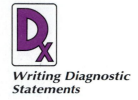

Writing Diagnostic Statements

data analysis employed the NANDA Human Response Patterns, you would look for your labels under the Exchanging pattern in that table (see inside front cover). There are quite a few titles under this pattern, but certainly fewer than the 100 listed in the alphabetical table. Of the labels under Exchanging, the only ones with possible connections (and some are remote, indeed) to Cluster 5 are the following:

Constipation   Diarrhea
Constipation, Colonic   Incontinence, Bowel
Constipation, Perceived

Of course, the most likely titles are ones that pertain to constipation, so check the *Nursing Diagnosis Guide* for those first. Does the label definition of Constipation match your explanation of the cue cluster? Do your client's cues match the defining characteristics of that label? How about Colonic Constipation?

For Ms. Winters, we can definitely eliminate all but Constipation and Colonic Constipation. Ms. Winters does not *at present* have any of the defining characteristics for either of these diagnostic labels; this makes sense because in Chapter 4 we concluded that this set of cues represents a *potential* problem for her. But look at the related factors for Colonic Constipation; several of these are identical to Ms. Winters's cues. Although Ms. Winters does not have the defining characteristics for colonic constipation, she does have some of the risk factors, which indicate that she is *likely* to develop the problem if there is no nursing intervention. Therefore, you would choose the title High Risk for Colonic Constipation. If you use the risk factors to describe the etiology, the entire nursing diagnosis would be as follows: "High Risk for Colonic Constipation related to history of inadequate exercise and fluid and fiber intake, postoperative effects of anesthesia, narcotic analgesics, and post-op decreased mobility."

The diagnostic statements for Ms. Winters's other cue clusters are given below. Compare the cue clusters in Table 4–4 to the definitions and defining characteristics in your *Nursing Diagnosis Guide*. Notice that the NANDA labels can be used for both problems and etiologies.

Cluster 1   Medical problem; no formal statement needed.

Cluster 1   Moderate, Chronic Pain (Abdominal cramps and back-
            ache) secondary to disease process (endometriosis).
            (*Note:* This applies to the preoperative period only.)

Cluster 2   Medical problem; no formal statement needed.

Cluster 3   Altered Health Maintenance possibly related to lack of
            knowledge about cardiac disease risk factors and other
            health-seeking behaviors (such as breast self-exam,
            balanced diet, and regular exercise program).

Cluster 4   Possible Low Self-Esteem related to complex factors and
            possibly related to threats to sexual identity 2° disease
            (endometriosis) symptoms.

The following potential complications complete the list of diagnoses for Ms. Winters.

Potential complication of hysterectomy:

1. Vaginal bleeding (hemorrhage)
2. Urinary retention
3. Thrombophlebitis
4. Trauma to the ureter, bladder, or rectum
5. Incision infection

Potential complication of intravenous therapy:

1. Inflammation
2. Phlebitis
3. Infiltration

Potential complication of indwelling catheter: Urinary tract infection

The potential complications of intravenous therapy and indwelling catheter do not require collaboration unless they develop into actual problems. They can be prevented by independent nursing actions. However, because Ms. Winters is not at higher risk for these problems than the usual population of hysterectomy patients, an individualized nursing diagnosis of High Risk for Infection is not written for these problems. They will be prevented by the usual routines and standards of nursing care and will require no special interventions. This will be explained further in Chapter 9, "Creating a Patient Care Plan."

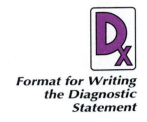

FORMAT FOR WRITING THE DIAGNOSTIC STATEMENT

As you have already learned, a diagnostic statement describes the patient's problem and the related or risk factors. This basic *Problem + Etiology* format varies slightly depending upon whether you are writing a nursing diagnosis or a collaborative problem, and depending upon problem status (actual, high-risk, or possible). Briefly, the *basic* components of a diagnostic statement are the following:

1. Problem. The problem part of the statement describes the client's health state clearly and concisely. Remember that it identifies what should be changed about the client's health status, so it should suggest client goals. Use the list of NANDA labels for this part of your statement when possible.

2. Etiology. The etiology describes factors causing or contributing to actual problems. For potential problems, it describes the risk factors that are present. It may be a NANDA label, some of the defining characteristics, a NANDA risk factor or related factor, or something entirely outside the NANDA standardized language. The etiology enables you to individualize nursing care for a client. Even though the problem is the same, Impaired Verbal Communication related to *inability to speak English* would suggest different interventions than Impaired Verbal Communication secondary to *tracheostomy*.

3. "Related to" (r/t). This phrase connects the two parts of the statement. The phrase *due to* is not used because it implies a direct cause-and-effect relationship, which does not always hold for etiological factors in a nursing diagnosis.

Writing Diagnostic Statements

Actual Nursing Diagnosis

Problem related to *Etiology* (r/t)

Actual Nursing Diagnoses

When a client's signs and symptoms match the defining characteristics of a label, an actual diagnosis is present. Note that the word *actual* is assumed and not written in the diagnostic statement.

Basic Format: Two-Part Statement

The basic format for an actual nursing diagnosis consists of two parts: the problem and the etiology.

Problem	*r/t*	*Etiology*
↓		↓
(NANDA label)	r/t	(Related factors)
↓		↓
Self-Esteem Disturbance	r/t	Being rejected by husband

Some NANDA labels contain the word *Specify*. For these you need to add words to indicate more specifically what the problem is.

> **Example:** Noncompliance (*specify*)
>
> Noncompliance (*diabetic diet*) r/t unresolved anger about having diabetes

The NANDA labels in most listings are arranged with the qualifiers after the main word (Infection, High Risk for) for ease of alphabetizing. Do not write your diagnoses in that manner; write them as you would say them in normal conversation.

> **Example:** *Incorrect:* Airway Clearance, Ineffective r/t weak cough reflex
>
> *Correct:* Ineffective Airway Clearance r/t weak cough reflex

---

P.E.S. Format

Problem r/t *Etiology*
A.M.B. *Symptoms*

P.E.S Format

Besides Problem + Etiology, you may wish to include the defining characteristics as a part of your diagnostic statement. This is called the *P.E.S. format,* for "problem, etiology, and symptom" (Gordon, 1987). This method makes the statement more descriptive and adds the concept of validation to the diagnosis. The P.E.S. format is especially recommended when you are first learning to write nursing diagnoses. If you use this method, simply add *as manifested by* (*A.M.B.*), followed by the signs and symptoms that led you to make the diagnosis. Use the following format:

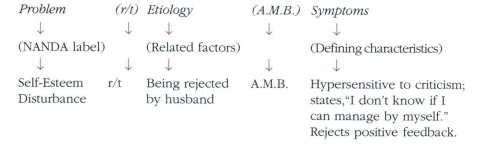

Problem	*(r/t)*	*Etiology*	*(A.M.B.)*	*Symptoms*
↓	↓	↓	↓	↓
(NANDA label)		(Related factors)		(Defining characteristics)
↓	↓	↓	↓	↓
Self-Esteem Disturbance	r/t	Being rejected by husband	A.M.B.	Hypersensitive to criticism; states,"I don't know if I can manage by myself." Rejects positive feedback.

Another example of the P.E.S. format follows. Notice that this method creates a very long statement.

Example: Noncompliance (diabetic diet) r/t unresolved anger about diagnosis A.M.B. elevated blood pressure, 10-lb weight gain, and statements: "forget to take my pills," and "can't live without salt on my food."

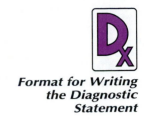
The signs and symptoms are often helpful in planning interventions for the nursing diagnosis, so it is important that they be easily accessible. If they result in a statement that is too long, you can record them in the nursing progress notes when you first make the diagnosis. This works especially well in a problem-oriented charting system. Another possibility, recommended for students, is to record the signs and symptoms *below* the nursing diagnosis, grouping the subjective and objective data.

Example: Noncompliance (diabetic diet) r/t unresolved anger about diagnosis.
S–"I forget to take my pills."
"I can't live without salt on my food."
O–Weight 215 (gain of 10 lb)
B/P 190/100

A common error among beginning diagnosticians who use the P.E.S. format is to write a vague, nonspecific problem and etiology, hoping that the client's health status will be explained by listing the signs and symptoms. Guard against this tendency by making the Problem + Etiology as specific and descriptive as possible before adding the signs and symptoms. Your diagnostic statement should present a clear picture of your client's health status even without the listing of symptoms.

Variations on the Basic Format

There are several variations of the basic Problem + Etiology format. For any of these, you can add signs and symptoms (A.M.B.) as in the preceding example.

One-Part Statements A few diagnostic statements can be made using the NANDA label (problem) without an etiology. As the diagnostic labels are refined, they tend to become more specific, so that the nursing interventions can be derived from the problem as well as from the etiology. Eventually all the labels may become so descriptive that it will not be necessary to include the etiology in the diagnostic statement. One label is already that specific: Rape-Trauma Syndrome.

For the following labels, it is difficult to think of an etiology other than a medical diagnosis, or if an etiology is written, it is somewhat redundant: Reflex Incontinence, Effective Breastfeeding, Post-Trauma Response, Defensive Coping. Reflex Incontinence, for instance, is fully described by its definition. The related factor is *neurological impairment* (e.g., spinal cord lesion that interferes with conduction of cerebral messages above the level of the reflex arc). As an etiology, this does not suggest nursing actions, nor does it really add to your

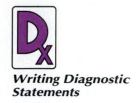

Writing Diagnostic Statements

understanding of the problem label, Reflex Incontinence. Similarly, the nursing interventions for Post-Trauma Response would be much the same regardless of whether the etiology is *related to war* or *related to earthquake.*

NANDA has specified that any new wellness diagnoses that are developed will be one-part diagnoses (for example, Potential for Enhanced Parenting).

"Secondary to"   Sometimes the diagnostic statement is clearer if the etiology is divided into two parts with the words *secondary to* (*2°*). The part following *secondary to* is often a pathophysiology or a disease process, as in "High Risk for Impaired Skin Integrity r/t decreased peripheral circulation *2°* diabetes."

Unknown Etiology   You can make a diagnosis when the defining characteristics are present, even if you do not know the cause or contributing factors. For instance, you might write, "Noncompliance (medication regimen) r/t unknown etiology."

If you have reason to suspect an etiology, but still need more data to confirm it, use the phrase *possibly related to*. When you have confirming data you can rewrite the diagnosis more positively. You might say, for example, "Noncompliance (medication regimen) *possibly r/t* unresolved anger about diagnosis."

Complex Etiology   Occasionally there are too many etiological factors, or they are too complex to be stated in a brief phrase. The actual causes of Decisional Conflict or Chronic Low Self-Esteem, for instance, may be long-term and complex. In such unusual cases, you can omit the etiology and replace it with the phrase *complex factors* (e.g., Chronic Low Self-Esteem *r/t complex factors*).

Three-Part Statements   Some diagnostic labels consist of two parts: the first indicates a general response, and the second makes it more specific. Adding an etiology to these labels creates a three-part diagnosis; adding *secondary to* makes it four parts.

> **Examples:** Labels: Ineffective Family Coping: Disabling
>   Altered Nutrition: Less than Body
>   Requirements
>   Feeding Self-Care Deficit (Level 3)
>
> Nursing Diagnosis: Altered Nutrition: Less than Body
>   Requirements r/t nausea 2°
>   chemotherapy

You may need to add a third part to other NANDA labels as well. Diagnostic statements must precisely describe the client's health concern because general concepts and categorizations are ineffective for planning nursing care. Not all NANDA labels provide this level of precision. You can sometimes make them more descriptive by using the P.E.S. format or by using a two-part etiology with *secondary to,* as in the preceding example. However, this is not always a satisfactory solution. In order to make the labels more specific, you may need to add a colon and third part, using your own words. Notice that the following example does not indicate the *degree* of mobility, even though the etiology is very descriptive. Can the patient turn himself in bed? Can he transfer to the chair unassisted? Or can he not move his legs at all? In some cases, the label definition makes the problem more specific, but in this instance it does not offer much help.

> **Example:**   Impaired Physical Mobility r/t knee-joint stiffness and pain secondary to muscle atrophy.

Label Definition: A state in which the individual experiences a limitation of ability of independent physical movement.

To make the nursing diagnosis more specific, you should add a third part (descriptor):

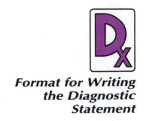

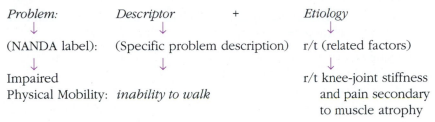

Problem:	*Descriptor*	+	*Etiology*
↓	↓		↓
(NANDA label):	(Specific problem description)		r/t (related factors)
↓	↓		↓
Impaired Physical Mobility:	*inability to walk*		r/t knee-joint stiffness and pain secondary to muscle atrophy

In the Impaired Mobility example, using the P.E.S. format does not help, because the signs and symptoms are the same as the etiology: inability to walk. The statement can be improved by adding *secondary to* to the etiology: *2° muscle atrophy.* However, inability to walk is really a *type* of mobility problem rather than the *cause* of a mobility problem; therefore, it should not be used on the right side of the diagnostic statement in the etiology phrase. The most logical way to write the diagnosis is to add a colon and a more specific description to the general problem of Impaired Mobility.

> **Example:** Impaired Mobility r/t inability to walk
>
> *P.E.S:* Impaired Mobility r/t inability to walk A.M.B. inability to walk
>
> *Better:* Impaired Mobility r/t inability to walk r/t muscle atrophy
>
> *Best:* Impaired Mobility: Inability to walk 2° muscle atrophy
>
> *Format:* **General Problem: (Specific Descriptor) r/t Etiology**

Pain is another label that often needs an added third-part descriptor. Even when considered with its etiology and definition, it does not always fully specify the client's problem. In the example below, you cannot tell how severe the pain is or where it is located. In the *Better* example, words are added to make the diagnosis thoroughly descriptive and specific to the client. Notice that in the *Better* example, the NANDA label describes the general area of the problem, and the descriptor describes the specific type of problem in that area.

> **Example:** Pain related to fear of addiction to narcotics
>
> *Better:* Pain: Severe Headache r/t fear of addiction to narcotics

You may see this diagnosis written as "Pain r/t severe headache." However, headache is a *type* of pain, not the *cause* of pain; the second part of the statement is supposed to consist of etiological factors, not problems. Furthermore, while this statement clarifies the location and severity of the pain, it does not indicate the cause.

High Risk for Infection and Altered Family Processes are other labels that may need a third part added to make them more specific. High Risk for Infection can often be made more specific by adding *secondary to.* However, in the following example, the first statement does not indicate whether the client is at risk for systemic infection or a localized infection of a wound or incision.

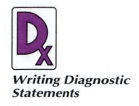

Writing Diagnostic Statements

Example: High Risk for Infection r/t susceptibility to pathogens 2° compromised immune system

Better: High Risk for Infection: Systemic r/t susceptibility to pathogens 2° compromised immune system, or

High Risk for Infection: Abdominal Incision r/t susceptibility to pathogens 2° compromised immune system

Remember that the diagnostic statement must thoroughly and specifically describe the problem and its causes (or risk factors). This is what dictates your format. In order to be fully descriptive, you will use *secondary to,* the P.E.S. format, qualifying words, a third-part descriptor, or a combination of these as needed.

High-Risk Problems

High Risk Problem (r/t) *Risk Factors*

High-Risk (Potential) Nursing Diagnoses

A high-risk (potential) nursing diagnosis is one that is likely to develop if the nurse does not intervene to prevent it. It is diagnosed by the presence of risk factors rather than defining characteristics. High-risk nursing diagnoses have the same Problem + Etiology format as actual diagnoses—the client's risk factors form the etiology.

Example: High Risk for Impaired Skin Integrity (pressure sores) r/t *immobility 2° casts and traction*

High-risk diagnoses may have most of the previously mentioned variations in format (e.g., one-part statement, three-part statement, multiple etiology). Of course the P.E.S. format cannot be used because the patient does not have signs and symptoms of the diagnosis—if signs and symptoms are present, the diagnosis is actual, not high-risk.

Possible Problems

Possible Problem (r/t) *Actual or Possible Etiology*

Possible Nursing Diagnoses

When you do not have enough data to confirm a diagnosis that you suspect is present, or when you can confirm the problem but not the etiology, write a *possible* nursing diagnosis. The word *possible* can be used in either the problem or the etiology. As in other kinds of diagnoses, the etiology may be multiple, complex, or unkown.

Examples: *Possible Low Self-Esteem* related to loss of job and rejection by family

Altered Thought Processes *possibly related to unfamiliar surroundings*

Possible Low Self-Esteem related to unkown etiology

Use *r/t unkown etiology* if you do not know the etiology; use *possibly r/t* if you suspect but cannot confirm the etiology. Remember, though, that etiologies are inferred, so you can never be *100%* certain an etiology is correct.

Collaborative Problems

Collaborative problems are complications of a disease, test, or treatment that nurses cannot treat independently. Nurses focus mainly on monitoring and preventing such problems. The etiologies of collaborative problems are likely to be diseases, treatments, or pathologies. Notice in the following example that with the usual Problem + Etiology format, the etiology does not suggest nursing interventions.

> *Example:* (Incorrect) Potential for Increased Intracranial Pressure r/t head injury

Carpenito (1992) suggests using the phrase *potential complication* to describe collaborative problems. The diagnostic statement should include both the possible complication you are monitoring for and the disease, treatment, or other factors that produce it. In the following example, you would monitor for signs and symptoms of increased intracranial pressure that might result from the patient's head injury.

> *Example:* Potential Complication of Head Injury: Increased Intracranial Pressure

Sometimes you will be monitoring for a *group* of complications associated with a disease or pathology. In that case, state the disease and follow it with a list of the complications.

> *Example:* Potential Complications of Pregnancy-Induced Hypertension:
>
> | | |
> |---|---|
> | Seizures | Hepatic or renal failure |
> | Fetal distress | Premature labor |
> | Pulmonary edema | CNS hemorrhage |

The P.E.S. format is not used for collaborative diagnoses because they are usually potential problems. The patient does not have the signs and symptoms—you are monitoring for them.

For some collaborative problems an etiology can be helpful in planning interventions; for example, the complication may be caused by something more specific than a disease process. While you are a student, you should write the etiology, as in the following examples, (1) when it clarifies your statement, (2) when it can be concisely stated, or (3) when it helps to suggest nursing actions.

> *Example:*

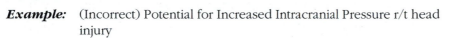

Disease/Situation	Complication	r/t Etiology
↓	↓	↓
Potential complication of *childbirth:*	Hemorrhage	r/t 1. uterine atony 2. retained placental fragments 3. bladder distention
↓	↓	↓
Potential complication of *diuretic therapy:*	Arrhythmias	r/t low serum potassium

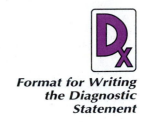

Format for Writing the Diagnostic Statement

Collaborative Problems

Potential Complication of disease or treatment: (Specify Complication)

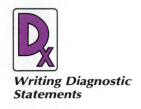

Writing Diagnostic Statements

EVALUATING THE QUALITY OF THE DIAGNOSTIC STATEMENT

In addition to using the correct format for your diagnostic statements, you must consider the quality of their content. They should, for example, be accurate, concise, descriptive, and specific.

Relationship of Nursing Diagnoses to Goals and Nursing Orders

The first part of the diagnostic statement (the problem) states what needs to change, thus it determines the goals needed to measure this change. In the example below, the goal would be to relieve the anxiety.

> *Example:*   Anxiety r/t lack of knowledge of scheduled venogram
> ↓
> **Goals**

The second part of the diagnostic statement (the etiology) identifies factors causing or contributing to the actual problem, or the risk factors for a high-risk problem. In many cases the etiology serves to direct the nursing interventions. In the preceding example, the etiology suggests a nursing order for patient teaching. In addition to teaching the patient about the venogram, though, the nurse would probably intervene more directly to relieve the anxiety—for instance, by helping the patient to recognize and express his anxiety. As you can see, nursing interventions can be directed by either part of the diagnostic statement.

> *Example:*   Anxiety   r/t   Lack of knowledge of scheduled venogram
> ↓   ↓
> **Nursing**   **Nursing**
> **Orders**   **Orders**

Like Anxiety, a few other problem labels call for particular nursing interventions regardless of the cause of the problem, for example: Decisional Conflict, Fear, Hopelessness, Ineffective Denial, and High Risk for Violence.

As the NANDA labels become more specific, you will probably discover more instances in which the etiology cannot be treated by independent nursing actions, and both the goals and nursing orders will be determined by the problem. In the example below, the nurse cannot treat a spinal cord lesion. Both the goals and nursing orders are suggested by "Reflex Incontinence."

> *Example:*   Reflex Incontinence   r/t   spinal cord lesion
> ↙   ↘
> **Goals & Nursing Orders**

When possible, you should rewrite the etiology so that it will provide direction for nursing intervention. Usually this means replacing a disease or medical condition with a principle or pathophysiology. This is not necessary for experienced nurses.

> *Example:*   High Risk for Infection r/t *surgical incision*
>
> *Rewritten:*   High Risk for Infection r/t *portal of entry for pathogen*s 2° surgical incision

138

In every case, the nurse should be able to prescribe definitive prevention and treatment for the *problem side* of a nursing diagnosis.

Criteria for Judging the Content of the Diagnostic Statement

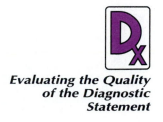

After writing your diagnostic statements, check them against the following criteria.

1. **The statement is precise and clear.** It uses terminology generally understood by other professionals and avoids jargon or abbreviations.

   Example:

   Incorrect: Self-Care Deficit: Toileting r/t inability to get *OOB w/o* help

   Correct: Self-Care Deficit: Toileting r/t inability to get *out of bed without* help

2. **The statement is accurate and valid.**
   a. Patient's signs and symptoms were compared to NANDA defining characteristics.
   b. For high-risk problems, patient's risk factors were compared to NANDA risk factors.
   c. The patient has validated the diagnosis.

3. **The statement is concise.** Using NANDA labels helps to keep the problem statement brief.
   a. If etiological factors are wordy and involved, use *r/t complex etiology.*
   b. If P.E.S. format produces a long statement, list the signs and symptoms under the diagnostic statement.

   Example: Self-Esteem Disturbance related to longstanding feelings of failure aggravated by recently being rejected by her husband as manifested by being hypersensitive to criticism, stating, "I don't know if I can manage by myself," rejecting positive feedback, and not making eye contact

   > *Better:* Self-Esteem Disturbance r/t complex factors
   > S–"I don't know if I can manage by myself."
   > O–Hypersensitive to criticism, rejects positive feedback, no eye contact.

4. **The statement is descriptive and specific.** The diagnostic statement should *fully* describe the client's problem. This criterion should be met even if it makes the statement longer than you would like. The NANDA label alone is usually very general (e.g., Parental Role Conflict); it is made more specific by
   a. knowledge of the label definition. (Check the NANDA definition to see if it makes the label more specific.)
   b. adding the etiology to make the complete problem statement.
   c. adding the patient's defining characteristics (P.E.S. format).

   If the statement is still not descriptive enough, make it more specific by
   d. adding qualifying words (e.g., *mild, moderate, intermittent*).
   e. adding *secondary to* in the etiology.

139

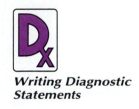

Writing Diagnostic Statements

f. adding a third part (a colon and a more specific problem).

> ***Example:*** Pain related to fear of addiction to narcotics.
>
> > *Better:* Pain: *Severe headache* r/t fear of addiction to narcotics

5. **Cause and effect are correctly stated**; that is, the etiology causes the problem, or the etiology puts the client at risk for the potential problem. To check this, insert the parts of your diagnostic statement in this sentence format (reading your statement backwards):

> "(*Etiology*) causes (*Problem*)."

> ***Example:*** Dysfunctional Grieving r/t inability to accept death of spouse

Read Backwards:
> Inability to accept death of spouse *causes* Dysfunctional Grieving
>
> (*Etiology*)   *causes*   (*Problem*)

> ***Example:*** High Risk for Infection r/t interruption of body's first line of defense 2° abdominal incision

Read Backwards:
> Abdominal incision *causes* interruption of body's first line of defense, *which then causes* High Risk for Infection
>
> (*Secondary*) *causes* (*Etiology*) *which then causes* (*Problem*)

If cause and effect are correctly stated, the sentence will make sense when read backwards.

6. **At least one side of the statement provides direction for nursing actions.**

a. Nursing diagnoses suggest independent nursing actions to treat or prevent.

Example:

> *Incorrect:* Sensory/Perceptual Alteration (Auditory) r/t progressive hearing loss 2° nerve degeneration

> *Correct:* Impaired Social Interaction r/t embarrassment at being unable to follow conversations r/t progressive hearing loss 2° nerve degeneration

b. Collaborative problems suggest nursing interventions to detect and prevent.

7. **The statement uses nonjudgmental language.**

> ***Example:*** *Incorrect:* High Risk for Injury: Falls r/t *poor housekeeping*
>
> > *Better:* High Risk for Injury: Falls r/t *cluttered floors*

8. **The statement uses legally advisable language.** It should not affix blame or refer negatively to aspects of patient care.

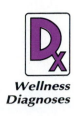

Wellness Diagnoses

Example:

Incorrect

Impaired Skin Integrity: Pressure Sores r/t *not being turned frequently enough*

High Risk for Infection: Knee Incision r/t *poor handwashing and breaks in sterile technique*

Correct

Impaired Skin Integrity: Pressure Sores r/t *inability to turn self*

High Risk for Infection: Knee Incision r/t *interruption of body's first line of defense*

9. **The complete list of nursing diagnoses and collaborative problems reflects the client's health status.** Although collaborative problems are not always written on the nursing care plan, the master problem list for the client should include all the client's collaborative problems, as well as the actual, high-risk, and possible nursing diagnoses. A complete list will enable you to plan all the nursing care the client requires.

10. **The statement does not include any of the errors described in Table 5–2.**

WELLNESS DIAGNOSES

Wellness diagnoses are especially useful for essentially healthy clients, such as school children or new parents, who require teaching for health promotion, disease prevention, and personal growth. Presently, there are a number of ways to label healthy responses. The approach you choose depends somewhat on the type of client you are working with.

Using NANDA Terminology to Write Wellness Diagnoses

Because the NANDA diagnostic labels primarily describe health problems, they do not work well for labeling healthy responses. NANDA does, however, include wellness as a nursing focus, and encourages nurses to submit new wellness diagnoses for approval. Following is the NANDA definition of a wellness diagnosis.

A wellness diagnosis is a clinical judgment about an individual, family or community in transition from a specific level of wellness to a higher level of wellness. (*Taxonomy I—Revised, 1990*, p. 117)

New wellness diagnoses will be preceded by the phrase *Potential for Enhanced,* and will be one-part statements (e.g., Potential for Enhanced Parenting).

Using NANDA Wellness Labels

There are presently only four NANDA labels that reflect healthy functioning: *Health-Seeking Behaviors; Family Coping: Potential for Enhanced; Effective Breastfeeding;* and *Anticipatory Grieving.* These labels are especially useful in settings such as occupational health clinics and birthing centers, where clients are asymptomatic but asking how to improve their health status. The NANDA label *Health-Seeking Behaviors* provides a clear focus for planning interventions without indicating that a problem exists. This is a specific diagnosis, however, to be used for those with "expressed or observed desire to seek a higher level

Table 5–2. Common Errors in Writing Diagnostic Statements

Error	Incorrect Example	Correction
Stating need instead of response	Needs suctioning r/t decreased cough reflex	Ineffective Airway Clearance r/t decreased cough reflex
Identifying as problem or etiology medical diagnoses, treatments, or diagnostic tests	High Risk for Impaired Skin Integrity r/t diabetes mellitus	High Risk for Impaired Skin Integrity r/t lack of knowledge of special skin care needed 2° diabetes
	Cardiac Catheterization r/t chest pain on exertion	Anxiety r/t unknown outcome of cardiac catheterization
	Potential Pneumonia r/t shallow breathing 2° incision pain	Ineffective Breathing Pattern r/t incision pain A.M.B. shallow breathing
Identifying symptom of illness as a problem	Dysuria r/t urinary tract infection	Altered Patterns of Urinary Elimination r/t urinary tract infection A.M.B. dysuria
Identifying nursing action as a problem	Relieve Anxiety r/t cardiac catheterization	Severe Anxiety r/t unknown outcome of cardiac catheterization
Statement has more than one diagnostic label (problem) related to same etiology	High Risk for Fluid Volume Deficit and Constipation r/t inadequate oral fluid intake	High Risk for Fluid Volume Deficit r/t inadequate oral fluid intake *and* Constipation r/t inadequate fluid intake
Etiology is a restatement of the problem	Chronic Pain r/t headache	Chronic Pain: Headache r/t unknown etiology
Identifying as problem or etiology factors that cannot be changed	Impaired Physical Mobility r/t casts, traction, and prescribed bedrest	High Risk for Impaired Skin Integrity r/t impaired physical mobility 2° casts, traction, and bedrest
Reversing cause (etiology) and effect (problem)	Fluid Volume Deficit r/t altered oral mucous membrane A.M.B. zerostomia and oral lesions	Altered Oral Mucous Membrane r/t fluid volume deficit A.M.B. zerostomia and oral lesions
Using nursing diagnosis label without validating presence of defining characteristics	Diagnosing as follows for all NPO patients: Fluid Volume Deficit or Altered Nutrition:Less than Body Requirements	Do not use label unless defining characteristics are present.

of wellness" (NANDA, 1990). Health-Seeking Behaviors—like Enhanced Family Coping and Effective Breastfeeding—is essentially for use with well clients, but these labels might be used for clients with chronic diseases who have the required defining characteristics.

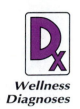

Wellness Diagnoses

Expressing NANDA Problem Labels in Positive Terms

One way to write wellness diagnoses is to use the NANDA diagnostic labels but express them in positive terms, using *Potential for Enhanced, Maintenance of,* or other positive qualifiers (e.g., Maintenance of Positive Body Image, Potential for Enhanced Parenting, Effective Individual Coping). This works well for clients who are ill and who have only a few healthy responses; expressing all the healthy responses of a well person in this fashion would produce an unmanageable number of diagnoses.

Using this method to describe healthy responses in ill clients presents difficulties. Hospitalized clients usually have many nursing diagnoses and collaborative problems. From a practical standpoint, you can address only a limited number of diagnoses during the course of a workday; so you will usually prioritize a patient's diagnoses and address the high-priority ones first. Because wellness diagnoses are usually lower in priority than actual and potential health problems, they may never be addressed. A better approach for ill clients may be to precede a NANDA problem-label with *Potential for . . .* A potential problem would likely be of a higher priority than a *Maintain Wellness* statement.

Example: Ms. Singh presently has no symptoms of or risk factors for noncompliance with her medication regimen. If you wished to focus assessments and supportive teaching on this area, you might diagnose *"Potential Noncompliance* related to usual side effects of antihypertensive medications."

This approach should be used cautiously, and only for those patients you definitely believe need nursing interventions. Any patient could be considered to be at *some* risk for noncompliance; *Potential for* should be reserved for those having a greater than normal need for nursing support of their health-promotion activities. Do not use the term *High-Risk* (instead of *Potential*) because this would convert the statement from a wellness to an illness diagnosis. (Recall that High Risk is used when risk factors are present.)

Modifications of the NANDA Taxonomy

The Bureau of Community Health Nursing, Missouri Department of Health, uses the NANDA labels, but with special modifiers that reflect wellness. Box 5–3 presents this taxomony of wellness diagnoses. The community health nurses in Multnomah County, Oregon, have also modified the NANDA taxonomy by adding wellness diagnoses based on Gordon's Functional Health Patterns (e.g., "Intake of nutrients sufficient but not in excess of metabolic need") (Multnomah County Health Services Division, 1987).

Non-NANDA Labeling Systems

Some nurses have developed wellness diagnoses that do not use the NANDA labels; additionally, healthy responses can be described in terms of framework patterns or in terms of patient strengths.

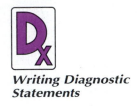

Writing Diagnostic Statements

Houldin et al.

Houldin et al. (1987) have developed a set of wellness-oriented nursing diagnoses that can be used for both well and ill clients. They organize their diagnoses according to Gordon's Functional Health Patterns. For each of their diagnostic concepts they have developed a label, definition, health status, contributing factors, and defining characteristics. Following is an example of a wellness diagnosis that might be written using Houldin's system:

Example: Effective Home-Maintenance Management associated with ability to cope with illness of child, proper hygienic practices and appropriate motivation of caregivers, as evidenced by maintenance of household, adequate family coping patterns and knowledgeable caregivers (parents)

A disadvantage of this system is that the diagnostic statements are lengthy, even when they do not include defining characteristics.

Box 5–3. Missouri Department of Health—Modified NANDA Taxonomy of Wellness Diagnoses

Activity/Rest
Diversional Activity, Adequate
Sleep Pattern, Healthy

Circulation
Cardiac Output, Adequate
Tissue Perfusion, Adequate

Elimination
Bowel Elimination, Adequate
Urinary Elimination, Adequate

Emotional Reactions
Coping, Effective Individual
Fear, Freedom From
Grieving, Appropriate
Self-Esteem, Healthy
Social Interaction, Effective

Family Pattern Alterations
Coping, Effective Family
Parenting, Adequate

Food/Fluid
Fluid Volume, Adequate
Nutrition, Adequate to Meet Body
    Requirements

Growth and Development
Growth and Development, Appropriate

Hygiene
Self-Care, Adequate (specify)

Neurologic
Communication, Effective Verbal
Sensory Perception, Appropriate
Thought Processes, Appropriate

Pain/Comfort
Pain Free

Safety/Protection
Injury Prevention Activities
Mobility, Adequate Physical

Sexuality/Reproductive
Sexual Function, Adequate

Teaching/Learning
Compliance (specify)
Health Maintenance, Adequate
Home-Maintenance Management,
    Adequate
Knowledge, Adequate (specify)

Ventilation
Airway Clearance, Effective
Breathing Patterns, Effective
Gas Exchange, Adequate

Used by permission of Bureau of Community Health Nursing: Nursing Diagnosis Taxonomy. Jefferson City, MO: Missouri Department of Health.

Using Framework Patterns for Wellness Statements

Another approach is to indicate positive or effective responses in the various categories of your chosen framework (e.g., the NANDA Human Response Patterns or Gordon's Functional Health Patterns). This label could be used when there are no problems in a pattern, but you wish to plan teaching or other measures to support healthy functioning in that area. If the category is large, like the NANDA Exchanging pattern, you can indicate which part of it is functioning effectively. Some examples of this approach follow:

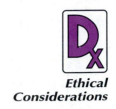

NANDA Human Response Patterns	Gordon's Functional Health Patterns
Effective Exchanging Pattern: Nutrition	Positive Health Perception
Effective Exchanging Pattern: Elimination	Effective Health Management
Effective Knowing Pattern	Positive Role/Relationship Pattern
Positive Feeling Pattern	Positive Sexuality/Reproductive Pattern

This approach can be used for either well or ill clients, but because the patterns are broad, it does not provide very specific direction for nursing interventions. Its usefulness is limited to situations that require very little intervention. The advantage of this approach is that you might need fewer diagnostic statements than if you used the method of expressing the more specific NANDA problem labels in positive terms.

Using Patient Strengths

For ill clients, perhaps a better way to describe healthy responses is to identify strengths to use in planning interventions for the other problems you identify. Concluding that there is no problem in a pattern does not necessarily indicate the need for a diagnostic statement. It is quite acceptable to identify healthy responses as strengths rather than writing them as wellness diagnoses. Especially in short-term situations, it is better to label a pattern with "No problem," since there may not be time to carry out the health-promotion interventions a wellness diagnosis would suggest. Following are some examples of patient strengths:

Pattern	Strength
Communicating	Communicates adequately in dominant language
Relating	Stable family situation
	Adequate financial support (works only part-time)

ETHICAL CONSIDERATIONS

With regard to ethics there is, first of all, the possibility of objectifying patients by overemphasizing the need to label their problems. This can be avoided if you make a conscious effort to think holistically, treating the patient rather than the problem.

The diagnostic process is not value-free. The nurse's values may lead her to emphasize or ignore certain data during assessment, affecting her choice of diagnoses. The resulting diagnoses direct the care the patient will receive and the way the patient is viewed and treated by others. Furthermore, if biased data result in missed or inaccurate diagnoses, the patient will not receive proper care.

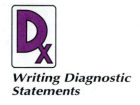

Writing Diagnostic Statements

Example: A nurse values safety over autonomy. When he cares for an elderly client, he is quick to diagnose "Altered Thought Processes r/t aging A.M.B. confusion and disorientation." The nurse did not take into account that confusion is a side-effect of one of the client's medications. As a result of this diagnosis, other nurses perceive the client as needing more supervision than he actually does. Gradually, the client loses his autonomy and becomes more dependent.

Even if the diagnostic process could be value-neutral, the phrasing of a statement can have ethical implications. A diagnosis that is stated in value-laden terms may influence other caregivers in their treatment of the patient. The etiology is the part of the diagnosis most likely to harbor negative or judgmental terms, because it is often complex and not stated in standardized language.

Examples: Ineffective Family Coping r/t *sexual promiscuity of the mother*

Anxiety r/t *unrealistic expectations of others*

Only by being aware of your values and biases can you recognize when they are creeping into your etiological statements.

The problem side of the diagnostic statement can also cause difficulty, because the NANDA diagnostic labels themselves are not entirely value-free. *Noncompliance* implies to some people that the patient is not cooperating as he should; this can negatively affect the attitude of other nurses toward that patient. Carpenito (1989, p. 42) points out that a well-written etiology can remove some of the stigma from such labels, as in the following: "Noncompliance related to the negative side-effects of the drug (reduced libido, fatigue)." Geissler (1991) suggests *Nonadherence* as a less value-laden term than *Noncompliance.*

Some diagnostic labels can be perceived as negative because of the nurse's values. *Anxiety* carries a negative connotation for nurses who value strength and self-control; they may see the patient as weak or unworthy of attention. *Knowledge Deficit* may imply lack of ability or lack of motivation to learn, either of which could evoke a negative reaction from those caregivers who place a high value on learning. To diagnose in an ethical manner, you must be aware of your values and their influence on the diagnostic process. You must realize the possible effect of your diagnostic statements on other caregivers and try to phrase them in neutral, nonjudgmental language.

LEARNING TO RECOGNIZE THE NANDA LABELS

As you become familiar with the diagnostic labels, it will be easier to recognize cue clusters in your patients—it is always easier to see something if you know what you are looking for. The best way to learn the labels is by using them; however, like most clinical skills, you need a certain degree of familiarity in order to use them. "Applying the Nursing Process," at the end of this chapter, will help you learn what the labels mean. Refer to your *Nursing Diagnosis Guide* frequently. It includes definitions and defining characteristics for each of the labels, as well as suggestions for situations in which they may or may not be useful. Detailed discussion of problematic labels is included.

RECORDING THE DIAGNOSES

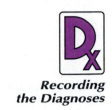
After validating and labeling the nursing diagnoses, you will write them in priority order in the appropriate documents: either the client's chart or the care plan. In some documentation systems, nursing diagnoses are recorded on a multidisciplinary problem list at the front of the client record (chart). In many agencies the care plan becomes a part of the client's permanent record upon dismissal, so diagnoses should be written in ink. When a diagnosis is resolved or changed, you can draw a single line through it or mark over it with a highlighter pen. Some care plans include a space beside the diagnosis to write the date the diagnosis is resolved or discontinued.

Prioritizing Diagnoses

Prioritizing is sometimes considered a part of the planning step of the nursing process, but if the diagnoses are to be recorded in priority order, then prioritizing must occur in the diagnosis step. Priorities are assigned on the basis of the nurse's judgment and the client's preferences. You can rank the diagnoses from highest to lowest priority (i.e.,1, 2, 3, etc.), or you can assign each problem a high, medium, or low priority. Prioritizing problems helps to assure that care is given first for the more important problems. This noes not necessarily mean that one problem must be resolved before you address another.

Example: Self-Care Deficit (Bathing) might be a long-term problem for a patient. This does not mean you should wait until the patient can bathe himself before addressing the next highest priority, High Risk for Constipation.

You should also consider high-risk problems when setting priorities. It is often as important to prevent a problem as it is to treat an actual one.

Example: For a poorly nourished, immobile patient, High Risk for Impaired Skin Integrity is of higher priority than Actual Diversional Activity Deficit.

If you use *preservation of life* as a criterion, you would rate the client's diagnoses high, medium, or low based on the amount of threat they pose to the client's life. Life-threatening problems would take priority over those that cause pain or discomfort. A **high-priority problem** is one that is life-threatening, such as severe fluid and electrolyte loss or respiratory obstruction. A **medium-priority problem** does not directly threaten life, but it may produce destructive physical or emotional changes (e.g., Rape-Trauma Syndrome). A **low-priority problem** is one that arises from normal developmental needs, or requires only minimal supportive nursing intervention (e.g., Altered Sexual Patterns related to knowledge deficit). After assigning high, medium, and low priorities, you can rank the diagnoses from most to least important.

Example:

Rank	Diagnosis	Priority
1	Fluid Volume Deficit related to vomiting	Medium
2	Sleep-Pattern disturbance . . .	Low
3	Diversional Activity Deficit . . .	Low

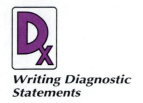

Writing Diagnostic Statements

Maslow's Hierarchy of Human Needs also provides a good framework for prioritizing nursing diagnoses. Recall from Chapter 3 that in Maslow's model there are five levels of human needs. Starting with the most basic (highest priority) need, they are: physiologic, safety/security, social, esteem and self-actualization. As a rule, the more basic needs must be met before the client can deal with the higher needs.

Kalish (1983) has made Maslow's system even more useful by dividing the physiological needs into survival and stimulation needs. Survival needs are the most basic; only when they are satisfied can the client be concerned about higher-level needs. When survival needs are met, the client tries to meet stimulation needs before moving up the hierarchy to safety, social, and other higher needs. Kalish's division of physiological needs includes the following:

Survival Needs: Food, air, water, temperature, elimination, rest, pain avoidance

Stimulation Needs: Sex, activity, exploration, manipulation, novelty

In this framework, diagnoses involving survival needs have priority over those involving stimulation needs.

Example: The following diagnoses are ranked from highest to lowest priority:

Need	Nursing Diagnosis
Survival	Altered Nutrition: Less Than Body Requirements related to fatigue
Stimulation	Diversional Activity Deficit related to infectious disease isolation
Esteem	Low Self-Esteem related to inability to perform role functions

As much as possible, *patient preference should be considered in priority setting.* You should give high priority to the problems the patient feels are important, as long as this does not interfere with survival needs or medical treatments. Because she is exhausted after delivery, a new mother's first priority may be to sleep. However, you must observe her closely for signs of postpartum hemorrhage, so you cannot safely follow her priorities in this situation. If you explain your priorities, you may be able to persuade the patient to agree with them.

Attending to problems that are high priorities for the patient increases the likelihood that they will be successfully resolved: the patient will cooperate most enthusiastically to solve problems she considers important. As in the following example, she may not be motivated to address other problems until her main concerns are dealt with.

Example: Pat Sams is an 18-year-old who has just had her first baby. The nurse knows she must teach Ms. Sams how to bathe her infant before she is dismissed—within 24 hours after delivery. The nurse has given highest priority to Ms. Sam's Knowledge Deficit diagnosis. However, Ms. Sams finds it difficult to concentrate on the bath demonstration. She is hoping the baby's father will come to visit, and has been washing her hair and putting on makeup. She has not heard from him since coming to the hospital, and she is worried he will not want to see her and the baby.

SUMMARY

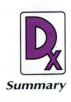

Summary

Diagnostic statements

✓ use North American Nursing Diagnosis Association (NANDA) labels—reviewed and modified at biannual meetings.

✓ use the format of Problem related to (r/t) Etiology (or the P.E.S.variation).

✓ are varied by one-part statements, use of *secondary to,* unknown and complex etiologies, and three-part statements.

✓ should be descriptive, accurate, and specific, using nonjudgmental, legally advisable language.

✓ are not value-free and require nurses to be aware of their own values and the perceptions of others.

✓ may describe wellness states as well as health problems.

✓ should be recorded on the care plan in priority order.

Skill-Building Activities

Scientists often make mental models to describe particular aspects of nature and to help us better understand various phenomena. For example, in the Bohr model of the atom, electrons orbit the nucleus much as moons orbit a planet. To cite a more familiar example, the nursing frameworks discussed in Chapters 3 and 4 are models that describe particular aspects of nursing. In the Roy model, for instance, nursing activity is described as promoting adaptation of the individual.

Practice in Critical Thinking: Comparing and Contrasting

You might create a model to understand something you encounter in everyday life. For instance, a model for an ideal teacher should include things like what kinds of lessons the teacher designs, what he lets students do in class, how he encourages you to think about the subject you are studying, or whether the tests are based on the stated objectives for the course. Such a model could provide a reference point to help you describe and understand a real teacher.

Here are some steps you might use when comparing real occurrences to a model:

1. List the important characteristics or behavior of the model.

2. Ask yourself if the real thing behaves like the model with regard to these same characteristics.

3. Considering the characteristics you identified in Step 2, determine what features of the real occurrence make it different from the model.

Learning the Skill

Use the three steps outlined above to compare your model of an ideal nurse with the behavior of real nurses.

1. *Use Step 1.* List the important characteristics that you think describe the ideal nurse.

2. *Use Step 2.* Considering each of the points you listed in (1), compare the behavior of someone you consider to be a typical nurse to the ideal nurse—perhaps someone you have observed during your clinical experiences.

3. *Use Step 3.* In (1) and (2) you have compared the behavior of typical and ideal nurses in a number of ways. Considering each of these points, explain why your typical nurse behaves differently from your ideal nurse.

Applying the Skill

1. This chapter presented several models of ideal diagnostic statements. The basic format of a nursing diagnosis is **Problem r/t Etiology.** List the variations of this model.

2. The chapter section "Criteria for Judging the Content of the Diagnostic Statement" provides another model of a diagnostic statement. List the qualities of an ideal diagnostic statement provided by this model.

3. Borrow a care plan from another student or copy at least six nursing diagnoses from a care plan in your clinical agency. Discuss whether or not real diagnoses are the same as the ideal diagnoses with regard to qualities listed in Steps 1 and 2 of this section.

4. If you did note a difference in Step 3, explain why a typical diagnosis might be different from the ideal diagnoses.

Adapted from Wilbraham et al., *Addison-Wesley Chemistry Critical Thinking Worksheets,* (Menlo Park, CA: Addison-Wesley, 1990).

Applying the Nursing Process

(Answer Key, p. 377)

Refer to your *Nursing Diagnosis Guide* as often as necessary when working the following exercises. Many of the exercises are designed to help you become familiar with the *Guide* and with NANDA labels.

1. In what year was the first national conference on nursing diagnosis held? _____

2. Each NANDA diagnosis has four components, some of which are subdivided. Write the name of the component beside its description. (Refer to *Nursing Diagnosis Guide* as needed.)

   a. _____ The component that expresses a clear, precise meaning for the diagnostic concept and differentiates it from all others.

   b. _____ The clinical criteria that validate the presence of a diagnostic label. Can be signs, symptoms, or risk factors.

   c. _____ These serve as defining characteristics of potential diagnoses.

   d. _____ These *must* be present in order to make the diagnosis.

   e. _____ A concise phrase or term describing the state of the client's health.

   f. _____ Clinical or personal situations that can change health status or influence actual problem development.

3. Identify the underlined parts of the nursing diagnoses by writing the correct terms beneath them. Use these terms:

   Label   Related Factors   Qualifying term
   Defining characteristics   Risk Factors

   a. High Risk for <u>Body Image Disturbance</u> r/t amputation of right leg

      _____

   b. High Risk for Body Image Disturbance r/t <u>amputation of right leg</u>

      _____

c. Severe <u>Chronic Pain</u> r/t knowledge deficit (effects of exercise and rest)

_____

d. <u>Severe</u> Chronic Pain r/t knowledge deficit (effects of exercise and rest)

_____

e. Severe Chronic Pain r/t <u>knowledge deficit (effects of exercise and rest)</u>

_____

4. Choose the most likely etiology for each of the following problems from the numbered list.

a. High Risk for Infection r/t ___
b. Activity Intolerance r/t ___
c. Altered Parenting r/t ___
d. Fluid Volume Deficit r/t ___
e. Possible Sexual Dysfunction r/t ___

1. insufficient oxygenation for activities of daily living
2. compromised immune system
3. increased fluid loss secondary to vomiting
4. delayed parent-infant contact 2° illness of infant
5. body image disturbance 2° mastectomy

5. Place a *C* beside the correctly written diagnoses.

a. ___ High Risk for Infection Transmission r/t lack of knowledge about communicable nature of the disease
b. ___ Altered Oral Mucous Membrane r/t dry mouth
c. ___ Elevated Temperature r/t infectious process
d. ___ Constipation r/t inadequate fiber intake and prolonged bedrest
e. ___ High Risk for Impaired Skin Integrity r/t prescribed bedrest
f. ___ Impaired Skin Integrity r/t prescribed bedrest
g. ___ Rape-Trauma Syndrome
h. ___ Acute Back Pain r/t unknown etiology
i. ___ Impaired Skin Integrity r/t not being repositioned often enough
j. ___ Crying r/t anxiety

6. Circle the risk factors. Underline the related factors.

a. Fear r/t progressive loss of vision
b. High Risk for Anxiety r/t possibility of going blind
c. Possible Fluid Volume Deficit r/t post-op NPO
d. Pain r/t effects of surgery
e. Grieving r/t recent loss of job

7. Write a diagnostic statement for each of the following cases. Refer to *Nursing Diagnosis Guide*.

   a. A hypertensive client states that she hasn't been taking her medication because it doesn't make her feel any better. Also, she says she has difficulty remembering to take it.

   b. An elderly patient with left-side paralysis has a red, broken area in the skin over his coccyx. The patient cannot turn himself in bed.

   c. The client is 45 pounds overweight. He states that he is in a high-stress job and doesn't have time to cook regular meals—he tends to eat fast food and snacks a lot. His job is sedentary, and he does not engage in any type of physical exercise or sport. For fun, he likes to "eat at a nice restaurant."

   d. A client is two hours post-operative vaginal hysterectomy. Her blood pressure has dropped from 130/80 to 100/60, and her pulse is 90. She is slightly pale, but not cyanotic. She has a 4 cm x 4 cm spot of blood on her vaginal pad. Her abdomen is firm and tender to the touch, but not distended.

   e. A client with pelvic inflammatory disease has just tested positive for gonorrhea. She states that she has unprotected sex.

8. Circle the labels that are NANDA-approved terminology.

Altered Nutrition: More Than Body Requirements	High Risk for Infection	Anorexia
Altered Body Temperature	Altered Bowel Elimination	Constipation
Diarrhea	High Risk for Aspiration	Altered Protection
	Social Isolation	Activity Intolerance

9. Circle the labels that require additional words to make the problem more specific (e.g., Feeding Self-Care Deficit, Level 3).

   a. Activity Intolerance

   b. Stress Incontinence

   c. Sensory-Perceptual Alteration

   d. Chronic Pain

   e. Impaired Physical Mobility

   f. Fatigue

   g. Ineffective Breastfeeding

   h. Colonic Constipation

10. For each of the labels you circled in item 9, write an example of words you might add to make the problem more specific.

11. Supply the label that fits the following definitions. Refer to the *Nursing Diagnosis Guide* in the back of this text as needed.

a. _____ A state in which an individual experiences a change in normal bowel habits characterized by involuntary passage of stool

b. _____ A state in which an individual experiences a change in normal bowel habits characterized by the frequent passage of loose, fluid, unformed stools

c. _____ Impairment of adaptive behaviors and problem-solving abilities of a person in meeting life's demands and roles

d. _____ The state in which an individual is at risk for entry of gastrointestinal secretions, oropharyngeal secretions, or solids or fluids into tracheobronchial passages

e. _____ A state in which an individual is unable to clear secretions or obstructions from the respiratory tract to maintain airway patency

12. Match the diagnostic label with the defining characteristics.

- **a.** Ineffective Airway Clearance
- **b.** Ineffective Breathing Patterns
- **c.** Sensory-Perceptual Alterations (specify)
- **d.** Social Isolation
- **e.** Impaired Social Interactions
- **f.** Impaired swallowing

____ **1.** Abnormal breath sounds, tachypnea, ineffective cough (with or without sputum), cyanosis, dyspnea, changes in rate or depth of respiration

____ **2.** *Major:* Inaccurate interpretation of environmental stimuli
Minor: Restlessness

____ **3.** Expressed feelings of aloneness
Feels rejected; says time passes slowly

____ **4.** Changes in respiratory rate and pattern; change in pulse; orthopnea

____ **5.** Reports inability to establish stable, supportive relationships; poor impulse control

____ **6.** *Major:* Observed evidence of difficulty in swallowing (e.g., stasis of food in oral cavity, coughing/choking)

13. Write the label that fits the following cue clusters. Compare the cue clusters to the defining characteristics in the *Nursing Diagnosis Guide*. You do not need to write etiologies.

a. _____

Mr. Maier has been hospitalized with a heart attack. He has been told he needs to rest and avoid stress. He says his advertising agency cannot run without him, and he phones the office several times a day to check on things and give instructions. He tells them he will be back to work "in a few days." He says he doesn't believe this is really a heart problem; "it feels like indigestion to me." He says he does not intend to change to a low-fat diet: "I'm too old to change my ways now." He does not seem anxious: he laughs and jokes a lot.

b. _____

Althea Harper has severe, chronic arthritis in her hands. When the nurse makes a home visit, Ms. Harper meets her at the door in a robe and slippers. Her hair is uncombed. She apologizes to the nurse for her appearance, saying, "I'm sorry I'm such a mess. It's just too hard to get dressed; I can't seem to work the buttons and zippers, or even tie my shoes. It hurts even to hold a hairbrush."

c. _____

Ms. Turner has been blind in her right eye for several years. Lately, her nurse has noticed that Ms. Turner does not seem to hear him when he speaks to her while standing to her right. The aide has reported several times that Ms. Turner ate only about half the food on her tray. The nurse observes that the food remaining is on the right side of the tray. To validate his findings, he pats Ms. Turner's right shoulder; Ms. Turner does not respond.

d. _____

The client reports that she must wear a vaginal pad because she leaks urine when she laughs or lifts heavy objects.

e. _____

The client reports that he must void every 30 minutes, but only small amounts. When he feels the need to void, he must hurry to the bathroom because he cannot wait. He also reports that he gets up three or four times during the night to void.

f. _____

A 70-year-old client has a medical diagnosis of arteriosclerosis. His left foot is blue and cold to the touch. The nurse finds a weak pedal pulse. She validates the findings by elevating his leg. It becomes pale, and the color does not return when she lowers it to a dependent position. She notes that the skin is shiny on both his lower legs.

g. _____

Lorraine Richards' three-week old son has a temperature of 104°. She says he has been having diarrhea and is not nursing well. His fontanels are still firm, and his skin turgor is good.

h. _____

Mr. and Ms. Welytok have a baby with myelomeningocele. They have been attempting to care for the baby at home for the past two weeks. Ms. Welytok confides to the visiting nurse that she doesn't feel she can care for the baby adequately. "I feel guilty, but I'm afraid to touch her, much less turn her. My husband just comes home from work and goes straight to bed, so he's no help at all. I can't give the other kids the attention they need now because I have to spend all my time with Jill. I don't feel like a very good mom right now."

i. _____

Tresa Liu is twelve weeks pregnant. She is 17 years old. She says, "I want to keep the baby, but my parents won't let me. They think I need to finish school. They want me to have an abortion. I think maybe they're right, but then I've heard sometimes you can't ever get pregnant after that. But I hate to quit school and miss all the basketball games and stuff. So I want to do it and then I don't. I should have made up my mind before this, I know."

j. _____

The client has been on prolonged bedrest. While ambulating, he complains of fatigue and dyspnea; he leans on the nurse for support. When she checks his vital signs, his heart rate is 120 and irregular.

14. Circle the related factors identified by NANDA for the label Hopelessness.

Long-term stress   Loss of belief in God

Multiple caretakers   Prolonged activity restriction creating isolation

Pain   Decrease in circulation to the brain

15. Circle the correct client in each situation. Consult your *Nursing Diagnosis Guide*.

   a. All clients have the appropriate defining characteristics: body weight 20% under ideal and total calorie intake less than RDA. For which client(s) should you use the problem label Altered Nutrition: Less Than Body Requirements?

      Mr. Jonas, who cannot swallow because of paralysis

      Ms. Petrie, who is depressed and says she is not hungry

      Bobby George, who is NPO for two days after surgery

   b. For which child should you diagnose High Risk for Poisoning?

      Billy, who is 6 months old and has a babysitter

      Jana, who is an active 2-year-old

      Jill, whose mother keeps her cleaning supplies under the sink

   c. For which client should you diagnose Impaired Skin Integrity?

      Mr. A, who has a sacral decubitus ulcer

      Mr. B, who has an abdominal incision

      Mr. C, who has self-inflicted razor cuts on his wrists

16. Write a diagnostic statement for each set of defining characteristics and related (or risk) factors. Focus on good format. Some of the statements are collaborative problems; others are nursing diagnoses. Use P.E.S. format only when directed to do so.

   a. *Use P.E.S. format.*

Defining Characteristics	Overuse of laxatives and suppositories
	Expectation of a daily bowel movement
Related Factors	Impaired thought processes

b. Defining Characteristics

Decreased frequency of bowel movement
Dry, hard stool; abdominal distention

Related Factors

There is no apparent reason for this problem.
Diagnostic tests are normal; diet appears normal.

c. Defining Characteristics

Decreased frequency of bowel movement
Dry, hard stool; abdominal distention

Related Factors

Inadequate fluid intake
Inadequate fiber intake
Inadequate physical activity

Medical Factors

Client is too weak to eat, drink, or exercise much because of advanced chronic lung disease.

d. *Use P.E.S. Format*

Defining Characteristics

Verbalizes inability to cope
Observed to be unable to solve problems

Related Factors

Related factors occupy 35 pages of history notes in the chart and show development of this problem over several years.

e. Defining Characteristics
Risk Factor

None
Intravenous therapy

f. Defining Characteristics

Possession of destructive means (gun)

Increased motor activity

(May be suicidal, but do not have adequate data to be sure)

Related Factors

Suspect toxic reaction to medications; not sure yet

g. Defining Characteristics

Expressed desire to seek higher level of wellness; has asked nurse to suggest an exercise regimen.

17. Assign high, medium, and low priorities to the following diagnoses, using a "preservation of life" criterion.

a. _____ Decreased Communication between husband and wife related to use of blaming and withdrawal

b. _____ Anxiety related to lack of knowledge of impending surgery and pre- and post-op routines

c. _____ Fluid Volume Deficit related to fever and vomiting secondary to gastroenteritis

d. _____ Fluid Volume Excess: Right Arm related to dependent position and effects of mastectomy

e. _____ Altered Nutrition: Less Than Body Requirements r/t refusal to eat secondary to dysfunctional grieving

f. _____ High Risk for Injury (falls) related to weakness and decreased vision

g. _____ Nonadherance (to diabetic diet) related to unresolved anger

h. _____ Unrelieved Incisional Pain related to hesitance to "bother" nurses

18. Use the Kalish/Maslow Hierarchy of Needs to prioritize the following diagnoses. Assign priorities as follows (1 being highest priority):

1—Survival   4—Love/Belonging
2—Stimulation   5—Esteem
3—Safety   6—Self-Actualization

a. ___ Decreased Communication between husband and wife related to use of blaming and withdrawal

b. ___ Anxiety related to lack of knowledge of impending surgery and pre- and post-op routines

c. ___ Fluid Volume Deficit related to fever and vomiting secondary to gastroenteritis

d. ___ High Risk for Injury (falls) related to weakness and decreased vision

e. ___ Unrelieved Incisional Pain related to hesitance to "bother" nurses

f. ___ Altered Health Maintenance (breast self-exam) related to lack of knowledge of how to do the procedure, and of its importance

g. ___ Ineffective Airway Clearance related to copious, thick secretions and weak cough effort

REFERENCES

Abdellah, F. (1957). Methods of identifying covert aspects of nursing problems. *Nursing Research, 6*(1): 4–23.

American Nurses Association. (1973). *Standards of Nursing Practice.* Kansas City, MO.

Bureau of Community Health Nursing. (1985). *Nursing Diagnosis Taxonomy.* Jefferson City, MO: Missouri Department of Health.

Carpenito, L. (1992). *Nursing Diagnosis: Application to Clinical Practice.* 4th ed. Philadelphia: J. B. Lippincott.

Carroll-Johnson, R., ed. (1989). *Classification of Nursing Diagnoses: Proceedings of the Eighth Conference.* North American Nursing Diagnosis Association. Philadelphia: J. B. Lippincott.

Carroll-Johnson, R., ed. (1991). *Classification of Nursing Diagnoses: Proceedings of the Ninth Conference.* North American Nursing Diagnosis Association. Philadelphia: J. B. Lippincott.

England, M. (1989). Nursing diagnosis: A conceptual framework. In Fitzpatrick, J., and Whall, A., eds., *Conceptual Models of Nursing: Analysis and Evaluation.* 2nd ed. Norwalk, CT: Appleton-Century-Crofts, pp. 347–69.

Fitzpatrick, J. (1990). Conceptual basis for the organization and advancement of nursing knowledge: Nursing diagnosis/taxonomy. *Nursing Diagnosis, 1*(3): 102–6.

Gebbie, K. (1976a). Development of a taxonomy of nursing diagnosis. In Walter, J., et al., *Dynamics of Problem-Oriented Approaches: Patient Care and Documentation.* Philadelphia: J. B. Lippincott.

Gebbie, K., ed. (1976b). *Summary of the Second National Conference: Classification of Nursing Diagnoses.* St. Louis: Clearinghouse—National Group for Classification of Nursing Diagnoses.

Geissler, E. (1991). Transcultural nursing and nursing diagnoses. *Nursing & Health Care, 12*(4): 190–92, 203.

Gordon, M. (1987). *Nursing Diagnosis: Process and Application.* 2nd ed. New York: McGraw-Hill.

Guzzetta, E., et al. (1989). *Clinical Assessment Tools for Use with Nursing Diagnosis.* St. Louis: C. V. Mosby.

Henderson, V. (1964). The nature of nursing. *American Journal of Nursing, 64*(8): 62–68.

Houldin, A., Saltstein, S., and Ganley, K. (1987). *Nursing Diagnoses for Wellness: Supporting Strengths.* Philadelphia: J. B. Lippincott.

Hurley, M., ed. (1986). *Classification of Nursing Diagnoses: Proceedings of the Sixth Conference.* North American Nursing Diagnosis Association. St. Louis: C. V. Mosby.

Kalish, R. (1983). *The Psychology of Human Behavior.* 5th ed. Monterey, CA: Brooks/Cole.

Kim, M., McFarland, G., and McLane, A. (1984). *Proceedings of the Fifth National Conference.* North American Nursing Diagnosis Association. St. Louis: C. V. Mosby.

Kobert, L., and Folan, M. (1990). Coming of age in rethinking the philosophies behind holism and nursing process. *Nursing & Health Care, 11*(6):308–12.

Kritek, P. (1985). Nursing diagnosis: Theoretical foundations. *Occupation Health Nursing,* (August): 393–96.

McLane, A., ed. (1987). *Classification of Nursing Diagnoses: Proceedings of the Seventh Conference.* North American Nursing Diagnosis Association. St. Louis, MO: C. V. Mosby.

Multnomah County Health Services Division (1987). *Nursing Diagnosis Classification Codes.* Portland, OR: Multnomah County.

North American Nursing Diagnosis Association (NANDA). (1990). *Taxonomy I—Revised, 1990.* St. Louis, MO.

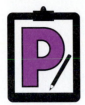

CHAPTER 6

PLANNING

OBJECTIVES

Upon completing this chapter, you should be able to do the following:
- Describe the nursing activities that occur in the planning step of the nursing process.
- Explain the relationship between planning and the other steps of the nursing process.
- Discuss the importance of initial, ongoing, and discharge planning.
- Explain how to derive measurable, observable, individualized client goals from nursing diagnoses.
- Discuss the purpose of a goal statement.
- Explain the process of developing and selecting nursing interventions.
- Identify the different types of nursing orders (i.e., observation, prevention, treatment, health promotion).
- Develop client goals and nursing orders for wellness diagnoses.
- Discuss the ethical considerations involved in developing client goals and nursing orders.

PLANNING: THE THIRD STEP OF THE NURSING PROCESS

This chapter discusses planning as a step of the nursing process, compares various types of planning, and explains how to write individualized goals and nursing orders. Figure 6.1 presents an overview of the planning step.

Planning is the third step of the nursing process. After diagnosing the patient's health problems and strengths, the nurse works with her to develop a plan to prevent, eliminate or reduce the problems. The American Nurses Association supports planning as a professional nursing responsibility (see Box 6–1). Certain nursing activities may be delegated to other caregivers (e.g., the nursing assistant may take the admission vital signs), but the registered nurse is responsible and accountable for planning the client's care.

Activities in the Planning Step

In the planning step the nurse develops the patient-care plan. With patient and family input, the nurse derives goals from the diagnostic statements, and identifies nursing measures to achieve those goals. The purpose and end product of this step is a written, holistic plan of care tailored to the patient's problems and strengths. The planning step ends when this plan has been written.

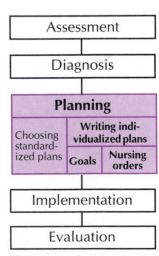

Figure 6-1. The Planning Step in the Nursing Process

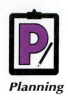

Planning

During planning, the nurse engages in the following activities:

1. Deciding which problems need individually developed plans and which can be addressed by standards of care, policies and procedures, and other forms of preplanned, routine care.

2. Choosing and adapting preplanned, preprinted interventions and care plans where appropriate. (This activity is explained in detail in Chapter 9, "Creating a Patient Care Plan.")

3. Writing individualized goals and nursing orders for problems that require nursing attention beyond preplanned, routine care.

Relationship to Other Nursing Process Steps

Remember that the nursing process steps are interdependent and overlapping; the planning step is no exception. Its effectiveness depends directly upon the assessment and diagnosis phases. If assessment data (assessment step) are complete and accurate and the diagnostic statements are correct (diagnosis step), the goals and nursing orders flow logically (planning step) and are likely to be effective. In the same way, implementation and evaluation depend on the planning phase. The goals and nursing orders written during planning serve to guide the nurse's actions during implementation. Furthermore, the goals developed during planning are the criteria used in evaluating whether patient care has had the desired effects (more about this in Chapter 8).

The steps overlap when nurses do **informal planning** while carrying out the activities of the other steps. For example, while listening to a patient's lung sounds (assessment), the nurse may be making a mental note (planning) to notify the physician of her findings. Although planning can be informal, this chapter emphasizes **formal planning,** which is a conscious, deliberate activity involving decision making, critical thinking, and creativity.

Box 6–1. ANA Standards for Planning	
Standard III.	The plan of nursing care includes goals derived from the nursing diagnoses.
Standard IV.	The plan of nursing care includes the priorities and the prescribed nursing approaches or measures to achieve the goals derived from the nursing diagnoses.
Standard V.	Nursing actions provide for client/patient participation in health promotion, maintenance, and restoration.
Standard VI.	Nursing actions assist the client/patient to maximize his health capabilities.

(From *Standards of Nursing Practice*, © 1973 by the American Nurses Association, Kansas City, MO. Reprinted with permission.)

Types of Planning

Planning begins with the first patient contact and continues until the nurse-patient relationship is ended, usually when the patient is discharged from the health-care agency. In addition to the planning involved in creating a nursing care plan, nurses use time-sequenced planning when they plan a patient's care for a shift or for a 24-hour period. For instance, you would use it

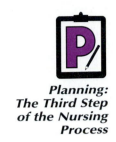

***Planning:
The Third Step
of the Nursing
Process***

1. to plan the timing and order of your nursing interventions for a patient (for example, giving pain medication before a painful dressing change).

2. to coordinate the timing of your nursing care with the actions of other health team members, visits from family and friends, and the patient's circadian rhythms.

3. to plan your daily work schedule. In addition to planning care for *each* patient, you must structure your own time so that you can give care to *all* the patients assigned to you for that shift.

Initial Planning

The nurse who performs the admission assessment should develop the initial comprehensive care plan. She has the benefit of the client's body language and some intuitive kinds of information that are not available from the written data base alone; thus, she is best qualified to plan the care and has that responsibility in most institutions.

Planning should be initiated soon after the assessment is done, especially with the trend toward shorter hospital stays. Even a partially developed plan can be helpful in the early nurse-client contacts. Because of time constraints or the client's condition, the initial data base is sometimes incomplete. In such situations, you should develop a preliminary plan with the information available, and refine it as you are able to gather the missing data.

Ongoing Planning

Ongoing planning can be done by any nurse who works with the client. It is carried out as new information is obtained and as the client's responses to care are evaluated. The initial care plan can be individualized even more as the nurses get to know the client better.

Where primary nursing is practiced, the primary nurse is responsible for ongoing planning, even if she did not write the initial plan. Other nurses caring for the client direct new data or changes in the plan to the primary nurse. This helps ensure that new data will be analyzed in relation to existing data and problems. Otherwise, nurses who are not familiar with the client might not recognize the significance of new data, and important data could be lost.

Ongoing planning also occurs as you plan your nursing care at the beginning of each day. In your daily planning, you will use ongoing assessment data to do the following:

1. Determine whether the client's health status has changed.

2. Set today's priorities for the client's care.

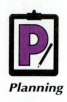

Planning

3. Decide which problems to focus on during this shift.

4. Coordinate your activities so that you can address more than one problem at each client contact.

Discharge Planning

Discharge planning concerns the process of preparing the client to leave the health-care agency. It includes preparing the client for self-care as well as providing for continuity of care between present caregivers and those who will care for the client after discharge. As with the rest of the care plan, the nurse who prepares the initial data base is in the best position to address discharge planning needs.

As a by-product of nationwide efforts to limit the cost of health care, an increasing number and variety of surgeries and treatments are being done in outpatient settings. Clients admitted to acute-care hospitals are being discharged earlier, often still in need of skilled nursing care. They may be placed in an intermediate-care facility, nursing home, or other continued-care setting, or they may be sent home to continue complicated treatments and therapies such as apnea monitors, intravenous therapies, and even mechanical ventilation. Clients and their families must also learn to manage basic hygiene and comfort needs and arrange for in-home professional help as necessary. If they are not well prepared, the client may develop complications and need to be rehospitalized. Clearly, discharge planning is an important nursing responsibility and is essential in every client-care plan. According to the American Nurses Association,

> continuity of care planning in an organized care system establishes a process designed to meet the needs of the patient or client during every phase of care. The process involves admission planning, discharge planning, referral and follow up. (ANA, 1975)

Effective discharge planning begins with admission and continues until discharge. It includes assessment of the level of problem resolution, the home environment, the availability of family and friends who can help with care, and family and community resources. Nurses make referrals for home care and to other community agencies, but a physician's order may be necessary in order to obtain third-party reimbursement (e.g., Medicare or private insurance). The client's learning needs are an important part of the discharge plan.

Critical Thinking in the Planning Step

After deciding which of the client's problems can be addressed by routine interventions contained in standards of care and model care plans, the nurse develops goals and nursing orders for the problems that require an individualized approach. This requires critical thinking skills, as does every step of the nursing process. The goals developed in the planning step serve later as criteria for evaluating patient progress. Developing evaluative criteria is a critical thinking skill in and of itself.

When generating nursing interventions, nurses use the skills of generalizing, explaining, and predicting, as well as the ability to make interdisciplinary connections and use insights from subjects such as physiology and psychology. Generating nursing interventions is similar to generating hypotheses in the scientific method, in that the nurse predicts the interventions most likely to achieve the client's health goals.

WRITING CLIENT GOALS

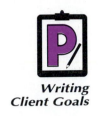

A **goal** is the desired outcome of a nursing intervention. On a care plan, the goals describe, in terms of observable client responses, what you hope to achieve by implementing the nursing orders. The terms *goal, expected outcome, outcome criterion,* and *predicted outcome* are used interchangeably by most nurses and in this book. You should be aware, however, that some literature does differentiate between the terms, defining *goals* as broad statements about the desired effects of the nursing interventions, and *expected outcomes, predicted outcomes,* or *outcome criteria* as the more specific, measurable criteria used to evaluate whether the goal has been met. An example follows:

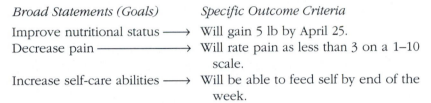

Broad Statements (Goals)	Specific Outcome Criteria
Improve nutritional status ⟶	Will gain 5 lb by April 25.
Decrease pain ⟶	Will rate pain as less than 3 on a 1–10 scale.
Increase self-care abilities ⟶	Will be able to feed self by end of the week.

When goals are defined broadly, as in the above examples, the patient-care plan must include *both* goals and outcome criteria. In fact, they are sometimes combined into one statement; the broad goal is stated first, followed by *as evidenced by,* and then a list of the observable responses that demonstrate achievement of the goal. Do not confuse *as evidenced by* with the phrase *as manifested by,* used in writing nursing diagnoses.

Example:

Correct	Incorrect
Nutritional status will improve *as evidenced by* Weight gain of 5 lb by 4/25	Nutritional status will improve *as manifested by* Weight gain of 5 lb by 4/25

While you are learning, writing the broad, general goal first may help you to think of the specific outcomes that are needed. Remember, though, that while broad goals can be a starting point for planning, the specific, measurable outcomes *must* be written on the care plan.

Purpose of the Goal Statement

Goal statements guide the planning and evaluation of patient care and serve as motivators for both nurse and patient. Planning proceeds more easily if the goals state precisely and clearly what you wish to achieve; ideas for nursing interventions will then flow logically from the goals, and it will be relatively easy to select nursing orders to achieve the desired changes in client responses.

Although predicted outcomes are developed in the planning step, they serve an important function in the evaluation step as the criteria used to evaluate the effectiveness of the nursing interventions. Because the objectives are stated in terms of desired client responses, you simply look for those responses to know whether your nursing actions have been effective.

Goal statements also provide a sense of achievement for both the client and the nurse and motivate them in their efforts to improve health status.

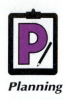

Example: Kay Stein has essential hypertension. She has a demanding career and family life, and she needs to lose 50 pounds. Even though she takes her antihypertensive medication faithfully, follows her low-calorie diet, and tries to decrease her stress, she still does not feel any better. In fact, she feels worse because the medication gives her a headache. However, she and her nurse have set measurable, achievable goals, such as "Loses 2 lb this week" and "B/P will be 130/80 by end of the week." When Kay's blood pressure reading is 120/80, and the scales show she has lost 4 pounds, she has proof that her efforts are really accomplishing something. This helps motivate her to continue making life-style changes that she finds very difficult.

Deriving Goals from Nursing Diagnoses

Diagnostic statements describe human responses that are problems for the patient. This suggests that the opposite response is preferred and is what you will try to achieve. The nursing diagnosis "Colonic Constipation r/t inactivity and inadequate fluid intake" indicates that the client's elimination status needs to change. An improvement in elimination status would be evidenced by an opposite (normal) response—that is, a regular, formed, soft bowel movement.

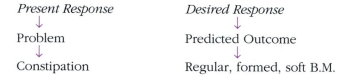

Present Response	*Desired Response*
↓	↓
Problem	Predicted Outcome
↓	↓
Constipation	Regular, formed, soft B.M.

Process

When developing goals, look at the problem and think what the alternative healthy response would be. To help describe the response in terms of specific behaviors, ask yourself the following:

1. If the problem is solved (or prevented), how will the client look or behave? What will I be able to see, hear, palpate, smell, or otherwise observe with my senses?

2. What must the client do to show that the goal is achieved? How well must he do it?

Goals describe desired, or normal, behaviors. Therefore, you can use any source that describes physiological, psychological, sociocultural, or spiritual norms to help you state the goals (e.g., physiology text, human growth and development text, hospital list of normal lab values).

Example: The nursing diagnosis is "Fluid Volume Deficit r/t insufficient fluid intake." The unhealthy response is *fluid volume deficit*; the alternative healthy response would be *adequate fluid volume*.

1. If the problem is solved (fluid volume is adequate), how will the client look or behave? One observable response you could see and palpate is *elastic skin turgor*.

2. What must the client do to demonstrate goal achievement? A possible answer to this is that he must *drink more fluids than he excretes.* Also, you might specify that he would drink *a minimum amount of fluids*, perhaps 100 cc/hour.

Therefore, your goal statement might be
  Will have adequate fluid volume, as evidenced by
a. elastic skin turgor
b. Intake = Output
c. drinks at least 100 cc/hour.

Goals, like nursing diagnoses, are concerned with a variety of human responses, including appearance, body functions, symptoms, knowledge, interpersonal functioning, and emotions (see Table 6-1).

Because goals are derived directly from the nursing diagnoses, they will be appropriate only if you have stated the nursing diagnosis correctly.

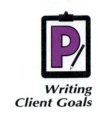

Writing Client Goals

Table 6-1. Examples of Alternative Healthy Responses

Nursing Diagnosis	Human Response	Predicted Outcome
Ineffective Airway Clearance r/t poor cough effort 2° incisional pain & fear of "breaking stitches loose"	Appearance	Within 24 hours after surgery, will have no skin pallor or cyanosis during post-op period.
	Body functioning	Lungs clear to auscultation during entire post-op period.
	Symptoms	Within 48 hours after surgery, states having no shortness of breath when ambulating to chair.
	Knowledge	After reteaching, states rationale for turn, cough, deep breathing after surgery.
	Emotions	Within 48 hours after surgery, states he is no longer afraid to cough.
Parental Anxiety r/t uncertainty of prognosis of newborn	Interpersonal functioning	By 3/1, parents will express their concerns to each other.
		Parents will avoid tendency to blame each other for baby's problems.

169

Planning

Example: Vincent Aarusa is highly anxious about the surgery he is to have. He does not have a good understanding of the procedure, nor of its risks and benefits. Worse, his father died after having a similar surgery 20 years ago. His admitting nurse failed to perceive the severity of his anxiety and wrote a nursing diagnosis of "Knowledge Deficit (Surgical Procedure) r/t no prior experience or teaching." The goal for this problem was stated as follows: "Will describe surgical procedure in general terms, and discuss risks and benefits prior to surgery." When Mr. Aarusa was able to perform these behaviors, the nurse on the next shift discontinued the Knowledge Deficit problem, and no further discussion of his surgery was attempted by the nursing staff. Mr. Aarusa was sent to surgery with adequate information, but with no relief of his anxiety.

Relationship to Nursing Diagnosis Clauses

The first clause (problem) of a nursing diagnosis contains the unhealthy response. This tells you what should change. The *essential* patient goals are derived from the problem clause. The second clause sometimes suggests some goals as well.

Problem + Etiology
↓

Goals

> Every nursing diagnosis must have at least one goal that demonstrates resolution of the problem response.

Goals derived from the etiology are different from those derived from the problem. Their achievement may help to resolve the problem, but they might also be achieved *without* resolving the problem. In that case, the care plan might be terminated because the goals had been met, but the client would still have the problem.

Example:

	Nursing Diagnosis	*Goals/Predicted Outcomes*
Problem:	Altered Nutrition: ⟶	**1.** Will gain 5 lb by 12/14.
	Less Than Body Requirements for Calories	**2.** Will consume at least 2,000 calories per day.
	↓	
	r/t	
	↓	
Etiology:	Lack of appetite 2° depression →	**3.** Will state his appetite is better within 3 days.
		4. Will be hungry at mealtimes by 12/1.
		5. By 12/1, will be less depressed, as evidenced by
		a. no more than one crying spell per day.
		b. participation in unit activities.

Achieving goals No.1 and 2 would actually show problem resolution. If the client gains 5 lb and consumes 2,000 calories per day, then he cannot have "less than body requirements for calories." This is not true for goals No. 3, 4, and 5. The client's depression might lift, and he might regain his appetite but still continue to lose weight. If you discontinued the nutritional problem after measuring only objectives No. 3, 4, and 5, you would do the client a disservice. Therefore, for every nursing diagnosis you must write at least one goal that, when achieved, shows direct resolution of the problem.

Writing Client Goals

Components of a Goal Statement

Every specific, measurable goal statement should contain a subject, an action verb, performance criteria, and a target time. A component for special conditions may also be necessary. See Table 6–2 for examples of goal statement components.

Subject

The subject of the goal is a noun. It is the client, any part of the client, or a property or characteristic of the client.

> **Examples:** Client
> Ms. Atwell
> Lung sounds
> Mucous membranes
> Vaginal discharge

The subject is the client unless otherwise stated. Think, "Client will . . ." as you begin the goal statement, but do not write it.

> **Example:**
>
> *Incorrect:* *Client will* describe pain as < 3 on a scale of 1–10.
>
> *Correct:* *Will* describe pain as < 3 on a scale of 1–10.
> *Describes* pain as < 3 on a scale of 1–10.

Action Verb

The verb describes the desired client action (for example, what the client is to learn or do). Using actions that can be seen, heard, smelled, felt, or measured will help make your goals specific and observable. Action verbs create a picture of the desired client condition or performance. Each goal should describe only one desired client condition; therefore, each goal should contain only one action verb.

Examples of Action Verbs

Apply
Breathe
Choose
Communicate
Define
Demonstrate
Describe
Design
Drink
Explain
Express
Identify
Inject
List
Move
Prepare
Report
Share
Sit
Sleep
Talk
Transfer
Turn
Use
Verbalize
Walk

Table 6–2. Components of Goal Statements

Subject	Verb	Special Conditions	Performance Criteria	Target Time
Patient	will list	(after attending nutrition class)	two low-fat foods from each of the Four Basic Food Groups	before discharge.
Patient's lungs	will be	—	clear to auscultation	within 24 hours.
Client	will walk	(using walker)	to bathroom and back without shortness of breath	within 3 days.

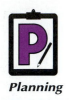

Planning

Example:

Correct: Will *describe* the Four Basic Food Groups . . .

Incorrect: Will *describe* the Four Basic Food Groups and *choose* a balanced diet . . .

Performance Criteria

Performance criteria are the standards used to evaluate the quality of the client's performance. They describe the *extent* to which the client is expected to perform the behavior. The performance criteria suggest nursing orders for meeting the goal and indicate what should be measured in evaluating goal achievement. Performance criteria may specify amount, quality, speed, distance, accuracy, and so forth—they tell *how, what, when, or where.*

Examples:

		What	**When**
Amount	Will lose	5 lb	during the first week.

		How	**What**
Accuracy	Will draw up	correct amount	of insulin.

		What	**How**
Quality	Will inject	insulin	using sterile technique.

		Where	**When**
Distance and Amount	Will walk	to the end of the hall	three times a day.

Target Time

Each goal should specify the time by which you realistically expect a change in patient response (e.g., by discharge, by April 2, prior to surgery, within 12 hours, at all times). The target time helps to pace the patient's care and motivates both the patient and the nurse by focusing on the future. It also provides a deadline for evaluating patient progress.

Example: Will name the Four Basic Food Groups *within 24 hours* after receiving pamphlet.

The target time is a type of performance criterion, since it specifies the speed with which a goal is to be accomplished. In the example above, the client's progress would not be satisfactory if he took longer than 24 hours to learn the basic food groups.

Nursing knowledge and experience are needed for setting realistic target times. You will need to know the usual rate of progress for clients with the identified medical and nursing diagnoses and consider the client's particular capabilities and resources.

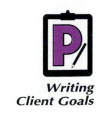

Example: Esther Brady has just had an abdominal hysterectomy. Review of usual progress after this surgery indicates that most patients require intravenous or intramuscular narcotic analgesics for 24–48 hours and are then able to obtain relief from milder, oral analgesics. However, Ms. Brady is very anxious and has a history of poor pain tolerance. It would not be realistic to set a target time of 48 hours for resolution of her Pain diagnosis. A more achievable goal might be "Will obtain adequate pain relief from p.o. analgesics within 72 hours post-op, as evidenced by patient's statement that pain is < 3 on a 1–10 scale."

Potential (High-Risk) Problems   Predicted outcomes for high-risk problems do not need target times. The broad goal is to prevent the problem from occurring, so in a sense the target time is *at all times*.

Example:

Nursing Diagnosis: High Risk for Impaired Skin Integrity r/t immobility . . .
Predicted Outcome: Skin will remain intact, with no redness over bony prominences.
(Target time: At all times)
(Evaluate plan: Daily)

In the example above, the target time is assumed, so you would not need to write it on the care plan. However, you may wish to schedule times for evaluating the predicted outcomes and the accompanying plan of care.

Special Conditions

If it is important to describe the conditions under which a client is to perform a behavior, you may need to add modifiers to the performance criteria. **Modifiers** describe the amount of assistance the client will need, available resources, environmental conditions, or experiences the client should have before being expected to perform the behavior. Like performance criteria, modifiers describe *how, when, where,* and *how much*.

Examples:

Type of assistance

How   Will walk to the end of the hall three times a day, using a walker, by April 8.

Prior experience

When   Will list foods high in cholesterol after consulting with dietitian.

Environmental conditions

Where   In one-to-one session, will express fear of abandonment by Friday.

Not all goals need special conditions; they are included only if they are important. If the performance criteria clearly specify the expected performance, special conditions are not necessary.

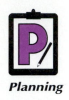

Planning

Short-Term and Long-Term Goals

Goals may be either short-term or long-term, depending on the length of time you think it will take for the client to achieve the specified behavior. Short-term and long-term goals are frequently combined, especially on teaching plans.

Short-term goals identify outcomes that can be achieved within a few days or a few hours. Goals dealing with survival needs may even be stated in terms of minutes. For this reason, short-term goals are useful in acute-care settings, such as hospitals, where nurses often focus on the client's more immediate needs. Also, the client may be discharged before the nurse can evaluate progress toward long-term goals. Some examples of short-term goals follow:

Examples:

Voids within 6 hours after delivery of infant.
States relief of pain within one hour after receiving p.o. oxycodone.
Walks to end of hall and back, unassisted, by day 3 post-op.

Short-term goals must usually be accomplished before the client can achieve long-term goals, and they are often used to measure the client's progress toward long-term goals. Achieving several short-term goals also provides frequent reinforcement for the client, encouraging him to keep working on the problem. The long-term goal for Constipation might be "Will have daily B.M. without use of laxatives within two months." The nurse would not want to wait for two months to determine whether the client's problem was improving, so a series of short-term goals should be used.

Example:

Long-Term Goal   Will have daily B.M. without use of laxatives *within two months.*

Short-Term Goals   After administration of enema will have bowel movement *within 4 hours.*
Will have next B.M. *within 36 hours* without aid of p.o. laxatives.
Will use chemical or mechanical stimulation for B.M. not more than two times *this week.*
Immediately, diet changes include prune juice and oatmeal (or other high-fiber cereal) for breakfast, and substituting whole grain for white bread.
Within one week reports he is eating at least one good source of fiber at every meal.

As a student, you will probably care for a patient for only a few hours at a time. You should write short-term goals to measure what you can realistically accomplish while you are with the client, so that you can evaluate the results of the care you have given. In a comprehensive care plan you should also include longer-range goals that other nurses can use to evaluate patient progress when you are not there.

Long-term goals describe changes in client outcomes over a longer period—usually a week or more. The ideal long-term goal aims at restoring normal functioning in the problem area. When normal functioning cannot be restored, the long-term goal describes the maximum level of functioning that can be achieved given the client's health status and resources. Long-term goals are especially useful for clients with chronic health problems and those in home health care, rehabilitation centers, and other extended-care facilities. Some examples of long-term goals follow:

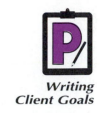

Writing
Client Goals

Examples:

> After attending six weekly childbirth-education classes, will correctly
>   demonstrate abdominal and shallow chest breathing.
> By 12 weeks post-op, will have full range of motion of right shoulder.
> Within 3 months (12/24), will feed self using fork or spoon.

Goals for Actual, High-Risk, and Possible Nursing Diagnoses

Goals may reflect promotion, maintenance, or restoration of health, depending on the type of nursing diagnosis (see table 6-3). For an *actual nursing diagnosis*, goals focus on restoring healthy responses and preventing further complications. They specify patient behaviors that demonstrate resolution or reduction of the problem and that patients should be able to achieve with the aid of independent nursing interventions.

Table 6-3. Goals for Different Problem Types		
Type of Problem	**Patient Response Demonstrates:**	**Nursing Focuses on:**
Actual nursing diagnosis	Resolution or reduction of problem	Resolution or reduction of problem
		Prevention of further complication
Potential nursing diagnosis	Problem has not developed	Prevention and detection of problem
Possible nursing diagnosis	No patient responses	Confirming or ruling out problem
Collaborative problem	Problem has not developed	Detection and prevention of problem
Wellness diagnoses		
Health maintenance	Continuation of healthy functioning	Health maintenance
Health promotion	Achievement of a higher level of wellness	Health promotion

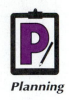

Planning

Examples:

Actual Nursing Diagnosis	*Goal Statement*
Calf Pain with Exercise r/t muscle ischemia 2° peripheral arterial disease	Reports pain is gone after 10 minutes of rest with legs dependent.
Impaired Skin Integrity: Dermal Ulcer over coccyx r/t inability to move self in bed	Ulcer will not extend to deeper tissues.
	Ulcer will not become infected, as evidenced by absence of purulent exudate.
	By 12/1 healing will be evidenced by decreased redness and appearance of granulation tissue in wound bed.

Goals for *high-risk nursing diagnoses* focus on preventing the problem; the client responses should demonstrate a problem-free level of functioning, or if that is not possible, maintenance of the present level of functioning. Achievement of these goals should mean that the problem is not occurring.

Examples:

High-Risk Nursing Diagnosis	*Goal Statements*
High Risk for Ineffective Breast-feeding r/t breast engorgement	Infant will be observed to "latch on," suck, and swallow at each feeding.
	Mother will state satisfaction with breastfeeding.
	Infant will regain birth weight within 14 days after birth.

Possible nursing diagnoses present an exception to the rule; they are *not* written in terms of desired patient response. A possible diagnosis is written when the nurse does not have enough data to know whether or not the patient has the problem. The goal for a possible nursing diagnosis is really a *nursing* goal: that the presence of the diagnosis will be confirmed or ruled out. It is not necessary to write goals for possible diagnoses. However, to help assure that follow-up assessments will be done, you may wish to set a target time for confirming or ruling out the problem. If so, you could write a nursing goal. Nursing goals should *not* be written on the care plan for actual or potential problems.

Example:

Possible Problem:	Possible Hopelessness r/t abandonment by significant other after onset of chronic illness
Nursing Goal:	Confirm or rule out Hopelessness by 6/12.

Goals for Collaborative Problems

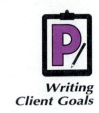

Writing Client Goals

Collaborative problems are a type of potential problem. Independent nursing care focuses on prevention and early detection of the complication. Predicted outcomes for *collaborative problems* should describe the patient responses that will be seen as long as the problem has not developed. The goals may describe normal functioning or problem symptoms that you do *not* want to occur.

Examples:

Collaborative Problem	Goal Statements
Potential Complication of Childbirth: Postpartum Hemorrhage	Postpartum hemorrhage will not occur, as evidenced by **1.** saturating less than 1 vag. pad per hour during first 24 hours. **2.** fundus firm and below umbilicus during first 24 hours. **3.** pulse and B/P in normal range for patient.
Potential Complication: Incision Infection	Incision will not become infected, as evidenced by **1.** no redness. **2.** no pus formation. **3.** edges approximated, sutures intact.

On working care plans for professional nurses, goal statements are not necessary for collaborative problems. It is understood that the broad goal is early detection of the problem, and nurses in practice usually do not need to have the problem symptoms listed. Student care plans, however, should include goals for collaborative problems, as in the examples above. This assures that the student knows precisely what symptoms to monitor for and can recognize whether or not the problem is developing.

Goals for Wellness Diagnoses

Recall that wellness diagnoses describe essentially healthy responses that the client wishes to maintain or improve. Goals for these diagnoses describe client responses that demonstrate health maintenance or achievement of a higher level of healthy functioning (health promotion). The following are examples of predicted outcomes for a wellness diagnosis described in Houldin et al. (1987, pp. 174–75).

Examples:

Wellness Nursing Diagnosis	Predicted Outcomes
Spiritual strength associated with an adaptable belief system as evidenced by: **1.** regular attendance at church services.	Over next 2 months, Ms. K will continue to receive spiritual support. Over next 2 months, Ms. K. will continue practicing religious activities.

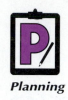

2. expressed satisfaction with religious affiliation.

Over next 2 months, Ms. K will continue to maintain her spiritual support.

Goals for Patient Teaching

Some patients may need a special teaching plan to address their learning needs (see Chapter 9). Teaching objectives describe in behavioral terms what the patient is to learn or how he will demonstrate learning. You should write objectives to reflect whether the learning is to take place in the cognitive, psychomotor, or affective domain. **Cognitive** learning involves perception, understanding, and the storing and recall of new information. **Psychomotor** learning involves physical skills. **Affective** learning involves changes in feelings, attitudes, and values.

Examples:

Cognitive domain	Learner will *explain* the effect of weight on B/P.
Psychomotor domain	Learner will *apply* B/P cuff correctly.
Affective domain	Learner will state that he *feels* confident with his ability to obtain correct B/P readings.

As with any objective, choose active verbs for learning objectives; they will help you to think of teaching strategies and make it easier to evaluate whether learning takes place. Table 6-4 provides a few suggestions for active verbs in each of the learning domains.

When writing objectives for the affective domain, keep in mind that you cannot directly observe a feeling or an attitude. Therefore, you could not write an objective such as "Learner will feel happier by May 2." You can, however, observe behaviors (cues) that *indicate* the client's feelings or moods. The following examples allow you to infer that the client is happy:

Examples: By May 2, will state that he feels happier than before.
By May 2, will be observed smiling at least twice a day.
By May 2, will resume past habit of singing in the shower.

Table 6–4. Active Verbs for Learning Objectives

Cognitive Domain	Psychomotor Domain	Affective Domain
Compare	Arrange	Choose
Define	Assemble	Defend
Describe	Construct	Discuss
Differentiate	Manipulate	Express
Explain	Organize	Help
Identify	Show	Justify
List	Start	Select
Name	Take	Share
State		

Guidelines for Writing Goal Statements

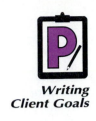

Writing Client Goals

The following guidelines may help you to improve the quality of your outcome statements. Ask the following questions about each of the goals you write. (Guidelines 1, 2, and 3 were discussed in detail earlier in the sections, "Goals for Actual, High-Risk, and Possible Nursing Diagnoses," and "Components of a Goal Statement."

1. For each actual nursing diagnosis, *does at least one goal clearly demonstrate resolution of the problem clause?* Goals *b* and *c* in Figure 6–2 demonstrate this guideline.

2. *Is the goal appropriate to the nursing diagnosis?* Achievement of the goal should clearly demonstrate that the problem is resolved (actual problems), that healthy responses have been supported (wellness diagnoses), or that potential problems are not occurring.

3. *Does each goal have all the necessary components*: subject, action verb, performance criteria, special conditions (when needed) and target time (usually)?

4. *Is each goal derived from only one nursing diagnosis?* A goal derived from more than one nursing diagnosis is likely to include more than one client behavior, making evaluation difficult. In Goal *a* in Figure 6–2, suppose the client had no urge incontinence but was still having pain when voiding. Would you say the goal was met or not met?

5. *Is the goal valued by the client and family?* The plan of care is more likely to be effective if it is designed to help the client achieve goals that he values. For example, knowing that obesity aggravates hypertension, your goal may be that the client lose 40 lb. However, if eating is the client's only pleasure, he

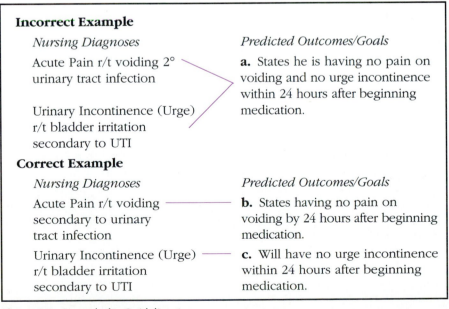

Figure 6-2. Example for Guideline 1

179

Planning

may not share your goal; he may prefer to accept the risks of hypertension rather than deprive himself of the pleasure of eating. If his goals do not include losing weight, then no matter how well you plan and carry out your nursing orders, the plan will probably fail.

When nurse and client goals conflict, it may help to explore the client's reasoning with him, provide a rationale for your goals, and look for alternative approaches. This has the advantage of involving the client in decisions about his care and keeping communication open.

Involve the client and family to the extent of their interest and abilities. Be sure they agree that the problem is one that requires change and that the goal is worth achieving. This will ensure that your time and energy are spent on plans that meet the unique needs of each client and are likely to succeed.

6. *Is the goal congruent with the total treatment plan?* The goal "Will demonstrate correct technique for bathing baby by postpartum day 2" would not be compatible with the medical treatment plan for a mother whose newborn is too ill to be bathed.

7. *Is the goal stated in terms of client responses, rather than nurse activities?* Thinking "Client will . . ." at the beginning of each goal may help you to focus on what the client will be able to do rather than on your own actions. However, do not actually write "Client will." Always assume that the goal refers to the client or some part of the client.

Example:

Nurse Activity (Incorrect)	Prevent infection of incision.
Client Response (Correct)	Incision will not become infected, as evidenced by
	1. absence of redness and drainage.
	2. edges approximated.

8. *Are the predicted outcomes phrased in positive terms*—that is, in terms of what you hope will occur rather than what you hope will not occur?

Example:

Negative Wording:	Skin will not become broken or ulcerated.
Positive Wording:	Skin will remain intact.

For potential problems, it may be difficult to think of positive terms to describe your predicted outcomes. It is easier to write "No redness" than to describe exactly the color of normal skin. You cannot say, "Skin color will be normal," because *normal* is too vague. In such instances, you may use negative terms. A measurable, negatively worded goal is actually a list of the signs and symptoms you are trying to prevent.

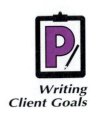

Example:

Problem	High Risk for Infection of Surgical Incision . . .
Predicted Outcomes	Incision will not become infected, as evidenced by

    1. No redness (negative wording).
    2. No purulent drainage (negative wording).
    3. Edges approximated (positive wording).

9. *Is the outcome directly observable or measurable?* Observable, measurable outcomes use action verbs to describe what the client will be able to do and *to what extent.* This assures that other nurses can make observations to determine whether the goal has been met and the problem resolved. In the following example, you cannot observe what Ms. Fretsch *knows.* However, you could observe whether Ms. Fretsch can *name* the high-sodium foods.

Example:

   Incorrect   By 11/30 (Ms. Fretsch) will *know* which foods to avoid.

     Correct   By 11/30 (Ms. Fretsch) will *name* the high-sodium foods to avoid in each food group.

    You cannot directly observe such actions as *understands, knows, feels,* or *appreciates.* If you cannot avoid using such verbs, make them measurable by adding the phrase *as evidenced by* followed by the signs and symptoms you wish to reduce or the positive responses you wish to achieve (e.g., Will *experience* relief of pain *as evidenced by* rating of < 2 on a 10-point scale, absence of facial grimace, and walking erect).

10. *Is the outcome specific and concrete?* Other nurses reading the goal should have no doubt about the focus for nursing care. Vague, general words that can be interpreted in several ways can lead to disagreement about whether the goal has been met. Avoid performance criteria such as *normal, adequate, sufficient, more, less,* and *increased.* Does a goal of "Increased activity tolerance" mean that the client can run a mile in four minutes or does it mean that he can ambulate from the chair to the bed with no shortness of breath? Action verbs, performance criteria, special conditions, and target times increase goal specificity.

    When possible, make goals more specific by individualizing them to describe the client's normal baseline measurements. The upper limit of normal blood pressure for most people is 140/90, and a goal of "B/P within normal limits" would imply this number. However, for a client who usually has a blood pressure of 90/50, the normal limit is probably too high.

Planning

Example:

   Incorrect: Blood pressure will be *within normal limits.*

More specific: Blood pressure will be *less than 130/80.*

    It may not be possible to write specific goals for an initial care plan, but as you continue to work with the patient you will gain a clearer idea of his health status and abilities. You will then be able to write more specific, individualized goals. Of course, you will continue to revise the goals as the patient's status changes. The following example shows how goals may be individualized and revised for a patient with a nursing diagnosis of Activity Intolerance r/t prolonged immobility.

Example:

Initial Goal: (General)	Ability to tolerate activity will improve, as evidenced by **1.** walking progressively farther each day. **2.** increased ability to perform self-care (hygiene, feeding, etc.).
Revised Goal: (More specific)	Ability to tolerate activity will improve, as evidenced by the following: **1.** by 5/12, walks to chair (8 ft.) without shortness of breath. **2.** by 5/12, assists with bath by washing own hands and face.
Revised Goal: (After condition change)	Ability to tolerate activity will improve, as evidenced by the following: **1.** by 5/18, walks to bathroom (20 ft.) without shortness of breath. **2.** by 5/18, washes hands, face, and upper torso.

11. *Are the predicted outcomes realistic and achievable* in terms of the client's internal and external resources? The client's physical and mental status, coping mechanisms, support system, finances, and available community services should be considered. The goal "Will demonstrate desire to comply with treatment by keeping all clinic appointments," may not be realistic for a client with no car and no money for cab fare. Clients are not motivated to achieve goals they perceive to be impossible.

    Consider also whether the capabilities of the nursing staff and the resources of the agency are adequate to achieve the goals. "Uses individualized relaxation techniques to achieve pain relief" is not achievable unless staffing is adequate to allow time for teaching and supervised practice.

12. *Is there an adequate number of goals to address each nursing diagnosis?* Ask yourself, "If these predicted outcomes are achieved, will the problem be resolved?" If they are written in very specific terms, several outcomes may be needed for each diagnosis in order to determine that the problem has been resolved or prevented. For the diagnostic label of Anxiety, none of the following outcomes by itself would show that the anxiety was sufficiently relieved:

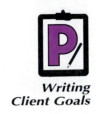

Writing Client Goals

Example:

Nursing Diagnosis	Severe Anxiety r/t unresolved role conflicts (mother-wife-attorney)
Predicted Outcomes	After one-on-one interaction, will be less anxious, as evidenced by

    1. statements that she feels better.
    2. fewer than two episodes of tearfulness in the next 24 hours.
    3. smoking no more than one cigarette per hour.

13. *Is the goal concise?* Predicted outcomes should be stated in as few words as possible without sacrificing clarity.

Example:

Wordy	By April 15, the client will demonstrate adequate knowledge of an appropriate low-calorie diet by listing foods to avoid and foods allowed in each of the Four Basic Food Groups.
More Concise	By 4/15, lists for each food group foods to avoid and foods allowed on low-calorie diet.

Occasionally the goal will refer to behaviors of someone other than the client, for instance, a parent or spouse. Specify who is to perform the behavior only when it is *not* the client. You might write, for example, "By dismissal, *Ms. Rauh* will demonstrate ability to change Mr. Rauh's dressing according to the printed guidelines given to her."

14. Remember that *goals can be written for an individual, family,* or *community.* For example, the U.S. Public Health Service (1990) has published the following overarching goals for the health of the nation:

    Increase the span of healthy life for Americans.
    Reduce health disparities among Americans.
    Achieve access to preventive services for all Americans. (p. 43)

Following are examples of some more specific and measurable objectives that contribute to those broad, general goals:

    To eliminate elevated blood lead levels in children under age 5 by the year 2000
    To reduce epidemic-related pneumonia and influenza deaths in people aged 65 and older by the year 2000

The preceding guidelines are listed for convenient reference in Box 6–2.

Planning

On the Care Plan

Nursing:
  order
  action
  intervention
  measure
  strategy

As an Activity

Nursing:
  action
  intervention

Box 6–2. Guidelines for Writing Goal Statements

1. Is each goal derived from only one nursing diagnosis?
2. For each actual nursing diagnosis, does at least one goal clearly demonstrate resolution of the problem clause?
3. Is the goal appropriate to the nursing diagnosis?
4. Does each goal have all the necessary components: subject, action verb, performance criteria, special conditions, target time?
5. Is the goal valued by the client and family?
6. Is the goal congruent with the total treatment plan?
7. Is the goal stated in terms of client responses rather than nurse activities?
8. When possible, are the predicted outcomes stated in positive terms?
9. Can the outcome be directly measured or observed?
10. Is the predicted outcome specific and concrete?
11. Is the predicted outcome realistic and achievable?
12. Is there an adequate number of goals to address each nursing diagnosis?
13. Is the goal concise?
14. Does the goal describe responses of an individual, family, or community as appropriate?

WRITING NURSING ORDERS

After writing the goals, the next step is to select and write nursing orders to help achieve those goals. **Nursing orders** (also called nursing *actions, interventions, measures,* or *strategies*) are the written, detailed instructions for performing nursing interventions. Nursing interventions or nursing actions are the activities and behaviors performed to change present client responses to the desired responses described in the goals. Nursing actions may be something you do for the client or something you help her to do for herself.

Nursing orders contain more specific, detailed instruction than physician's orders. A physician's order regarding a client's nutritional status might read "Diet as tolerated." Related nursing orders would specify how the diet is to progress, as well as assessments that need to be made. For example:

1. Auscultate bowel sounds q4h.
2. Observe for abdominal distention, nausea, or vomiting.
3. Limit ice chips to 1 cup per hour until bowel sounds are auscultated; then give clear liquids × 8 hours.
4. If no nausea or vomiting, progress to full liquids . . .

Purpose

Nursing orders provide specific direction and a consistent, individualized approach to the patient's care. They are written as instructions for others to follow, and other nurses are held responsible and accountable for their implementation. Since many different nurses are involved in caring for the patient, nursing orders must be detailed enough to be interpreted correctly by all caregivers. An order to "force fluids" could be interpreted in many ways. A nurse accustomed to working with young adults might expect this to mean 200 cc per hour; a gerontology nurse might think it means 50 cc per hour; another nurse might focus on total volume rather than a consistent hourly intake. A better nursing order would be "Give fluids hourly: Day shift = 1,000 cc; Evening shift = 1,000 cc; Night shift = 400 cc."

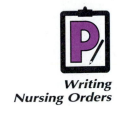

Nursing orders guide documentation as well as implementation of care. Using the preceding nutrition example, the nurse would know to chart the client's abdominal assessment as well as his tolerance of the fluids. For example:

> "0800—Abd. soft, not distended. Faint bowel sounds auscultated in all 4 quadrants.
>   Taking 50 cc ice chips/hour with no nausea since 0600.
> 0830— 50 cc carbonated beverage p.o.
> 0930— Complained of nausea at 0900. 30 cc clear emesis."

When nurses use the nursing orders as a guide for documentation, the nursing process is automatically reflected in the patient's chart. This is important in meeting standards set by agencies that accredit health-care institutions (e.g., Joint Commission on Accreditation of Health Care Organizations).

Types of Nursing Orders

Interventions are identified and ordered during the planning step; however, they are actually performed during the implementation step. Nursing interventions may be dependent, interdependent, or independent.

Independent interventions are those that the nurse prescribes and performs or delegates; they include physical care, emotional support and comfort, teaching, counseling, environmental management, and making referrals to other health-care professionals. Recall that nursing diagnoses are treated primarily by independent nursing interventions.

Dependent interventions are prescribed by the physician and carried out by the nurse. Medical orders commonly include orders for medications, intravenous therapy, diagnostic tests, treatments, diet, and activity. The nurse is responsible for explaining, assessing the need for, and administering the medical orders. Nursing orders may be written to individualize the medical order, based on the patient's status.

Example:

Medical Order	Progressive ambulation, as tolerated
Nursing Orders	**1.** Dangle for 5 min, 12 hr post-op.
	2. Stand at bedside 24 hr post-op; observe for pallor, dizziness, and weakness.
	3. Check pulse before and after amb. Do not progress if P >110.

Medical orders are usually transcribed to special sections of the care plan; however, you may sometimes wish to record a medical order in your individualized plan for a nursing diagnosis (see number 3 below).

Planning

Example:

> A nursing diagnosis of Pain includes interventions for helping the client to take less medication. The nursing orders follow:
> **1.** Coach client in using guided imagery. If ineffective,
> **2.** Try cutaneous stimulation.
> **3.** If pain is > 4 (on a 1–10 scale), *give Tylenol No. 3* (see Medication Record).

Interdependent interventions are the actions the nurse carries out in collaboration with other health team members, such as physical therapists, social workers, dietitians and physicians. For example, the physician might order physical therapy to teach the patient crutch-walking. As the nurse, you would be responsible for informing the physical therapy department and for coordinating the patient's care to include the P.T. sessions. You would be responsible for assisting the client to walk with his crutches when he is back on your unit, and you would also collaborate with the physical therapist to evaluate the client's progress.

Nursing Orders and Problem Status

Depending upon the type of patient problem, you will write nursing orders for observation, prevention, treatment, and health promotion.

1. *Observation.* This includes observations to determine whether a complication is developing, as well as observations of the client's responses to nursing, medical, and other therapies. Observation orders should be written for every problem: actual, high-risk, and possible nursing diagnoses and collaborative problems.

> *Examples*: Auscultate lungs q8h.
> Observe for redness over sacrum q2h.
> Assess for urinary frequency.
> Intake and output, hourly.

2. *Prevention.* Prevention orders prescribe the care needed to prevent complications or reduce risk factors. They are used mainly for high-risk nursing diagnoses and collaborative problems, but they can also be appropriate for actual nursing diagnoses.

> For example, if a client has Actual Impaired Skin Integrity: Pressure Ulcer, an order to turn the client and keep pressure off the affected area might prevent the ulcer from extending, even if it did not improve the condition. For well clients, disease-prevention orders aim at helping the client to *avoid* specific health problems.

> *Examples:*

Turn, cough, and deep breathe q2h.   (Prevents respiratory complication)
If fundus is boggy, massage until firm.   (Prevents postpartum hemorrhage)
Refer to county health department for   (Prevents specific disease
    measles immunizations.   (measles))

3. *Treatment.* This includes teaching, referrals, physical, and other care needed to treat an existing problem. Treatment measures are appropriate for actual nursing diagnoses. Notice that the same order may accomplish either prevention or treatment of a problem (compare examples below to preceding examples).

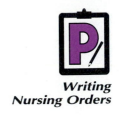

   Examples:

   Turn, cough, deep breathe q2h.   (Treat respiratory problem)
   If fundus is boggy, massage until firm. (Treat actual postpartum hemorrhage)
   Help client plan exercise regimen.   (Treat actual activity intolerance)

4. *Health Promotion.* When there are no health problems, the nurse helps the client to identify areas for improvement that will lead to a higher level of wellness. Health-promotion strategies encourage approach behaviors; that is, they help the client promote positive outcomes rather than avoid negative outcomes. Health promotion is not specific to any disease or problem, but aims to encourage activities that will actualize the client's general health potential.

   Examples:

   Discuss the importance of daily exercise.
   Teach components of a healthy diet.
   Explore infant-stimulation techniques.

   Table 6–5 shows how orders for observation, prevention, and treatment are related to the status of the patient's problems.

Table 6–5. Types of Nursing Orders in Relation to Diagnoses

Actual Nursing Diagnoses	High-Risk Nursing Diagnosis	Possible Nursing Diagnosis	Collaborative Problems
Observation for improvement or complications	**Observation** for onset of problem	**Observation** to confirm or rule out diagnosis	**Observation** for onset of complication
			Physician Notification of problem onset
Prevention of further complications	**Prevention** Reduce risk factors		**Prevention** Includes physician orders, nursing policies & procedures
			Collaborative treatments
Treatment Remove causal & contributing factors Relieve symptoms			

Planning

Generating and Selecting Nursing Orders

For any given problem, several nursing interventions might be effective. You will select the ones that are most likely to achieve the desired goal, taking into consideration the patient's abilities and preferences, the capabilities of the nursing staff, the available resources, and the policies and procedures of the institution. Creativity is needed for generating new and effective interventions. One of the dangers in using preplanned (standardized) care plans is the temptation to plug in ready-made solutions rather than look for different, more effective approaches for a particular patient. Even if an intervention has been useful in the past, always rethink it to be sure it is the best way for the patient with whom you are working.

The following decision-making process will guide you in reviewing the nursing diagnosis and goals, identifying all the possible interventions, and selecting the best options from among the alternatives.

Review the Nursing Diagnosis

You should first review the nursing diagnosis to be sure you understand the problem and etiology. Be sure you are familiar with the factors causing or contributing to actual problems, and the risk factors that predispose the client to high-risk problems. You should also know the signs and symptoms associated with any high-risk diagnoses or collaborative problems. Try to think of interventions to reduce or eliminate causal, contributing, and risk factors, or to relieve problem symptoms. In the following example, the nursing orders should reduce the contributing factor, breast engorgement.

Example:	*Nursing Diagnosis:*	Ineffective Breastfeeding r/t breast engorgement
	Nursing Orders:	**1.** Teach to massage breasts before feeding.
		2. Use hot packs or hot shower before nursing infant.

Nursing orders are individualized primarily from the second clause (etiology) of a nursing diagnosis. The etiology describes the factors that cause or contribute to the unhealthy response, and the nursing orders would specifically target these causal and contributing factors.

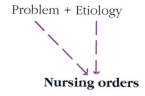

Problem + Etiology

Nursing orders

Any number of factors might contribute to a problem, but it would be inefficient and probably ineffective to address them all; individualized nursing orders address the etiological factors specific for a given client. For example, many factors could contribute to Chronic Constipation: lack of knowledge, lack of exercise, eating habits, long-term laxative use, or a schedule that causes the client to ignore the urge to defecate. A well-written nursing diagnosis states which factors are causing the client's problem, and suggests nursing interventions that deal directly with those factors. The following example illustrates how different etiologies suggest different nursing orders. Notice that in both cases, the *problem* is the same.

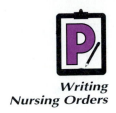
Example:

1. *Nursing Diagnosis:*   Chronic Constipation r/t *long-term laxative use*

   Nursing Orders: **1.** Working with the client to develop a plan for gradual withdrawal of the laxatives.

2. *Nursing Diagnosis:*   Chronic Constipation r/t *inactivity and insufficient fluid intake*

   Nursing Orders: **1.** Help client to develop an exercise regimen that he can follow at home.

   2. Help client plan for including sufficient amounts of fluids in his diet.

You may also need to write nursing orders (especially observation orders) for the problem clause of the nursing diagnosis. For a diagnosis of "Chronic Pain related to joint inflammation," nursing orders might include some pain-relief interventions that have nothing to do with relieving joint inflammation:

Observe level of pain before and after activity.
Give back rub (to promote general relaxation of tension).
Instruct client to take analgesic before pain becomes too severe.
Teach slow, rhythmic breathing as a pain control method.

Review the Goal

You should also review the goals to recall the patient outcomes you wish to produce. The goals will help you to develop nursing orders that are specific to the individual patient.

Example: *Nursing Diagnosis:* High Risk for Ineffective Breastfeeding r/t breast engorgement

Goals:

1. Infant will be observed to "latch on," suck, and swallow.

2. Infant will regain birth weight of 8 lb. 6 oz within 14 days after birth.

Nursing orders suggested by goals:

1. Observe infant at breast for effective latching on, sucking, and swallowing.

2. Teach mother to make these observations.

3. When sucking not long and rhythmic, institute massage of alternate areas of breast without removing infant from breast.

4. Weigh infant daily at 0600.

Identify Alternative Actions

Keeping goals and etiology in mind, think of all the nursing activities that might bring about the desired responses. Include unusual or original ideas. Don't try to predict at this point which ones would be best.

Planning

Perhaps you are wondering, "How will I be able to think of interventions to address the etiology? How will I know which actions will achieve the goals?" Principles and theories from nursing and related courses (e.g., anatomy, physiology, psychology) are good sources of ideas for nursing actions. You may also wish to consult resources such as model care plans, agency procedure manuals, nursing texts, journal articles, instructors, and practicing nurses. Remember to consult the patient and his family about the care they find to be most helpful.

To begin thinking of interventions, ask yourself two broad questions: (1) What should I watch for? and (2) What should I do? Branch out to consider all the possible activities that might address the etiology or achieve the goals. Depending upon the type of problem, include both independent and collaborative activities from the following categories, discussed previously in "Types of Nursing Orders."

Observation of patient status	Treatments
Preventive measures	Health-promotion measures

Specific nursing activities in each of those categories might include the following:

Physical care	Emotional support
Teaching	Making referrals
Counseling	Managing the environment

Teaching Orders   Not all teaching requires a separate, formal teaching plan. Informal teaching is an intervention for many, if not most, nursing diagnoses. You may do specific teaching to enable the patient to do some of his own care (e.g., how to take his own pulse and blood pressure), and you will find that you are teaching almost constantly as you explain to clients what you are doing for them and why. Informal teaching may include such activities as explaining the expected effects and side-effects of a medication you are giving, explaining why the client should not ambulate without help, or clarifying the need to remain NPO.

Teaching orders should include the teaching strategies to use in presenting the new information or skill. The appropriate strategy depends on the client's needs and the learning outcome you are working toward. Cognitive content is usually taught through discussion, lecture, printed materials, and audiovisuals. Psychomotor skills need to be demonstrated and discussed, and then reinforced with practice. Affective goals generally require role-modeling, discussion, and counseling to help the client gain insight. An example of a teaching order would be "Demonstrate technique for drawing up insulin."

Counseling and Emotional Support Orders   Counseling includes the use of therapeutic communication techniques to help clients make decisions about their health care and perhaps make life-style changes. It also involves techniques for helping clients recognize, express, and cope with feelings such as anxiety, anger, and fear. Counseling includes emotional support—but emotional support may occur on a less complex level: it may be given simply by the nurse's touch, presence, or apparent understanding of the patient's situation. An example of a counseling order would be "Help client to recognize when she is anxious by pointing out symptoms as you observe them."

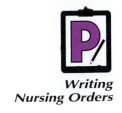

Referral Orders You should make referrals when the client needs in-depth interventions for which other professionals are specifically prepared. For instance, while the nurse may counsel an anxious patient, long-term treatment of severe anxiety would be referred to a psychotherapist or counselor. Nurses often make referrals for follow-up care after dismissal. An example of a referral order is "Refer to Social Service Department for transportation to clinic."

Environmental Management Orders Nursing orders are often created to provide for a safe, clean, therapeutic environment. Environmental management includes removing hazards for clients who are particularly at risk for injury—for instance, children, the elderly, and those with a decreased level of consciousness.

Examples: Teach mother to check temperature of formula with back of hand.

Remain at bedside while client is smoking.

Keep crib rails up at all times.

Selection Grid Figure 6–3 is a grid you might use to be sure you have considered all the various types of nursing orders for a patient. First think of the observation orders that apply to the problem. If one of the orders is to auscultate the patient's lungs, you would place an *X* in the box under "Observation" and beside "Physical Care." You might wish to teach a client to assess her own blood glucose level; if so, place an *X* in the box under "Observation" and beside "Teaching." Probably none of the other actions in the vertical column would fit under "Observation." Next consider what kind of physical care, teaching, and so on would be involved in preventive nursing orders. Continue to move across the top of the grid in this manner.

	Observation	*Prevention*	*Treatment*	*Health Promotion*
Physical Care	×			
Teaching	×			
Counseling				
Emotional Support				
Activities of Daily Living				
Environmental Management				
Referrals				

Figure 6–3. Grid for Identifying Alternative Nursing Orders

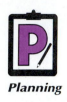

Planning

Select the Best Options

Selecting the best interventions is a matter of hypothesizing that certain actions will bring about the desired outcome. The best options are those you expect to be most effective in helping the client to achieve the goals. To determine this, ask yourself the following questions:

1. What nursing orders have been successful in solving this problem in the past?
2. Which nursing orders are especially appropriate for the client's knowledge, abilities, and resources?
3. Which actions directly address the cause of the client's problem?

Your knowledge, experience and intuition will help you make these judgments, as will the "Guidelines for Writing Nursing Orders" that conclude this section.

Even carefully selected nursing orders do not guarantee success in meeting client goals. A successful intervention for one client may not work at all for another. In fact, for the same client, an intervention may be effective at one time and not at another. Nursing research has established the probability of success for some interventions. Use nursing orders based on scientific principles and sound research, when possible, to improve the likelihood of success.

Components of a Nursing Order

After selecting the appropriate nursing interventions, write them on the nursing care plan in the form of nursing orders (see Table 6–6). A well-written nursing order contains the following components:

1. *Date the order was written.* The date will be changed to reflect review or revisions.
2. *Subject.* The subject is implied, not written. Nursing orders are written in terms of *nurse* behaviors; so the subject of the order is *the nurse.* As you learn to write nursing orders, think "The nurse will . . ." or "The nurse should . . ." at the beginning of the statement, but do not write it.

Table 6–6. Examples of Nursing Orders

Subject	Action Verb	Descriptive Phrase	Time Frame	Date and Signature
(Nurse)	(will) Monitor	for verbalization of interest in group activities	With each patient contact	4-14-92 J. Jonas, RN
(Nurse)	(will) Instruct	to avoid drinking liquids with meals if nausea occurs	Evening shift 4/14	4-14-92 J. Jonas, RN
(Nurse)	(will) Pad	side rails	During periods of restlessness and confusion	4-14-92 J. Jonas, RN
(Nurse)	(will) Discuss	with family their need for assistance with client's care at home	on Friday	4-14-92 C. Van, RN
(Nurse)	(will) Palpate	uterine fundus for firmness	hourly x 2, then q4h	3-8-92 L. Taylor, RN

192

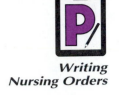

Example:

Goals	*Nursing Orders*
Patient behaviors	**Nurse behaviors**
↓	↓
(Pt. will) Walk to the door with help beginning on 2/12.	*(Nurse will)* Assist pt. to ambulate to the door t.i.d.

3. *Action verb that directs what the nurse is to do.* Examples of action verbs are *offer*, *assist*, *instruct*, *refer*, *assess*, *auscultate*, *change*, *give*, *listen*, *demonstrate*, and *turn*.

Examples: *Auscultate* lungs at 0800 and 1600 daily.
Assist to chair for 30 min. t.i.d.

4. *Descriptive qualifiers.* This is the phrase that tells the nurse how, when, and where to perform the action. It may also describe the action in more detail (*what*). When one activity depends on another, the descriptive qualifier also includes the sequence in which actions are to be done.

Examples:

	What	**When**
Give	written instructions for incision care	before dismissal.

	What	**Sequence/When**
Take	B/P	before and after ambulating.

5. *Specific times.* State when, how often, and how long the activity is to be done.

Example: Assist to chair *for 30 minutes b.i.d.*
Change dressing at *0800 and 1400 daily.*

When scheduling times for the nursing actions, be sure to consider the patient's usual rest, visiting hours, mealtimes, and other activities of daily living. Also coordinate the times with collaborative tests and treatments (e.g., physical therapy).

Because you must document nursing interventions, the times and frequencies written in the nursing orders actually specify when and how often you will chart information about each problem. If the documentation interval is *not* the same as the frequency of the nursing care, you should indicate both on the care plan. Some forms have a separate column in which to write the documentation interval.

6. *Signature.* The nurse who writes the order should sign it, indicating acceptance of legal and ethical accountability. A signature also allows other nurses to contact the writer for questions or feedback about the order. Nursing orders should be followed only if all components are present. You would not follow an unsigned physician's order; the same should be true of a nursing order. You would not follow an imprecise medical order such as, "Give an analgesic occasionally"; nor should you implement an imprecise nursing order such as, "Give emotional support."

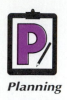

Planning

Formal Teaching Plans

Nursing orders for formal teaching plans are written in the same format as other nursing orders. They contain the content to be covered by the nurse, the teaching strategy to be used, and the learner activities assigned or used in the session.

Teaching orders and strategies should be based on principles of teaching and learning. You may wish to refer to a basic nursing text for more information about various teaching strategies, such as role modeling, discussion, demonstration, and use of audiovisual materials. Teaching is likely to be more effective under the following conditions.

1. *The learner's knowledge and abilities are assessed first.* Many factors affect a client's ability to learn, including existing knowledge, previous experience, education, age, and state of health. Misconceptions and misinformation may interfere with learning new facts. Illness or sensory-perceptual deficits may make it difficult for the client to process or remember information.

2. *The learner has no unmet physical or emotional needs* that interfere with learning (e.g., pain, fatigue, hunger).

3. *Teaching proceeds from simple to complex.* This makes the content easier to understand. Learning is a sequential process, in which new information builds on previous knowledge and experience.

4. *The learner is ready and motivated to learn.* People learn best when they can see a need to learn. A client with hypertension may not be ready to learn about a low-calorie diet until he begins having symptoms of the disease. Denial is a common psychological defense mechanism for persons who develop serious illness. Clients who have not yet worked through their denial do not learn well because they cannot see the need to learn about a problem they do not yet acknowledge having. If the client is not ready, the nurse may need to direct the teaching to significant others.

5. *The learner is actively involved.* A learner who is involved in an activity learns and retains more than one who is listening passively. Encourage the client to ask questions, and periodically ask him to summarize his understanding of what you have said. Supervised practice, feedback, and positive reinforcement are other forms of active involvement that promote learning.

6. *The environment is conducive to learning.* It should be quiet, at a comfortable temperature, appropriately lighted, and free from distractions.

7. *The emotional climate is favorable.* Very little learning occurs in the presence of intense emotions such as anger, anxiety, and fear. When such emotions are present, the nurse should use therapeutic communication to help the client deal with these emotions before attempting to teach.

8. *Rapport exists between patient and nurse.* A positive relationship, in which the client trusts and perceives the nurse as caring, promotes client cooperation and learning.

9. *Repetition and reinforcement are used.* Continued practice helps the client to retain new information. Rewards may be internal (personal) or external (praise). Pride in accomplishment can be a good learning incentive.

Guidelines for Writing Nursing Orders

After choosing the nursing orders, evaluate them by applying the following criteria. Each nursing order should meet most, if not all, of these criteria.

The nursing orders should	Example or Comments
1. be written in terms of nurse behaviors.	*Incorrect*: Needs to be suctioned. *Correct*: (Nurse will) Suction oropharynx prn.
2. be individualized for the client's specific needs.	*Incorrect*: Encourage fluids *Correct*: Offer fluids qhr. Ct. likes orange juice.
3. be specific and detailed enough to be interpreted the same by everyone.	*Incorrect*: Encourage fluids. *Correct*: Give 2400 cc/24 hr 7–3, 1000 cc 3–11, 800 cc 11–7, 600 cc
4. be concise.	*Incorrect*: Complex, routine procedures written on care plan. *Correct*: See Unit 6 Procedure Manual for tracheal suctioning procedure. (*Note*: If modifications need to be made to adapt the procedure to the client, these changes *should* be noted in the nursing orders; e.g., "Use alcohol; client allergic to Betadine.")
5. be consistent with standards of care.	ANA, JCAHO, the health-care agency.
6. be realistic in terms of client abilities and resources.	It would be unrealistic to order "Refer to home health agency for aide," if the client had no money to pay for this service.
7. be realistic in terms of nursing and institution resources and abilities.	"Turn hourly" may not be a realistic order on a unit that is short-staffed.
8. be congruent with the client's values, beliefs, and psychosocial background.	Even if a client were protein-deficient, you would not write an order to add meat to the diet if she were a strict vegetarian.
9. be safe.	A nursing order for range-of-motion exercises that specifies "Do not force beyond the point of resistance."

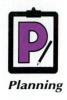

Planning

10. be compatible with medical and other therapies.	*Incorrect*: A nursing order to assist the patient with ambulation to prevent constipation, when there is a medical order for bed rest.
11. be complete. (All components present: date, signature, action verb, descriptive qualifiers, specific times.)	Who, what, where, when, how, how often, how much.
12. be moral (ethical).	A nursing order to withhold information in order to prevent emotional upset may be morally questionable because it does not respect the patient's autonomy.
13. be based on scientific rationale or research.	Research shows that axillary temperatures for newborns are accurate and safer than rectal temps.
14. address all aspects of the etiology.	Remove or decrease causal, contributing, or risk factors.
15. include independent and collaborative actions as appropriate.	
16. address observation, prevention, treatment and health promotion as appropriate.	(See grid, Figure 6–3)
17. include a variety of approaches.	For example, teaching, counseling, referring (see grid, Figure 6–3).

NURSING INTERVENTIONS FOR WELL CLIENTS

Nursing interventions for well clients stress self-responsibility and active client involvement. The nurse may suggest health-promotion strategies, considering the client's age, sex, life-style, education, sociocultural background, and other variables. However, the client is the primary decision maker; the nurse functions mainly as teacher and health counselor. Activities needed for goal achievement may be written in terms of what the nurse is to do or what the client is to do.

Nursing orders on wellness care plans may take the form of specific behavioral changes the client wishes to make (e.g., "I would like to stop smoking") and strategies for reinforcing the new behaviors. The most effective rewards are self-rewards rather than reinforcement from the nurse.

Example: A moderately overweight client wishes to lose weight.

Specific Behavioral Changes	*Rewards*
I will walk for 45 minutes every day for the next two weeks	I will buy myself a new jogging suit.
I will not eat between meals for one week.	I will treat myself to dinner out at my favorite seafood restaurant.

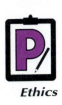

Ethics

Most disease-prevention/health-promotion strategies involve life-style changes such as diet changes, regular exercise, stress reduction, or cessation of smoking. Motivation for change is sometimes difficult when no actual problem exists. A number of behavior-change strategies are available for helping clients to modify health behaviors, for example, self-confrontation, cognitive restructuring, modeling, and operant conditioning. Pender (1987, Chapters 9 and 10) may be useful if you wish to develop detailed nursing interventions to promote high-level wellness.

ETHICS

Ethical issues in the planning step involve decisions about the extent to which a client should be involved in planning her own care and about whether or not she is truly able to make free and informed decisions about her care. Goals are not value-neutral—not even the goals that nurses and clients set together. Merely by stating a goal in the direction of health, the nurse and client declare that health is something they value. Most people probably do value health, but the situation is not so clear with all goals.

Obligation to Inform

The first tenet of the American Nurses Association *Code for Nurses* (1985) states that "The nurse provides services with respect for human dignity and the uniqueness of the client . . ." Respect for human dignity derives from the moral principle of autonomy. An autonomous person is one who is both free and able to choose. This suggests that nurses should provide clients with information so that they can make informed choices about their care, that is, about the goals for improving their health and the means for achieving those goals (nursing interventions and treatments). Clients may not be aware of what goals are possible for them to achieve, nor of what is required in order to achieve them.

Obligation to Respect Choices

From a practical standpoint, involving clients in goal setting increases their motivation to achieve healthy outcomes. Client involvement is also a moral obligation. Mutual goal setting and care planning demonstrate respect for clients' values and for their dignity and worth as persons. Clients in the health-care system are in a vulnerable and dependent state. They often feel that caregivers are more capable than they are to make decisions about their care, and their decision-making abilities may actually be diminished by their illness. When clients are experiencing conflict about choices, or when they are too ill to choose, it is appropriate to propose alternatives. In your eagerness to help, however, you can, without even realizing it, impose your own values on the client. Unless you are very sensitive, clients may defer to what they believe you want them to do, without making their true preferences known. Nurses must be aware of their power to influence patient decisions and make sure the choices are truly the client's.

Planning

Summary

Planning
✓ begins when the client is admitted to the institution and continues until dismissal.

✓ may include special teaching or discharge planning.

✓ insures the efficacy and moral aspects of nursing care.

✓ provides a written framework necessary for individualized care and third-party reimbursement.

Goals
✓ are guides to planning and evaluation that motivate client and nurse by providing a sense of achievement.

✓ are stated in terms of observable, achievable client behaviors.

✓ are comprised of subject, action verb, performance criteria, target time, and special conditions.

✓ may be short-term or long-term.

Nursing orders
✓ provide specific direction and a consistent, individualized approach to patient care.

✓ should address observation, prevention, treatment, and health promotion.

✓ are composed of date, subject, action verb, descriptive qualifiers, specific times, and signature.

✓ may address dependent or independent nursing interventions (i.e., teaching or environmental manipulation).

Ethical issues
✓ in planning center around the principle of autonomy, implying a moral obligation to inform and involve clients in planning their own care.

Skill-Building Activities

In everyday life you often analyze complex situations. You might watch a football game and try to understand the plays. Analyzing football plays is easy for some people because they have learned to see the relevant information. They know, for instance,

Practice in Critical Thinking: Recognizing Relevant Information

that watching the quarterback just after the play starts can help them understand whether the play is a run or a pass. If you want to learn to analyze football plays you must learn how to find the relevant information.

Learning the Skill

Example A. Recognizing football plays is a two-step process.

Step 1. Learn the names used to identify the various plays. The meanings of these names help you to remember what the plays are. For instance, there are *running* plays; during a running play, what is the player doing?

Step 2. Learn to focus your attention on the relevant aspects of the play—the people involved and the situation at hand. At the beginning of a football play, which player should you watch most carefully?

Example B. Recognizing the presence of a client's nursing diagnosis uses the same two-step process.

Step 1. Learn the names and definitions of the various NANDA labels.

In the *Nursing Diagnosis Guide* you will find labels like Anxiety, Fear, and Personal Identity Disturbance. These names may be familiar to you. Which one means inability to distinguish between self and nonself?

Which one means a vague, uneasy feeling with a nonspecific source?

Step 2. Learn to focus your attention on important aspects of the nursing diagnosis—the defining characteristics or risk factors. If you do not know which signs and symptoms are associated with a particular label, you may not realize the significance of the client's signs and symptoms. In fact, if you do not know what signs and symptoms to look for, you may not even be aware of the cues, much less the existence of a problem.

Nurses often misdiagnose Fear and Anxiety because some of the physical and emotional manifestations may be the same. If you focus only on the relevant cues, however, you can make the distinction. Use your *Nursing Diagnosis Guide* as needed.

1. For which label is the feeling one of *dread*?
   For which label is the feeling *vague and uneasy*?
   Write a rule you could use to tell these two labels apart.

2. In which label is the source of the feeling known to the client?
   In which label is the source of the feeling nonspecific or unknown to the client?

   Write another rule you could use to tell these two labels apart.

3. Which of these labels has only one defining characteristic?
   What is the defining characteristic?
   Write another rule you could use to differentiate between Anxiety and Fear.

4. In the following case study, your client is exhibiting physical and emotional signs of distress. Circle the cues that are *relevant* to a diagnosis of Fear.

   Mr. Cheng has pneumonia. His I & O record shows he has not been drinking fluids. When you auscultate his lungs, you hear bilateral crackles and rales. His temperature is 100°, and his B/P is 140/90. He says he is very weak. He states, "I just feel like something awful is going to happen to me." He is perspiring, and his hands are shaking. He has just been started on oxygen therapy, and he tells you the mask makes him feel that he is suffocating. You check his data base and find he has a history of claustrophobia.

Applying the Skill

The same process is used in identifying collaborative problems. You must know the complications that may occur with medical diagnoses and therapies and the signs and symptoms of the complications.

1. Read the following case study. Refer to a basic nursing text or a medical-surgical nursing text if you need to.

   Katie O'Hara has severe vomiting and diarrhea because of gastroenteritis. Because she needs fluids and antibiotics, her physician has prescribed intravenous therapy, which she will need for several days.

a. What are the two obvious potential complications of intravenous therapy?

b. What are the symptoms of those complications?

(1)

(2)

c. If you are assessing Katie for Complications of Intravenous Therapy: Infiltration and Phlebitis, which data would be relevant? (Circle the relevant data.)

B/P 110/80, pulse 80, temperature 100° F. Katie states that she feels afraid, but "just can't put my finger on what it is." She remains NPO. Her output for the shift is 350 cc emesis, 150 cc of urine, and six unmeasured liquid stools. Her hands are warm and dry; the skin turgor is good on her forearms. Her IV is infusing at 100 cc per hour, but it is positional (i.e., it sometimes stops running when she changes the position of her arm). You have opened the roller clamp completely, but it will not run at the prescribed rate of 150 cc per hour. There is no redness at or above the insertion site. The area around the insertion site is pale and cool to touch. Katie states that it is a little tender to touch. When you hang her piggyback antibiotic, she complains that it burns her arm. Katie's data base shows no allergy to any medications.

2. Suppose you were assessing a patient for Impaired Tissue Integrity (Decubitus Ulcer). List the relevant data (i.e., what signs, symptoms, and risk factors would you look for?).

---

* Adapted from *Critical Thinking Worksheets*, a supplement of *Addison-Wesley Chemistry*, by Wilbraham et al. (Menlo Park, CA: Addison-Wesley Publishing Company, 1990).

(Answer Key, p. 378)

1. Place a check (✔) beside the examples of activities performed during the planning step of the nursing process.

   a. ____ Conducting a client interview

   b. ____ Placing a "Protocol for Oxytocin Induction" in Mrs. Freidrich's care plan

   c. ____ Discussing with the client whether a goal should be included on the care plan

   d. ____ Changing the bed linens

   e. ____ Writing a nursing order, "Intake and Output q8hr"

   f. ____ Measuring a client's urine output

   g. ____ Choosing nursing orders from a computer menu

   h. ____ Checking to see if the nursing unit has standards of care for preeclampsia patients

   i. ____ Writing a nursing diagnosis

   j. ____ Deciding which of the client's problems need to be written on the care plan

2. Write the type of planning next to the appropriate definitions or examples.

   Formal   Initial   Discharge

   Informal   Ongoing

   a. _____ Conscious, deliberate activity involving decision-making, critical thinking, and creativity.

   b. _____ As the nurse is admitting the client, she is beginning to plan how she will conduct the rest of the admission interview.

   c. _____ The admitting nurse uses the admission data base to create a new care plan.

   d. _____ The nurse is planning the work she must accomplish during her shift.

   e. _____ Planning that is done as new information is obtained and as the patient's responses to care are evaluated.

   f. _____ Writing a nursing order to assess the availability of family and friends who can help care for the client at home.

3. List four benefits of having a written nursing care plan.

a.

b.

c.

d.

4. Circle the correct word: Predicted outcomes are stated in terms of (nurse)(client) behaviors.

5. Place a check mark beside the measurable, observable goals (for brevity, none of the goals has a target time).

___ Will be progressively less anxious.   ___ Rates pain as 3 on a 1–10 scale.

___ Eats fruit at least 3 times/day.   ___ States less anxious than before exercise.

___ Skin warm and dry to touch.   ___ Will not have foul-smelling lochia.

___ Temp. will be < 100.1.   ___ B/P will be normal.

___ Explains importance of exercise.   ___ Tolerates increased activity.

___ Normal skin color.   ___ Experiences increased confidence.

___ States he feels more confident.   ___ Verbalizes understanding of home-care instructions.

6. The problem responses are given for you. Write an opposite, normal response that might be used in an outcome statement. The first one is done for you.

	Problem Response	Desired (Opposite) Response
a.	Constipation	Regular, formed, soft bowel movement
b.	Impaired Skin Integrity: Pressure Sore	
c.	Hypothermia	
d.	Dressing Self-Care Deficit	
e.	Altered Oral Mucous Membrane	

7. Use the normal responses you wrote in Exercise 6 to create expected outcomes. Fill in the boxes with the necessary components. Since there is no actual client, target times have been omitted. The first one has been done for you.

Subject	Action Verb	Special Conditions	Performance Criteria
a. (Client)	will have	(none)	regular, soft, formed B.M.
b.			
c.			
d.			
e.			

8. Write predicted outcomes for the following nursing diagnosis:

Back Pain r/t incision of recent spinal fusion and muscle stiffness from decreased mobility

   a. An outcome derived from the *problem*:

   b. An outcome derived from the *etiology*:

9. A nursing diagnosis for Ms. Jackson follows: "High Risk for Impaired Skin Integrity (Pressure Ulcers) r/t long periods of lying in bed." Write predicted outcomes and nursing orders for this diagnosis.

Goals/Predicted Outcomes	Nursing Orders

10. Place a *G* by the goals and an *N* by the nursing orders.

   a. ___ Will verbalize anxieties about his surgery by 12/16.

   b. ___ Will rate pain as less than 3 on a scale of 1 to 10.

   c. ___ Keep head of bed elevated to 45°.

   d. ___ Turn patient every 2 hours.

   e. ___ Force fluids up to 250 cc per hour.

   f. ___ Circulation to left foot will be improved, as evidenced by pink color, warm skin.

   g. ___ Infection will be prevented, as evidenced by temp. < 100.1.

   h. ___ Wear sterile gloves for dressing change.

   i. ___ Take temperature hourly if elevated.

   j. ___ Will list foods allowed on low-fat diet by 12/16.

11. Circle the action verbs:

Apply   Improve   Be

Demonstrate   Have   Verbalize

12. Both short-term and long-term goals are used on nursing care plans. Which type of goal is most important to include on student care plans? Why?

13. Label the following objectives, *A*—Affective, *C*—Cognitive, *P*—Psychomotor

a. ___ (Learner will) draw up the correct amount of insulin.

b. ___ (Learner will) explain the syringe markings correctly.

c. ___ (Learner will) discuss his fear of needles openly.

d. ___ (Learner will) list four foods that can be used as bread exchanges.

e. ___ (Learner will) express anger appropriately.

f. ___ (Learner will) inject himself, using sterile technique.

g. ___ (Learner will) state the relationship between exercise and insulin requirements.

h. ___ (Learner will) insert needle at a 45° angle.

14. Circle the letter of the correctly written outcomes. If it is incorrectly written, state what is wrong with it (refer to Box 6–2 and "Guidelines for Writing Goal Statements"). Some of the predicted outcomes address potential problems, so do not count it as an error if no time frame is given.

	Predicted Outcome	Errors (Guideline Violated)
a.	Client will develop adequate leg strength by 9/1.	
b.	Will have no signs of hemorrhage: VS-WNL, Hct and Hbg WNL, uses < 1 vag. pad per hour.	
c.	Will state the signs and symptoms of angina by 9/1.	
d.	Will feel better by morning.	
e.	Improved appetite.	
f.	Will be able to feed self by 9/1.	
g.	(On a 30-bed unit with only 2 wheelchairs) Will spend 4 hours each day in a wheelchair.	
h.	Client will discuss expectations of hospitalization and will relate the effects of a high carbohydrate diet on blood-sugar levels with a basic knowledge of exchange diet for diabetes.	
i.	After second teaching session, will demonstrate correct technique for testing blood for glucose.	
j.	Injects self with insulin.	
k.	Will state adequate pain relief from analgesics and will take at least 100 cc of p.o. fluids per hour.	
l.	IV will remain patent and run at 125 cc/hr.	
m.	By 7/15 expresses a desire for social contact and interaction with others.	
n.	Reports no numbness or tingling in left hand.	
o.	Voids at least 150 cc within 4 hr after removal of catheter.	

15. Read the following list of nursing actions. Classify them (e.g., Dependent/Independent) by writing the letters beside the appropriate category in the chart. Interventions can be classified in several ways, so most will belong in more than one category. (The first one has been done for you.)

Nursing Orders

a. Review booklet on post-mastectomy exercises with Ms. Petrie on evening of 7/13.

b. Spend at least 10 minutes per shift sitting with Ms. Adkins; encourage her to express her feelings about her husband's death.

c. Give acetaminophen gr. 500, p.o. q3h if temp. >101.2.

d. Remove staples from abdominal incision today.

e. Minimize environmental stimuli: dim lights, restrict visitors, speak and move slowly and quietly.

f. DO NOT take rectal temperatures.

g. Cut food for patient. Allow at least an hour for meals. Reheat food as needed.

h. Palpate uterine fundus for firmness q hr until saturating < 1 pad/hr.

i. B/P q4h unless elevated. If >150/94, take q hr.

j. Pad side rails with blankets or rubber pads.

k. Teach patient to wash hands carefully before handling infant.

l. Refer to Public Health Dept. for Rubella immunization.

m. Give pamphlets on "Basic Four Foods" and "Foods for Healthy Living."

Independent: *a*   Dependent:
Observation: Treatment: *a*   Prevention: Health promotion:
Physical care: Teaching: *a*   Counseling: Referral: Environmental management:

Case Study. Exercises 16–18 pertain to this case.

Ms. Nancy Atwell is a 32-year-old, unmarried teacher who has been diagnosed as having rheumatoid arthritis for approximately 4 years. This change has made her knees painful and has limited the motion and weight-bearing ability of the knee joints themselves. Ms. Atwell's knee inflammation is aggravated by the fact that she is 75 lb overweight. Her diet history reveals that she eats when feeling depressed or stressed and that she snacks frequently on potato chips and colas.

She has recently been diagnosed as having endometriosis, and now enters the hospital on the evening shift to have a hysterectomy in the early A.M. On her previous admission for treatment of her arthritis, she had been quiet, withdrawn, and extremely concerned for her privacy. Now she seems more outgoing and less overtly concerned about privacy. When questioned, Ms. Atwell states that she has had no previous surgical experience, but denies feeling nervous about the operation.

Her preoperative orders follow:

1. S.S. enema at HS

2. Nembutal 100 mg. p.o. at HS

3. NPO after midnight

4. pHisohex shower in A.M.

5. Pre-op med: Demerol 50 mg. and Vistaril 25 mg. IM at 0600

The day-shift nurse has identified the following nursing diagnoses for Ms. Atwell. (*Note:* There are other appropriate nursing diagnoses; for simplicity, we consider only these five.)

    a. High Risk for Low Situational Self-esteem r/t unresolved feeling about inability to bear children after hysterectomy

    b. Chronic Pain r/t inflammation of knees 2° rheumatoid arthritis

    c. High Risk for Sleep-Pattern Disturbance r/t strange environment and possible anxiety regarding surgery

    d. Altered Nutrition: More Than Body Requirements for calories r/t excess calorie intake from "emotional eating"

    e. High Risk for Noncompliance with NPO Order r/t lack of understanding of its importance for anesthesia

16. Prioritize the nursing diagnoses. Number them in order, giving #1 to the highest priority. Put an asterisk beside the ones that the evening nurse *must* address today.

17. Underline the portion of each of the nursing diagnoses for which you *must* write a goal.

18. On the following chart, write goals, predicted outcomes, and nursing orders for the three top-priority nursing diagnoses. Include dependent nursing actions (e.g., medications) under nursing orders on this care plan.

Nursing Diagnoses	Goals and Predicted Outcomes	Nursing Orders

19. Refer to Figure 3–3 (Nikki Winters's date base in Chapter 3) and the problem list for Nikki Winters in Chapter 5.

   a. One of Ms. Winters's collaborative problems is Potential Complication of Hysterectomy.

   (1) List the complications that might develop as a result of Ms. Winters's hysterectomy. Refer to your medical-surgical text as needed.

   (2) Now rewrite the collaborative problem statement, using the format suggested in Chapter 5.

   (3) Write a predicted outcome for each of the complications you listed in (2).

b. Another of Ms. Winters's collaborative problems is Potential Complications of Intravenous Therapy: Inflammation,Phlebitis, Infiltration. Develop a care plan for this problem.

(1) List the signs and symptoms of each of the complications.

Inflammation:

Phlebitis:

Infiltration:

(2) In the columns below, write predicted outcomes and nursing orders for each of the complications.

Predicted Outcomes	Nursing Orders
For inflammation	
For phlebitis	

Predicted Outcomes	Nursing Orders
For infiltration	

REFERENCES

American Nurses Association. (1985). *Code for Nurses with Interpretive Statements.* Kansas City, MO.

American Nurses Association. (1975). *Continuity of Care and Discharge Planning Programs in Institutions and Community Agencies. A Statement of the American Nurses Association Division on Medical Surgical Nursing Practices and the Division of Community Health Nursing Practice.* Kansas City, MO.

American Nurses Association. (1973). *Standards of Nursing Practice.* Kansas City, MO.

Houldin et al. (1987). *Nursing Diagnoses for Wellness: Supporting Strengths.* Philadelphia: J. B. Lippincott.

Pender, N. (1987). *Health Promotion in Nursing Practice.* 2nd ed. Norwalk, CT: Appleton & Lange, Chaps. 9 and 10.

U.S. Department of Health and Human Services, Public Health Service. (1990). *Healthy People 2000.* DHHS Publication No. (PHS) 91-50212. Washington, DC: Superintendent of Documents, U.S. Government Printing Office.

CHAPTER 7

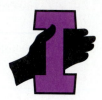

IMPLEMENTATION

OBJECTIVES

Upon completing this chapter, you should be able to do the following:
* Discuss the relationship of the implementation step to the other steps of the nursing process.
* Discuss preparations necessary before implementing patient-care activities.
* Follow guidelines for successful implementation of the nursing care plan.
* Compare four nursing care delivery systems: team nursing, primary nursing, functional nursing, and case management.
* Compare and contrast four methods of writing nursing progress notes: narrative, SOAP, focus charting, and charting by exception.
* Observe guidelines for documenting and reporting patient care and status.
* Explain how patient dignity and privacy can be maintained during implementation.

INTRODUCTION

Implementation is the nursing process step in which the nurse performs the activities necessary for achieving the client's health goals. Described broadly, the activities in this step are (1) doing, (2) delegating, and (3) recording (see Figure 7–1). During implementation the nurse performs or delegates the nursing orders that were developed in the planning step. The implementation step ends when nursing actions and the resulting client responses have been recorded in the client's chart.

Professional standards for nursing practice support client participation in implementation, as in all phases of the nursing process. The degree of participation in this step depends on the client's health status and resources, as well as on the type of action being considered. For example, an infant or an unconscious person cannot participate at all in implementation strategies; all interventions for such patients are carried out by nurses, significant others, or other caregivers. In the case of health-promotion strategies, the client alone might carry out the strategies.

Example: With the help of his nurse, David Mikos devised a plan for lowering his cholesterol intake. The plan is to follow a low-fat diet at home and reward himself with concert or theater tickets for each month of successful dieting. In this case, the nurse is not involved at all in the implementation step.

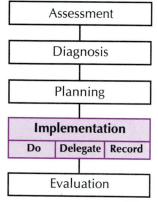

Figure 7-1.
The Implementation Step in the Nursing Process

RELATIONSHIP OF IMPLEMENTATION TO OTHER NURSING PROCESS STEPS

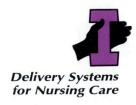

Delivery Systems for Nursing Care

Implementation depends on the first three steps of the nursing process: assessment, diagnosis, and planning. These steps provide the basis for the autonomous nursing actions performed during implementation. Without them, implementation (and nursing) would reflect only dependent functions—carrying out medical orders and institutional policies. In turn, the implementation step provides the actual interventions and client responses that are evaluated in the evaluation step.

Implementation is also interrelated to and overlaps with the other steps of the nursing process. Using data acquired during assessment, the nurse can individualize the care given during implementation, tailoring interventions to fit a specific client rather than applying them routinely to categories of patients (e.g., "All pneumonia patients . . . ") Ongoing assessment often occurs simultaneously with implementation. While implementing, you will continue to assess the patient at every contact, gathering data about her responses to the nursing actions and about any new problems that may develop. Ongoing assessment is not the *same* as implementation; it occurs *during* implementation.

> **Standard V.**
> Nursing actions provide for client/patient participation in health promotion, maintenance, and restoration.
>
> **Standard VI.**
> Nursing actions assist the client/patient to maximize his health capabilities (ANA, 1973).

Examples:

Implementation	Assessment
While bathing an elderly patient,	the nurse observes a reddened area on the patient's sacrum.
When emptying the catheter bag,	the nurse measures 200 cc and notices a strong odor.

The nurse also implements nursing orders that specifically *direct* ongoing assessment. For example, a nursing order might read, "Auscultate lungs q4h." When performing this activity, the nurse is both carrying out the nursing order and performing ongoing, focused assessment.

Data obtained during implementation activities is used to identify new diagnoses, or revise existing diagnoses (diagnosis step). It also enables the nurse to revise and adapt the original goals and nursing orders (planning step) as the patient's unique needs become more apparent.

DELIVERY SYSTEMS FOR NURSING CARE

Five models commonly used for implementing nursing care are (1) functional nursing, (2) team nursing, (3) primary nursing, (4) case management, and (5) differentiated practice. These systems, except for differentiated practice, differ in the way they allocate responsibilities, tasks, and authority; however, all can be used in a variety of settings (e.g., hospitals, clinics, home health).

In **functional nursing** a charge nurse (or head nurse) assigns caregivers to various tasks according to their level of knowledge and skill. For example, on a given shift, one RN might administer medications to all patients on the floor, another RN might perform the physical assessments and the patient teaching, a nursing assistant might take vital signs and make unoccupied beds for all the

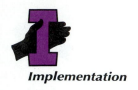

Implementation

patients, and an LPN might bathe patients and perform some of the treatments. This system is efficient but tends to fragment care, as each patient sees several different caregivers during the course of a day.

In **team nursing** a team of registered nurses, licensed practical nurses, and nursing assistants work together to care for a group of patients during a shift. In some settings the team keeps the same group of patients from day to day. The team leader, an RN, is responsible for planning and assigning care to team members (nursing assistants, LPNs and other RNs), who function under her direction. Although the team leader plans and directs care, she does not always give care under this model. The success of this model depends greatly upon communication between team members and the management abilities of the team leader.

In **primary nursing** a registered nurse is responsible for managing the care of a small group of patients 24 hours a day, 7 days a week. The primary nurse develops and implements the plan of care while she is at work. The RN gives total, direct care to a caseload of patients. When she leaves, the plan is followed by nurse associates on the other shifts. Although the primary nurse may be assisted by other levels of staff, she is responsible for planning and coordinating all aspects of the patient's care, including medications, treatments, hygiene, comfort needs, communication with other professionals, emotional support, and so on. An advantage of this model is the continuity of care it provides; each patient has one nurse who is accountable for and well informed about his care.

Case management has evolved from primary nursing as a response to the recent emphasis on shorter hospital stays. Third-party payers have begun to make payments based on the client's diagnosis, or *diagnosis-related group* (*DRG*), rather than on the number of days he stays in the hospital. Case management focuses on achieving specific client outcomes within the length of stay allowed by the client's DRG. The plan of care includes a client outcome timeline, which specifies the times at which predictable, key events must occur if the allowable length of stay is to be achieved (American Nurses Association, 1988). In this system, a case manager is responsible for a caseload of clients throughout their hospitalization. Case managers are professional nurses with expertise in a particular clinical area. Their caseloads may be organized geographically by hospital unit (e.g., surgical units), by diagnosis (e.g., cardiac rehabilitation), or by physician.

Unlike the preceding delivery systems, **differentiated practice** cannot be characterized by the way it allocates responsibilities, tasks, and authority. Differentiated practice is an attempt to reorganize nursing care within an institution so that quality care can be achieved in spite of a shortage of RNs. Its effect on staffing patterns and allocation of responsibilities varies from agency to agency, but it usually involves the analysis of tasks and the creation of new job descriptions. New levels of practitioners may be added, or new caregiver roles created (e.g., nurse aides may be used in new ways). Sometimes partnerships are created by permanently scheduling two caregivers to work together. Partnering may involve, for example, an RN and an aide, or a bachelor's degree RN and an associate degree RN. Differentiated practice tends to place the RN in a supervisory role. It is similar to functional nursing in that it distributes tasks among various levels of personnel. However, it includes careful consideration of client goals, using them as the criteria by which the system of care delivery is evaluated.

PREPARING TO ACT

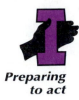

Preparation for patient-care activities actually begins in the planning step of the nursing process. When you use time-sequenced planning to set your work priorities and make your daily work schedule, you are actually taking the first step in delivering care to your assigned patients. Box 7–1 is a guide you may wish to use in organizing your nursing care for a clinical day. It may be helpful, especially for students, to create a time schedule around this guide to provide structure for the day and ensure that the patient's needs are met.

During a time when many institutions are experiencing staffing problems, it is important that each nurse-patient encounter be fully utilized. When possible, try to implement care for several goals simultaneously. While at the bedside taking vital signs and making physical assessments, for instance, you might use that time to talk with the patient, show interest and concern, or do patient teaching.

Preparing the Nurse

Before beginning an intervention, be sure that both you and the patient are prepared. Always review the care plan to familiarize yourself with the actions you are to take. This allows you to clarify any details and determine if you need help in performing any of the interventions. You may require assistance under the following conditions:

1. *You lack the skill or knowledge to implement a nursing order.* For example, if you have never taught a patient to crutch-walk, you should ask a colleague for help or review the written procedure before attempting the intervention.

2. *You cannot safely perform the action alone.* For example, you should obtain help when moving a large, immobile patient from a bed to a chair.

3. *Assistance would reduce the client's stress.* For example, having help in repositioning a patient who experiences pain when being moved will minimize her pain.

You are legally and ethically responsible for questioning nursing or medical orders that you believe to be inappropriate or potentially harmful. This should also be done as a part of your preparation.

Preparation includes determining points in the activity where you need to pause for feedback. The immediate feedback you obtain during an activity guides you in making on-the-spot alterations in the action. For example, when preparing to help a patient ambulate, you might plan to look for responses (feedback) after he sits on the side of the bed for a minute, after standing, after walking to a chair, and again after he has been sitting in the chair for 15 minutes.

Preparing the Client

Just before implementing, you should *reassess whether the intervention is still needed.* Never assume that an order is still necessary simply because it is written on the care plan; the situation or the client's condition may have changed. For example, a nursing diagnosis for Gayle Fischer is Sleep-Pattern Disturbance related to anxiety and unfamiliar surroundings. When the nurse makes rounds, she discovers that Gayle is sleeping, so she omits the back rub that was planned as a relaxation strategy.

Are You Prepared to Act?
- Have you reviewed the care plan?
- Do you have the necessary skills? Knowledge?
- Do you need help to perform the action safely?
- Do you need help to reduce stress on the client?
- Are there orders that seem inappropriate or potentially harmful?
- What are the feedback points?

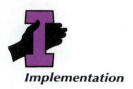

Implementation

Box 7–1. Student Guide for Organizing Clinical Activities

Client profile: Name_____ Age_____

    Admitting diagnosis_____Admit date_____

    Name client wishes to be called_____

    Significant other(s)_____

Current health status (today):

    Has the client's physical or emotional status changed since you received your assignment?

    Do you need to modify your care plan?

Basic Care Needs:

    Hygiene _____

    Elimination _____

    Feeding _____

    Dressing _____

    Other _____

    Special safety precautions _____

Medications and IVs:

Collaborative tests and treatments (for scheduling and observation)—e.g., physical therapy, X-ray.

Prioritized nursing diagnoses and strategies (that you can realistically address today):

New medical orders that need to be implemented (e.g., discontinue IV, ambulate):

Special teaching or counseling needs:

You should also *assess the client's readiness.* The client's behavioral cues will help you to choose a time when the activity will benefit her most. A great deal of time can be wasted in performing interventions when a client is not psychologically ready. For example, when the nurse goes to Ms. Fischer's room to teach her about diabetic foot care, she notices that Ms. Fischer has been crying. Realizing that the patient would probably not be receptive to new information at this time, the nurse decides to postpone the teaching.

Finally, *explain to the client what is to take place.* The client is entitled to an explanation of the action, the sensations he can expect, what he is expected to do, and the results the therapy or procedure is expected to produce. Preparation also includes provision for privacy, as well as any physical preparation, such as positioning.

Example: Before administering an enema to Jo Slevin, the nurse explains that this will prevent contamination of the surgical area during her bowel surgery. She shuts the door, pulls the curtain around the bed, helps Jo to assume a side-lying position, and drapes her with a bath blanket. She tells Jo she will feel pressure and perhaps some cramping as the fluid is instilled, and that she should retain the solution for 5 or 10 minutes, until she feels a strong urge to defecate.

Preparing Supplies and Equipment

Assemble all necessary equipment and materials before entering the room, so that you can proceed efficiently and with a minimum of stress to the patient. You may need supplies for dressing changes, equipment for removing staples from an incision, linen for a bath and bed change, or pamphlets for a teaching session. The following example demonstrates how inefficient and ineffective it is to stop in mid-procedure because the necessary supplies are not at hand.

Example: A nurse is inserting a urinary catheter. After draping the patient, opening the sterile kit, and donning sterile gloves, the nurse breaks sterility when one of her gloves brushes against the patient's leg. Because she did not think to bring an extra pair of sterile gloves into the room, she is faced with the choice of leaving the patient draped and positioned while she goes for another pair, continuing the procedure with an unsterile glove, or going for new gloves, opening a new cath kit, and redraping the patient to be sure sterility is maintained.

ACTION: DOING OR DELEGATING

After preparations are complete, activity begins. The nurse applies a wide range of knowledge and skills in performing or delegating planned nursing strategies. The number and kind of specific nursing activities is almost unlimited. They consist of every skill, process, and procedure you have learned as a student and as a practitioner.

Levels of Autonomy

The nursing process enables nurses to identify, evaluate, and emphasize their independent activities. However, the full nursing role encompasses dependent and collaborative functions as well. Most nurses provide care for ill clients, whose comprehensive health needs include attention to their medical

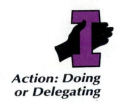

Action: Doing or Delegating

Is the Patient Prepared?

° Determine whether the action is still needed.

° Assess the patient's readiness.

° Explain what is to be done and what results to expect.

° Tell the client what sensations to expect.

° Tell the client what he is expected to do.

° Provide for privacy.

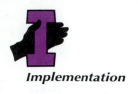

Implementation

condition. In the implementation step, you will implement both (1) the nursing orders on the patient's care plan and (2) physician's orders for the medical care plan.

Recall that **dependent interventions** are those performed when following physician orders or agency policies. Usually they relate directly to the client's medical diagnosis or disease processes.

Example: The nurse gives IV morphine sulfate for pain relief, according to a physician's written order.

These so-called dependent interventions are not performed mindlessly; nurses use critical thinking to make judgments about how, when, and to what extent they carry out medical orders.

The amount of time spent on dependent functions varies with the type of client, the employment setting, and the nurse's position, education, and experience. Critical-care nurses, for instance, spend more of their time on dependent functions than do home-health nurses and gerontology nurses (Guzzetta, 1987, p. 634). Some clinical nurse specialists perform few, if any, dependent interventions.

Collaborative (interdependent) interventions are performed either with other health professionals or as a result of decisions made jointly with them. Suppose, for example, that a nurse determines that a patient with a recent myocardial infarction needs concentrated teaching about his diet. She asks a dietitian to see the patient and reinforces the dietitian's instructions in her own interactions with the patient. The nurse and dietitian later use nursing observations to jointly evaluate the patient's progress toward understanding, accepting, and following diet restrictions.

Coordination of the patient's care is an important nursing activity that is related to, but not the same as, collaboration. This activity involves scheduling the client's contacts with other hospital departments (e.g., laboratory and X-ray technicians, physical and respiratory therapists) and serving as a liaison among the members of the health-care team. As the professionals who are in touch with the patient 24 hours a day, nurses are in the best position to receive all the fragments of information and synthesize a holistic view of the patient. By making rounds with other professionals, reading their reports, and interpreting their findings to patients and families, the nurses assure that everyone gets the "big picture" as well as the specialized one.

Independent (autonomous) interventions are performed when carrying out the nursing orders, and often in conjunction with medical orders. Bulechek and McCloskey (1985) group independent nursing interventions into the following categories:

Category	*Examples*
1. Stress management	Imaging; alternate muscle-relaxation techniques
2. Life-style alteration	Counseling, teaching, support groups
3. Acute-care management	Preoperative teaching, surveillance
4. Self-care assistance	Bathing, assisting with ambulation, positioning
5. Communication	Discharge planning, active listening

When working with well clients, the nursing focus is to promote self-responsibility and self-care. Health-promotion and disease-prevention activities consist mainly of educating and motivating clients to maintain healthy life-styles (Items 1, 2 and 5 above).

In addition to legally conferred autonomy, the nurse's knowledge and skills determine the degree to which an action can be considered autonomous; the same activity can be independent in one situation and dependent in another.

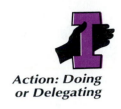

Action: Doing or Delegating

Example: Taking vital signs can be a dependent or independent activity. Mr. Rauh has a temperature of 100.1°. The nurse realizes that many things can affect body temperature, and asks Mr. Rauh if he had anything to eat or drink before his vital signs were taken. The medical order reads, "V.S. t.i.d;" but because the temperature represents an unusual reading for Mr. Rauh, and because the nurse knows he is at risk for infection, she retakes his temperature an hour later to establish whether this is a pattern or an isolated cue.

This nurse's actions are independent. If she had been functioning in a completely dependent manner, she would have recorded Mr. Rauh's vital signs without validating their accuracy or questioning their meaning. She might have telephoned the physician for instructions, or simply passed the data on to the next shift without checking to see if Mr. Rauh's temperature remained the same, continued to rise, or returned to normal.

Accountability is an aspect of autonomy. **Autonomy** implies that the nurse is answerable for her actions and can define, explain, and evaluate the results of her decisions. The nurse in the preceding example is answerable for the decisions she made (i.e., to wait an hour and retake Mr. Rauh's temperature before calling the physician) and would have been able to provide a rationale for her actions. Skilled use of the nursing process will enable you to expand the scope of your independent and collaborative functioning. Confidence in your clinical competence, knowledge, and skills, and a willingness to assume responsibility for your actions all add to the autonomous nature of your practice.

Skills Needed for Implementation

Nurses must have good cognitive, interpersonal, and technical skills in order to successfully implement the care plan. These skills are discussed individually in order to facilitate understanding; in practice, however, you will use them in various combinations and with different emphasis, depending upon the activity. For instance, when inserting a urinary catheter, you need cognitive knowledge of the principles and steps of the procedure, technical skill in draping the patient and manipulating the equipment, and interpersonal skills to inform and reassure the patient.

Cognitive (intellectual) skills include problem solving, decision making, critical thinking, and creative thinking. In the implementation step, nurses use these skills to apply theories and principles from nursing and related courses to each specific patient-care situation. When performing nursing strategies, the nurse may discover new problems that require quick identification and solution. For example, when helping a patient walk, a nurse identifies that the IV flow rate is too slow. She quickly checks to see that the tubing is not kinked and that the

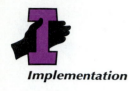

Implementation

insertion site is in satisfactory condition. If no mechanical problems are noted, she opens the roller clamp to regulate the flow rate. If it is still a little slow, she raises the bag higher to make use of gravity.

Critical thinking is especially important in making the quick, on-the-spot decisions that are characteristic of implementation. It enables the nurse to rapidly think of alternative courses of action when the planned strategies do not work as predicted and, as in the example of Mr. Rauh's elevated temperature, to decide whether, and when, to notify a physician about a client's status.

Nurses use **interpersonal skills** in nearly every contact with patients, families, and other health team members; for example, when they are listening actively, conveying interest, giving clear explanations, comforting, making referrals, and sharing attitudes, feelings, and knowledge. It is usually not possible for you to provide all the nursing care a client needs. You will use interpersonal skills to delegate some activities to other team members and to supervise and evaluate the performance of those interventions. The effectiveness of an intervention depends in part upon your ability to convey information to patients and other health team members so that they will know exactly what to expect and what to do.

Technical (psychomotor) skills are used during the implementation step in performing a variety of hands-on skills, such as changing dressings, giving injections, turning and positioning patients, attaching a monitor to a patient, and suctioning a tracheostomy. When procedures are done skillfully, the plan is more likely to be successful. Competent performance of technical skills also helps build rapport with the client. If, for instance, you can turn and reposition a client with minimal discomfort, the client will perceive you as someone who can help, and begin to trust you. Refer to Box 7–2 for a summary of guidelines to help you implement your nursing strategies successfully.

RECORDING

After doing or delegating, the nurse completes the implementation step by recording the nursing interventions and client responses. These nursing progress notes are a part of the agency's permanent record for the client. This section of the text describes different systems for organizing client records and then specifically describes nursing responsibilities for documentation.

The **client record (or chart)** is a permanent, comprehensive account of information about the client's health care. It consists of various forms on which information is recorded about all aspects of the client's care (e.g., physician's orders, results of laboratory and diagnostic tests, and progress notes written by physicians, nurses, and other caregivers). *Nursing* documentation in the permanent record is found on the following forms:

1. The initial, comprehensive nursing assessment (admission data base)
2. The individualized nursing care plan
3. Nursing progress notes
4. Flowsheets (e.g., graphic sheets, medication records)
5. The client discharge summary

Functions of Client Records

The written record *facilitates communication* between professionals from different disciplines and on different shifts, helping to coordinate care and avoid duplication of effort. Written notes about the client's progress and condition serve as a reference for nurses on other shifts who later need to refresh their memory or clarify the verbal report they received. Caregivers also refer to the chart as a reference point to help them assess new client responses.

Recording

Box 7–2. Guidelines for Successful Implementation

Prepare the Nurse

1. *Determine whether you need help* to perform the action safely and minimize stress to the client.

2. Be sure you *know the rationale* for the intervention, as well as any potential side effects or complications. When actions are based on practice wisdom, examine them critically.

3. *Question any actions you do not understand* or that seem inappropriate or potentially unsafe.

4. *Determine feedback points* and *assess the client's response* during the activity.

5. *Schedule activities* to allow adequate time for completion.

6. *Delegate interventions to other team members* in order to use your time efficiently.

7. *Improve your knowledge base* by continually seeking new knowledge.

Prepare the Client

8. *Determine that the action is still needed and appropriate.*

9. *Assess client readiness.*

10. *Inform the client* of what to expect and what is expected of him.

11. *Provide for privacy and comfort.*

Prepare Supplies and Equipment

12. *Gather and organize all necessary supplies.*

During Implementation:

13. *Adapt interventions to the individual's* age, values, and health status. Remain flexible and make creative modifications as you work.

14. *Encourage the client to participate actively.*

15. *Perform interventions according to professional standards* of care and agency policies and procedures.

16. *Perform interventions carefully and accurately.*

17. *Supervise and evaluate delegated interventions.*

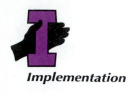

Implementation

As a *legal document*, the patient's record may be entered into court proceedings as evidence for a number of purposes (e.g., accident or injury claims by the client; malpractice charges against health professionals). The chart may be the only evidence that competent care was given. The chart itself is generally considered the property of the institution; however, courts recognize the client's right to the information contained in the record (Feutz, 1989).

Reimbursement from third-party payers (e.g., Medicare, private insurance companies) to clients and health-care institutions is tied directly to documentation. The chart is examined to see that all medical orders were carried out properly, that medications were given, that equipment charged for was actually used, and so on. For instance, if a client's hospital bill included a charge for a urinary catheter, the progress notes might be examined for an entry stating that the client had been catheterized.

Of course, health team members refer to the client's chart when *planning care*. For instance, the physician may change a client's anticoagulant dosage on the basis of blood-clotting times found in the laboratory reports, or a nurse may use blood gas values and progress notes from the respiratory therapist to evaluate the effectiveness of nursing strategies for improving pulmonary ventilation.

Formal evaluations of the quality of care that clients receive in an institution are usually done after the client has been discharged. Outside groups also perform audits for accreditation purposes (e.g., Joint Commission on Accreditation of Healthcare Organizations). Therefore, written records are essential sources of data.

In addition, client records *provide educational information* for students in health disciplines, *statistical information* for institutions and government agencies, and *data for research and tracing historical trends*. Administrators involved in *financial planning* for a hospital may use nursing documentation to help them estimate nursing costs in the institution. Nursing costs represent a significant part of a hospital's budget, so it is important to estimate them accurately.

Client Record Systems

Three systems commonly used to keep an ongoing and permanent record of the patient's health care are (1) source-oriented records, (2) problem-oriented records and (3) computer records. These systems differ in the way the information is organized and/or stored.

Source-Oriented Records

In this widely used, traditional system the client's record is divided into sections according to the source of the data. Each discipline records data on its own special form. For example, physicians use an order sheet, a medical history form, and physician's progress notes; nurses record data on a nursing history form and in the nursing progress notes; and results of blood and urine tests are found on a laboratory report. Source-oriented records are convenient because each discipline can easily locate the necessary forms on which to write its entries. It is also easy for each professional to track the data of specific interest to his or her discipline.

The disadvantage is that information about a particular problem is scattered throughout various sections of the chart, so it is difficult to track a client's progress with regard to a problem. For example, if a client has diarrhea, the physician's history and physical records trace the development of the symptom; the physician's progress notes describe the client's daily elimination and hydration status and the proposed therapy; the nursing progress notes describe the number and nature of the stools and related physical status; the activity flowsheet notes that the client is too weak to bathe herself; the graphic sheet reflects an elevated pulse and total intake and output; the laboratory report shows a negative stool culture. To find data about that particular problem, you would have to search through six different forms in different sections of the chart.

Problem-Oriented Records

In problem-oriented medical records (POMR), also called *problem-oriented records* (*POR*), information is organized according to the client's problems. All health professionals, regardless of discipline, record on the same forms. The entire team contributes to a master list of client problems and to the plan of care for each problem. The basic components of a POR follow:

1. *Defined data base.* The data base consists of all the *initial* information about the client's health: the nursing admission assessment, the medical history and physical examination, initial laboratory and diagnostic test results, and social and family histories if pertinent.

2. *Master problem list.* The initial problem list is developed from the data base. All health-care professionals contribute to the problem list, which may contain medical, psychological, sociocultural, and spiritual problems. The master list is usually at the front of the chart, and serves as an index to numbered entries on the progress notes. Problems are listed in the order in which they are identified (see Table 7–1).

3. *Problem-oriented plan of care.* An initial plan is developed for each problem on the master list. Physicians write plans (or orders) for medical problems; nurses write orders for nursing diagnoses. Note that in this system the nursing care plan is not a separate document, but is integrated within the progress notes in the client's chart.

4. *Multidisciplinary progress notes.* All health professionals involved in the client's care make narrative entries in these notes, which are numbered to correspond with the problems on the master list. To follow the client's progress in resolving a problem, one simply reads all the progress notes labeled with that problem number.

Table 7–1. Master Problem List

No.	Problem	Identified	Resolved
1	Appendicitis	1980	1980
2	Hysterectomy	12/4/91	
2A	Pain related to surgical incision	12/4/91	12/10/91
3	Grief related to loss of childbearing ability	12/4/91	

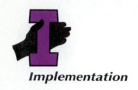

Implementation

The POR method promotes collaborative relationships between health professionals, who record on the same forms and work together to develop the master problem list and the plan of care. It also facilitates tracking a client's progress with regard to any particular problem and is likely to improve understanding of that problem, since each professional can observe what other disciplines have done. With all members of the health-care team addressing the same problems, quality of care should be improved.

The disadvantages of this method are that (1) time and money must be committed to teaching members of all disciplines to use the POR system; (2) some disciplines may resist the use of an integrated system; (3) the care plan is scattered throughout the progress notes.

Computer Records

As computers become more cost-effective, more and more agencies are using computerized information systems for all their records. This means that nurses use a computer to store the client's data base, add new data, create and revise care plans, and document client progress. Some institutions have a computer terminal at each client's bedside, enabling the nurse to document care immediately after it is given.

Information can be easily retrieved in a variety of forms (e.g., you could obtain the results of a blood test for a patient, a schedule of all patients on the unit having surgery today, a suggested list of interventions for a nursing diagnosis, or a printout of all the progress notes for a patient). Many systems can generate a work list for the shift, with a list of all the treatments, procedures, and medications needed by the client.

After the initial learning curve, computers make care planning and documentation relatively easy. Because computerized record keeping is fast, efficient, and thorough, nurses find it easier to plan and deliver individualized patient care. Nurses now entering practice will surely need to be computer literate at some time in their careers.

Nursing Responsibilities for Documentation

After caring for a patient, the nurse records the interventions and patient responses. Nursing documentation is a part of the patient's permanent legal record. It provides the most current assessment of patient status, as well as a chronological record of care and health status from admission through discharge.

Forms for Nursing Documentation

Institutions usually develop forms to meet their particular needs. Therefore, forms vary, and you will need to become familiar with new forms and record systems when you move to a different health-care agency. Whether the system is source-, problem-, or computer-oriented, three kinds of forms are usually used to record nursing progress notes: (1) flowsheets, (2) descriptive nursing progress notes, and (3) discharge summaries. They all provide for time-sequenced documentation of assessments, interventions, and client responses.

Flowsheets Several kinds of flowsheets are used as a quick way to record routine nursing care. A **medication record** is used to record all medications administered to the client. (Refer to a nursing fundamentals text for examples of medication records.) **Graphic flowsheets** are used to record routine measurements made at specified intervals (e.g., daily weights, vital signs). Graphic sheet data consists mainly of numbers. A **daily activity record** is a modified flowsheet for recording routine activities, especially those repeated frequently or at specified times (e.g., bath and skin care, diagnostic tests performed, activity level). In addition to daily activity flowsheets, most institutions design **special assessment flowsheets** for situations in which the same assessments are repeated routinely or frequently (e.g., hourly neurological assessments).

Figure 7–2 is an example of a graphic flowsheet; it also incorporates a few basic care activities, such as the bath and oral care. Figure 7–3, "Patient Care Notes," is a combined record of the patient's activities and assessments of patient status (to save space, one page of this form is omitted). Like most flowsheets, this one provides a list of descriptive words and phrases that the nurse simply circles. Notice that this form is organized according to Gordon's Functional Health Patterns (1987), as is the admission assessment form for this hospital (Appendix C). Such consistent use of a nursing framework throughout the entire set of nursing records promotes thorough, efficient data collection, analysis, and recording.

Figure 7–4 is an example of a Nursery Flow Record that is used to record assessments and care of normal newborns. This form combines a flowsheet format with space for brief narrative progress notes.

Nursing Progress Notes   Progress notes are a narrative description of patient progress toward goal achievement. They should include the following elements:

> Assessments of client's mental and physical condition
> Client activities and responses
> Nursing treatments and interventions, and client responses
> Visits by other caregivers or family members, if pertinent
> Treatments performed by the physician that affect nursing care

The form used and the manner of recording will vary, depending upon whether the hospital's record system is source-oriented or problem-oriented. In all systems, though, nursing progress notes, written in brief phrases and sentences, are used to augment (as needed) but not duplicate the data in the flowsheets.

Discharge Summary   A discharge summary is a special nursing progress note written at the time a client is dismissed from the agency. It usually includes the following:

> Current status of each client problem
> Teaching and counseling that was done to prepare the client for dismissal
> Current medications and treatments that are to be continued
> Activities of daily living and self-care abilities
> Support system, significant others
> Mode of discharge (e.g., walking, wheelchair)
> Person who accompanied the client
> Where client is going (e.g., home, nursing home, another unit in the hospital)

Figure 7–5 is an example of a discharge record that is used in conjunction with the nursing progress notes. This discharge record focuses on the information given to the patient at the time of dismissal; a copy is given to the patient. When this type of form is used, the description of the client's condition and the problem status are recorded as a final entry on the progress notes.

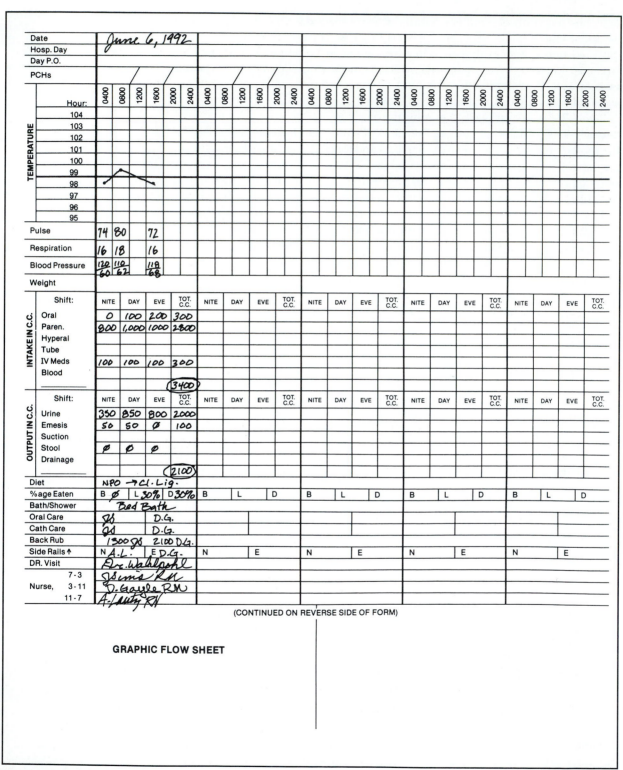

Figure 7–2. Graphic Flow Sheet.
Courtesy of Shawnee Mission Medical Center, Merriam, KS.

PATIENT CARE NOTES

TIME:			
Neuro	Alert Lethargic Unconscious Oriented X 3 Disoriented Speech: Clear Slurred Absent	Alert Lethargic Unconscious Oriented X 3 Disoriented Speech: Clear Slurred Absent	Alert Lethargic Unconscious Oriented X 3 Disoriented Speech: Clear Slurred Absent
Integument/Wound	Skin: warm ·cool dry moist color: IV location: N/A or Skin care: N/A Simple Extensive Skin breakdown: N/A or Wound Location: N/A or DSG Appearance: Dry or Wound Care: Drains: N/A or	Skin: warm cool dry moist color: IV location: N/A or Skin care: N/A Simple Extensive Skin breakdown: N/A or Wound Location: N/A or DSG Appearance: Dry or Wound Care: Drains: N/A or	Skin: warm cool dry moist color: IV location: N/A or Skin care: N/A Simple Extensive Skin breakdown: N/A or Wound Location: N/A or DSG Appearance: Dry or Wound Care: Drains: N/A or
Cardio-Vascular	Radial pulse: regular irregular Edema: N/A or _____	Radial pulse: regular irregular Edema: N/A or _____	Radial pulse: regular irregular Edema: N/A or _____
Respiratory	Resp: unlabored labored Lungs clear or Oz @ ____ per _____ Cough: nonproductive productive	Resp: unlabored labored Lungs clear or Oz @ ____ per _____ Cough: nonproductive productive	Resp: unlabored labored Lungs clear or Oz @ ____ per _____ Cough: nonproductive productive
Gastrointestinal	Abdomen: soft or Bowel Sounds: active or Nausea Vomiting Passing Flatus Stoma: N/A or Stool: None or continent incontinent x____ Supp/enema: N/A or Results: NG: N/A or Placement Verified Suction: Irrigation: Drainage:	Abdomen: soft or Bowel Sounds: active or Nausea Vomiting Passing Flatus Stoma: N/A or Stool: None or continent incontinent x____ Supp/enema: N/A or Results: NG: N/A or Placement Verified Suction: Irrigation: Drainage:	Abdomen: soft or Bowel Sounds: active or Nausea Vomiting Passing Flatus Stoma: N/A or Stool: None or continent incontinent x____ Supp/enema: N/A or Results: NG: N/A or Placement Verified Suction: Irrigation: Drainage:
Genitourinary	Urine continent incontinent x_____ catheter: N/A or Irrigation: N/A or Vag ding: N/A small mod. large Color: _____	Urine continent incontinent x_____ catheter: N/A or Irrigation: N/A or Vag ding: N/A small mod. large Color: _____	Urine continent incontinent x_____ catheter: N/A or Irrigation: N/A or Vag ding: N/A small mod. large Color: _____
SIG.			

NAME _____ HOSPITAL NO. _____ DATE _____

FORM OS-328 (10/89)

Figure 7–3. Patient Care Notes. © Department of Nursing, Bronson Methodist Hospital, Kalamazoo, MI. All rights reserved.

TIME:			
Psycho Social	Calm Resting Quiet Anxious Restless	Calm Resting Quiet Anxious Restless	Calm Resting Quiet Anxious Restless
Activity/ Rest	Bedrest/BRP chair ambulate Self Assist of _____ Gait: Steady Unsteady Immobility: N/A or 2^0 _____ Slept:	Bedrest/BRP chair ambulate Self Assist of _____ Gait: Steady Unsteady Immobility: N/A or 2^0 _____ Slept:	Bedrest/BRP chair ambulate Self Assist of _____ Gait: Steady Unsteady Immobility: N/A or 2^0 _____ Slept:
Equipment	Eggcrate Clinitron/Kinnair ____ °F warm/cool pad ____°F to ____ feeding pump Trapeze/frame IV Controller X ____ IV Volumetric X ____ Isolation:	Eggcrate Clinitron/Kinnair ____ °F warm/cool pad ____°F to ____ feeding pump Trapeze/frame IV Controller X ____ IV Volumetric X ____ Isolation:	Eggcrate Clinitron/Kinnair ____ °F warm/cool pad ____°F to ____ feeding pump Trapeze/frame IV Controller X ____ IV Volumetric X ____ Isolation:
Safety	Sensory deficit N/A or bed position: low or siderails: up down visual observation q: restraints: N/A or remove/ROM/reapply q: sitter: N/A or continuous ID Band on: Yes No Reapplied	Sensory deficit N/A or bed position: low or siderails: up down visual observation q: restraints: N/A or remove/ROM/reapply q: sitter: N/A or continuous ID Band on: Yes No Reapplied	Sensory deficit N/A or bed position: low or siderails: up down visual observation q: restraints: N/A or remove/ROM/reapply q: sitter: N/A or continuous ID Band on: Yes No Reapplied
Assessment	Time _____ Location/Type: Severity 1 2 3 4 5 6 7 8 9 10 Action/Results:	Time _____ Location/Type: Severity 1 2 3 4 5 6 7 8 9 10 Action/Results:	Time _____ Location/Type: Severity 1 2 3 4 5 6 7 8 9 10 Action/Results:
	Time _____ Location/Type: Severity 1 2 3 4 5 6 7 8 9 10 Action/Results:	Time _____ Location/Type: Severity 1 2 3 4 5 6 7 8 9 10 Action/Results:	Time _____ Location/Type: Severity 1 2 3 4 5 6 7 8 9 10 Action/Results:
Pain	Time _____ Location/Type: Severity 1 2 3 4 5 6 7 8 9 10 Action/Results:	Time _____ Location/Type: Severity 1 2 3 4 5 6 7 8 9 10 Action/Results:	Time _____ Location/Type: Severity 1 2 3 4 5 6 7 8 9 10 Action/Results:
Tests/ Procedures	Specimen: time: procedure: prep:	Specimen: time: procedure: prep:	Specimen: time: procedure: prep:
SIG.			

LABS							
TIME							
SUGAR INITIALS							
STOOL ACETONE							
CHEM BG HEMATEST							

NUTRITION:

	BREAKFAST	LUNCH	DINNER
DIET/SOLUTION:			
% AMT./RATE			
S—SELF A—ASSIST F-FEED TF—TUBE FEEDING			

HYGIENE: TIME: _____

BEDBATH   SHOWER   TUB/SITZ

SELF   ASSIST   COMPLETE

NAME _____ HOSPITAL NO. _____ DATE _____

Figure 7–3. (concluded)

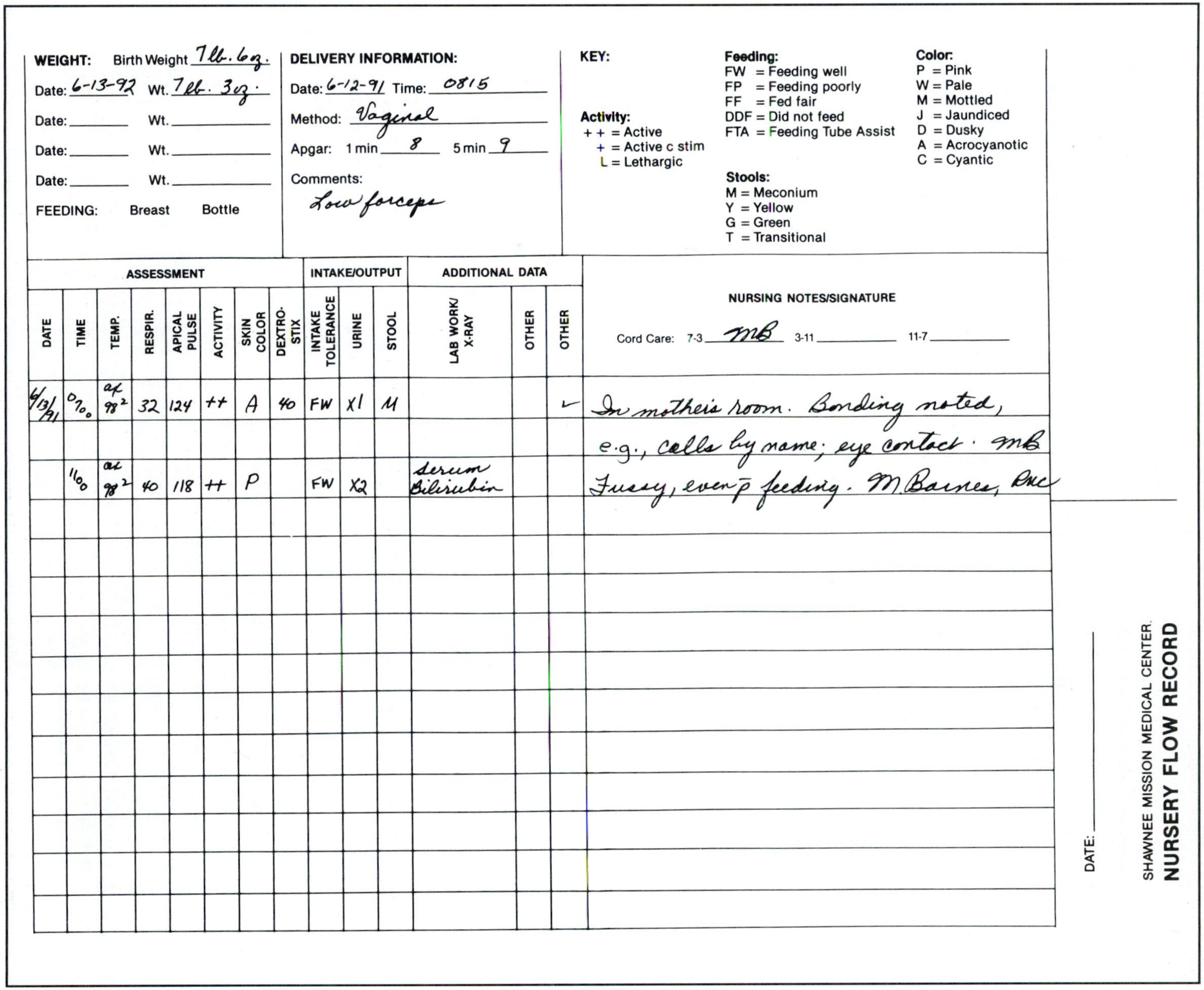

NURSERY FLOW RECORD

WEIGHT:
Birth Weight: 7 lb. 6 g.
Date: 6-13-92 Wt. 7 lb. 3 g.
Date: ___ Wt. ___
Date: ___ Wt. ___
Date: ___ Wt. ___

FEEDING: Breast   Bottle

DELIVERY INFORMATION:
Date: 6-12-91 Time: 0815
Method: Vaginal
Apgar: 1 min   8   5 min   9
Comments: Low forceps

KEY:

Activity:
++ = Active
+ = Active c stim
L = Lethargic

Feeding:
FW = Feeding well
FP = Feeding poorly
FF = Fed fair
DDF = Did not feed
FTA = Feeding Tube Assist

Color:
P = Pink
W = Pale
M = Mottled
J = Jaundiced
D = Dusky
A = Acrocyanotic
C = Cyantic

Stools:
M = Meconium
Y = Yellow
G = Green
T = Transitional

Cord Care: 7-3 ___ MB ___ 3-11 ___ 11-7 ___

ASSESSMENT / INTAKE/OUTPUT / ADDITIONAL DATA

DATE	TIME	TEMP.	RESPIR.	APICAL PULSE	ACTIVITY	SKIN COLOR	DEXTRO-STIX	INTAKE TOLERANCE	URINE	STOOL	LAB WORK/X-RAY	OTHER	OTHER
6/13/91	0200	98²	32	124	++	A	40	FW	X1	M	serum bilirubin		
	0600	98²	40	118	++	P	P	FW	X2	M			L

NURSING NOTES/SIGNATURE

To mother's room. Bonding noted, e.g., calls by name, eye contact. MB
Teaching, event p feeding. M Barnes, RN.

DATE: _____

SHAWNEE MISSION MEDICAL CENTER.
NURSERY FLOW RECORD

Figure 7–4. Nursery Flow Record.
Courtesy of Shawnee Mission Medical Center, Merriam, KS.

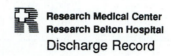

Research Medical Center
Research Belton Hospital
Discharge Record

Date _3-6-92_____ Time _1130_____

To: (HOME)   3W   2N   ECF
OTHER _____

By: AMBULATORY   (WC)   CART
AMBULANCE   OTHER _____

If discharged to 3W or 2N, Stop Here.

USE BALLPOINT PEN: PRESS FIRMLY AGAINST A HARD SURFACE

Name of Medication	Dose/Frequency	Purpose	Pharmacy Take Home	Prescription Given	At Home
Nitroglycerin	- tabs 1, as needed	- Chest Pain			✓
Tylenol #3	- 1 tab. every 4 hrs, as needed	- for general discomfort		✓	
Milk of Magnesia	- 2 oz.	- as needed for constipation			✓

Follow Up Care with Physician:

☑ Notify physician if you experience any of the following: _pain on urination._
☐ No Appointment Necessary   _inability to urinate._
☑ Make Appointment within _10 days_   _blood in urine._
☑ Card/Number Given   _____

After Discharge Instruction:

☑ Diet _Regular. As before surgery_
☑ Exercise/Activity _May walk ½ mile per day. No lifting._
☐ Dressing Changes/Special Equipment/Supplies _____
_____
_____

Other Information - (List Medications Already Administered)
Tylenol #3, one tab at 0900
_____
_____

I understand the Above Instructions.

Don Franklin
Patient/Other

Discharge Instruction By:

G. Gordon RN

Form #10-36-165 (Rev 8-90)

Form Dist.: Yellow - Patient, White - Chart, Pink - Physician

Figure 7–5. Discharge Record.
Courtesy of Research Medical Center, Kansas City, MO.

Methods for Writing Nursing Progress Notes

As mentioned above, all client record systems provide a section for writing descriptive progress notes about the patient's status and progress. The four prevalent methods of writing progress notes are (1) chronological narrative, (2) SOAP format, (3) focus charting, and (4) charting by exception.

Chronological Narrative Charting Narrative charting (e.g., Figure 7–6) is the traditional charting format. It is used primarily in source-oriented record systems. Nurses write notes in paragraph form for a given period of time (e.g., every two hours, or twice a shift). Events and client responses are recorded in chronological order. The disadvantage of this format is that it is not systematic; one entry may contain information about several problems or interventions. Because it is difficult to follow the progress of a specific problem without reading all of the recorded information, the narrative section is often combined with a flowsheet, as in Figure 7–4.

Figure 7–7 is a sample of a form that uses a nursing framework to impose structure upon the nursing notes. This form is divided into sections using a modification of Roy's Adaptation model (1980). (Appendix B is an admission assessment form using this model.) Interventions and patient responses are recorded in the appropriate box. It is still difficult to follow the progress of a particular problem, but the data can be easily traced by process categories (e.g., elimination, oxygenation) or modes (e.g., role function, self-concept, interdependence). Notes that are too long to fit in the boxes are charted in a section called "Nursing Progress Notes" on the back of the form.

SOAP Charting The SOAP method originated with the problem-oriented records system, but is now used in other systems as well. SOAP is an acronym for Subjective data, Objective data, Assessment, and Plan. SOAP charting is problem-oriented; that is, each SOAP note refers to a specific problem. Multiple problems require multiple SOAP notes. Most agencies require a SOAP note on each active problem every 24 hours, or more often if the problem status changes. An explanation of the SOAP elements follows.

S—Subjective data is information obtained from what the client says. It describes the client's perspectives, perceptions, and experience of the problem. When possible, quote the client's words; otherwise, summarize his statement. Include *subjective data* only when it is important and relevant to the problem.

O—Objective data consists of information that can be measured or observed by use of the senses (e.g., vital signs, bowel sounds, laboratory and X-ray results). The objective data section is also used to record interventions that have been carried out (e.g., "Taught correct procedure for drawing up insulin"). Note that this differs from the definition in Chapter 3, which states that *data* is information about the *client*. In the SOAP recording method, *objective data* refers to nursing interventions as well as client responses.

A—The **Assessment** is an interpretation or explanation of the subjective and objective data. During the *initial* assessment, the master problem list is created from interpretations and conclusions about the *S* and *O* data. At this time, the *Assessment* entry should be a statement of the problem. In all subsequent SOAP notes, the *A* should describe the client's condition and

DATE	TIME	NOTES	SIGNATURE
9-6-92	0800	Refused breakfast. States, "I feel too sick." abd. firm but not distended. No bowel sounds heard p̄ auscultating for 5 min. in ⓡ quadrant. Using PCA (morphine) frequently for incision pain (see med. Record).	S. Fried, RN
	0900	200 cc. clear, yellow emesis ————	S. Fried, RN
	0930	100 cc. clear, yellow emesis. c/o severe nausea. Compazine 5 mg. given I M in LVG area. Closed door & advised to lie still to decrease sensation of nausea.	S. Fried, RN
	1030	States still nauseated, but less severe. No further emesis. T.E.D. hose removed for 15 min & reapplied. No edema or redness on legs. Dangled @ bedside for 5 min. Moves c̄ much reluctance. States, "Hurts too much." ————	S. Fried, RN

Shawnee Mission Medical Center
PATIENT PROGRESS RECORD

Figure 7–6. Patient Progress Record
Courtesy of Shawnee Mission Medical Center, Merriam, KS.

		DATE 9-6-92	2300-0700	0700-1500	1500-2300
		SIGNATURE		*S Fried, RN*	
EXERCISE/REST		Type of activity How far? How long? Repositioned ROM Aides (walker, cane, crutches, etc.) Sleep	Sleeping _____ Reposition q 2 hrs _____ Checked q 1 hr _____ ____Help of ___	1030 ____Help of _1_ *Lying still most of a.m. to ↓ nausea. Dangled at bedside for 5 min. Moves c̄ much reluctance; States, "Hurts too much."*	____Help of ___
NUTRITION/ FLUID/ELEC		N/V Feeding assistance Tube feedings	No Problems Identified _____ Not Assessed/Sleeping _____	No Problems Identified _____ ____Feed ____Assist *0800 Refused break- fast. States, "I feel too sick. (See Nursing Prog. Notes)*	No Problems Identified _____ ____Feed ____Assist
ELIMINATION		Stool: freq/char Urine: freq/char Bowel sounds flatus, distention	No Problems Identified _____	No Problems Identified _____ *0800 - Abd. firm, but not distended. No bowel sounds heard p̄ auscultating 5 min. in ℞ quad.*	No Problems Identified _____
OXYGENATION		Breathing pattern Breath sounds Chest tubes Sputum O_2 Tissue perfusion	Eupneic _____	0800 Eupneic *SF*	Eupneic _____
CIRCULATION		Pulse quality/presence Heart sounds Edema	See Graphic _____ Not Assessed/Sleeping _____	1030 See Graphic ✔ *T.E.D. hose removed for 15 min + reapplied No edema or red- ness of legs.*	See Graphic _____
TEMP REGUL/ SKIN INTEGRITY		Skin assessment Wound/incision Rash Heparin Lock Site	Warm/Dry _____	0800 Warm/Dry *SF*	Warm/Dry _____

PATIENT DAILY ASSESSMENT SUMMARY FLOW SHEET

Figure 7–7. Patient Daily Assessment Summary Flow Sheet.
Courtesy of Shawnee Mission Medical Center, Merriam, KS.

	DATE 9-6-92	2300-0700	0700-1500	1500-2300
	SIGNATURE		S Fried RN	
SENSORY/ NEURO	Visual/hearing aid Communication aid Perceptual ability Pain Neuro assessment Level of conscious.	Alert/Oriented _____ No c/o pain _____	Alert/Oriented _____ No c/o pain _____ 0800 Using PCA Morphine frequently for incision pain (see MAR) 1030 — See Ns. Prog. Notes	Alert/Oriented _____ No c/o pain _____
ENDOCRINE	Uterine/prostate status Menstrual/lactation Pregnancy Endocrine status	See Diabetic Record _____ NA _____	See Diabetic Record _____ NA ✓ SF	See Diabetic Record _____ NA _____
SELF CONCEPT/ INTERDEPENDENCE	Emotional status Coping mechanisms Role of S.O.	Cooperative _____ Pleasant _____	Cooperative _____ Pleasant _____	Cooperative _____ Pleasant _____
ROLE FUNCTION	Knowledge deficit Learning abilities Discharge planning Adaptive difficulty to new roles			

	TIME	NURSING PROGRESS NOTES
NURSING PROGRESS NOTES	0900	NUTRITION: 200 cc clear, yellow emesis ——— S. Fried, RN
	0930	NUTRITION: 100 cc clear, yellow emesis. C/o severe nausea. Compazine 5 mg. given IM in LVG area. Closed door + advised to lie still to ↓ sensation of nausea ——— S Fried, RN
	1030	NUTRITION: States still nauseated, but less severe. No further emesis. ——— S Fried, RN

Figure 7–7. (concluded)

level of progress, not merely restate the diagnosis or problem. If a new problem develops later, it would be stated under the *A* at that time, but not in subsequent entries.

P—The **Plan** is the plan of care designed to resolve the stated problem. The person who enters the problem on the record writes the *initial* plan. For medical problems, the physician writes orders for diagnostic and treatment interventions; the nurse focuses on nursing interventions to monitor and support the medical treatment plan. Other disciplines, such as physical therapy, add their specific interventions to the plan. For nursing diagnoses, the nurse develops the primary treatment plan, and other disciplines add to the plan as needed. When writing subsequent SOAP notes for a problem, the plan is compared to plans in previous notes; then decisions are made about revising, continuing, or discontinuing previous interventions.

SOAPIE and SOAPIER are variations of the SOAP format. In these formats, the interventions (*I*) are written separately from the objective data (*O*), and an evaluation component (*E*) is added. The SOAPIER format adds a section for revision of the plan (*R*).

APIE is a similar format, developed by Groah and Reed (1983, p. 1184). In this format, the assessment (*A*) includes both subjective and objective data, as well as the nursing diagnosis; the plan (*P*) includes predicted outcomes with the nursing actions; and implementation (*I*) and evaluation (*E*) are the same as in the SOAPIE format. See Table 7–2 for a comparison of the SOAP, SOAPIER, and APIE formats. Compare these entries to Figures 7–6 and 7–7, which contain the same information about nausea.

Focus Charting® Like SOAP notes, Focus Charting uses key words to label and organize the progress notes, but the subject of the note is not necessarily a problem. According to Lampe (1985, p. 43), a focus can be any of the following:

A current client concern or behavior
A significant change in client status or behavior
A significant event in the client's therapy

A focus should be something that requires nursing care; therefore, it should not be a medical diagnosis. The focus can, however, describe needs and conditions that are *associated with* the medical diagnosis. For example, foci for a client with a medical diagnosis of fractured femur might include admission information, preoperative teaching, Pain, High Risk for Constipation, and cast/traction assessment.

The Focus method uses three columns: Date/Time, Focus, and Progress Notes. The progress notes column is organized in a DAR format.

D—The **data** includes the nurse's observations of client status and behaviors. This might include data from flowsheets (e.g., vital signs, intake, and output). It includes both subjective and objective data, but they are not labeled *S* and *O*. This section corresponds to the assessment step of the nursing process.

A—**Action** entries include interventions just performed as well as plans for further action. This step corresponds to the planning and implementation steps of the nursing process.

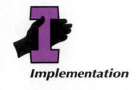

Implementation

R—Response entries describe the client's responses to nursing and medical interventions. The data in this section consists of client measurements and behaviors, many of which will be recorded on flowsheets and checklists. This section corresponds to the evaluation step of the nursing process.

Table 7–2. Comparison of the SOAP, SOAPIER, **and** APIE **Formats**

SOAP Format	SOAPIER Format	APIE Format
9/6/92 #5. Nausea 1030	9/6/92 #5. Nausea 1030	9/6/92 #5. Nausea 1030
S— Refused breakfast. "I feel too sick." c/o severe nausea during A.M. Stated less severe after IM Compazine.	S— Refused breakfast. "I feel too sick." c/o severe nausea during A.M.	A—Post-op nausea & vomiting. Refused breakfast. "I feel too sick." Abd. firm, not distended. No bowel sounds heard after auscultating 5 min. @ quadrant. Vomited x 2; total 300 cc clear, yellow emesis.
O—Abd. firm but not distended. No bowel sounds heard after auscultating for 5 min. @ quadrant. Vomited x 2: total 300 cc clear, yellow emesis. Closed door: advised to lie still to decrease sensations of nausea. Compazine 5 mg given IM in LVG area at 0930.	O—Abd. firm but not distended. No bowel sounds heard after auscultating for 5 min. @ quadrant. Vomited x 2: total 300 cc clear, yellow emesis.	
	A—Post-op nausea r/t decreased peristalsis; Compazine somewhat effective.	P— Decrease nausea: Instruct to lie still. Compazine per order.
A—Post-op nausea r/t decreased peristalsis; Compazine somewhat effective. Possible ileus.	P— Instruct to lie still to decrease sensations of nausea. Medicate with Compazine. Continue I&O. Continue to assess for N&V. Assess hydration q shift.	Prevent fluid deficit: Continue to assess N&V. Assess hydration q shift.Continue I&O. If nausea and vomiting continue, notify MD.
P— Continue to observe for N&V. If nausea unrelieved by Compazine, notify MD. Continue I&O. Assess hydration q shift. Offer fluids 40 cc/hr if no further emesis.	I— Instructed to lie still to decrease sensations of nausea. Compazine 5 mg given IM in LVG area at 0930.	I— Instructed to lie still. Compazine 5 mg given IM in LVG area at 0930.
	E— States still nauseated but somewhat relieved after Compazine. Lying still most of A.M. No emesis after Compazine.	E— Lying still most of A.M. No emesis since Compazine given. States still nauseated, but less severe.
	R— Offer fluids 40 cc/hr if no further emesis. If nausea unrelieved by Compazine, notify MD.	

Focus notes can be used in source-, problem-, or computer-oriented record systems. Like the SOAP method, Focus notes can be scanned to quickly find the desired subject; it is not necessary to read the entire set of notes, as in narrative charting. The Focus method is useful for health-promotion and disease-prevention activities because charting can be organized around positive headings instead of problems. Figure 7–8 is an example of a Focus note containing the same information about nausea that appears in Figures 7–6, 7–7, and Table 7–2.

Charting by Exception Charting by exception (CBE) is a method of documenting nursing care developed at St. Luke's Hospital in Milwaukee to save time and eliminate repetitive charting of insignificant information. CBE is a system of record keeping that can be applied just to nursing documentation or to the entire patient record. CBE incorporates three key components for the documenting interventions (Burke and Murphy, 1988, p. 7):

Recording

Date/Time	Focus	Progress Notes
1/6/92		
1430	Post-op nausea	D—Refused breakfast. Stated, "I feel too sick." c/o severe nausea throughout A.M. Vomited x 2, total of 300 cc clear, yellow emesis. Abd. firm but not distended. No bowel sounds auscultated after listening for 5 min. in @ quadrant.
		A—Closed door. Advised to lie still to decrease sensations of nausea. Compazine 5 mg given IM in LVG at 0930 per order. Continue to assess for N&V. If unrelieved by Compazine, notify MD. Continue I&O. Assess hydration x 1 per shift. Increase p.o. fluids to 40 cc/hr if no further emesis.
		R—Nausea somewhat relieved by Compazine. Stated "less severe." No emesis since Compazine administered. See flow sheet for I&O and VS.————R. Keeler, RN

Figure 7–8. Example of a Focus Charting® Note

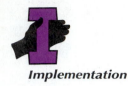

Implementation

1. *Unique flowsheets* that highlight significant findings and define assessment parameters and findings. Completed interventions are documented in the nursing progress notes or on one of the following four flowsheets: Nursing/ Physician Order Flowsheet, the Graphic Record, the Patient Teaching Record, and the Patient Discharge Note. Guidelines on the back of the flowsheets specify what each assessment should include and the norms for each. A check mark beside the assessment indicates that it was made as specified and that the findings were within normal limits. For an exception, the nurse makes an asterisk instead of a check mark, and writes a narrative note describing the unusual finding. Following is an example of guidelines and norms from the Nursing/Physician Order Flowsheet:

GASTROINTESTINAL ASSESSMENT

Guidelines: GI assessment will include abdominal appearance, bowel sounds, palpation, diet tolerance & stools.

Norms: The following will constitute a negative assessment: Abdomen soft, bowel sounds active (5-34/min). No pain with palpation. Tolerates prescribed diet without nausea & vomiting. Having BMs within own normal pattern & consistency. (Burke and Murphy, 1988, p. 11)

If a client needs GI assessments, the nurse writes "GI Assessment" on the Order/Flowsheet. A check mark beside this order indicates that everything in the guidelines was done and that the findings were as described in the norms. If diet tolerance was not assessed, however, the nurse would place an asterisk beside "GI Assessment" and write in the progress notes, "*NPO—Diet tolerance not assessed."

2. *Documentation by reference to Standards of Nursing Practice.* An agency using CBE must develop its own specific, detailed Standards of Nursing Practice that identify the minimum criteria for patient care regardless of clinical area. Some units also have unit-specific standards unique to their type of patient. The following are examples of standards related to hygiene patterns:

> The nurse shall ensure that the patient has oral care offered T.I.D.

> The nurse shall ensure that the patient has a bath and backrub offered daily and a shampoo offered weekly. (Burke and Murphy, 1988, p. 33)

A check mark in the "Routine Standards" box on the Graphic Record indicates that all appropriate standards were implemented. No comment is written unless there are exceptions to the standards. This eliminates the need to document routine interventions such as repositioning, traction care, and care of the IV site. Exceptions to standards are clearly described in the progress notes.

3. *Bedside accessibility of documentation forms.* In the CBE approach, all flowsheets are kept at the bedside. Care is documented as it is implemented, eliminating the need to chart from memory or transcribe information from a worksheet to the permanent record.

In this system, only significant findings or exceptions to norms are written in the descriptive nursing progress notes. The nurse writes a progress note, in SOAP format, when she (1) activates a nursing diagnosis, (2) evaluates a goal, (3) resolves or discontinues a nursing diagnosis, (4) writes a discharge summary, or (5) makes a major revision of the care plan.

Guidelines for Charting

Legal requirements for record keeping vary from state to state. In addition, each agency has its own standards and policies for record keeping. Such policies may describe which personnel are responsible for recording on certain forms, the frequency with which entries are to be made, which abbreviations are acceptable, and the preferred way to handle an error in recording. You should, of course, be familiar with legal and policy requirements. In addition, observe the following general guidelines.

When to Chart   Timing guidelines are critical for legal reasons as well as for their contribution to safe care.

1. *Date and time each entry.* Using the 24-hour (military) clock avoids confusion about whether a time is A.M or P.M. For example, 9:30 A.M. would be written as 0930 in military time; 9:30 P.M. would be 2130.

2. For each entry, *indicate both the time the entry was made and the time the observation or intervention occurred,* if different. For example, in a chart entry timed 1445, you might write, "Drank 150 cc water at 1245, vomited 200 cc clear fluid at 1310."

3. When possible, *record the nursing action or client response immediately after it occurs.* The longer you wait, the less accurate your memory. Immediate recording is especially important for medications and treatments because it helps insure that the client will not be medicated or treated a second time by a different nurse. It is usually acceptable to record routine repetitive nursing actions at the end of the shift (e.g., hourly position changes, mouth care).

4. *Never leave the unit for an extended break unless all important information has been charted.* (Rationale is similar to that for Guideline 3.)

5. *Do not document interventions before carrying them out.* The client might refuse the treatment or you might encounter an emergency situation that prevents you from carrying out the intervention. Another staff member, seeing it charted, might conclude the action has been done and not wish to repeat it. The result would be that the client does not get the care he needs.

What to Chart

1. *The nurse who makes the entry should sign it.* You should not sign someone else's notes. Remember that the person signing the entry is accountable for the entry.

2. In general, *you should not chart actions performed by someone else.* In some situations, it is permissible to chart an action you did not perform, but your note should identify the person who actually gave the care (e.g., "Assisted to car by nursing assistant. L. Woods, RN").

Recording

Comparison of Conventional and Military Time	
Conventional	Military
12:01 A.M.	0001
12:15 A.M	0015
12:45 A.M	0045
1 A.M	0100
2 A.M	0200
3 A.M	0300
4 A.M	0400
5 A.M	0500
6 A.M	0600
7 A.M	0700
8 A.M	0800
9 A.M	0900
10 A.M	1000
11 A.M	1100
12 NOON	1200
12:01 P.M.	1201
12:15 P.M.	1215
12:45 P.M.	1245
1 P.M.	1300
2 P.M.	1400
3 P.M.	1500
4 P.M.	1600
5 P.M.	1700
6 P.M.	1800
7 P.M.	1900
8 P.M.	2000
9 P.M.	2100
10 P.M.	2200
11 P.M.	2300
12 MIDNIGHT	2400

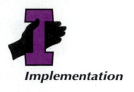

Implementation

3. *Progress notes must be accurate and correct.* Never write an assessment you are unsure of. If you are not absolutely sure the patient's lungs are "clear to auscultation," ask someone else to check before you chart.

4. *Progress notes should be factual and specific.* Chart what you see, hear, smell or observe; not opinions and interpretations. To improve the precision of your charting, think, "Exactly what happened, and how, when and where did it happen?" For example, you would chart, "Talking constantly, pacing the floor; pulse 120," rather than "Patient is anxious." An exception is that in SOAP charting, the A *is* an interpretation of the S-O data. Any time you think an interpretation should be charted, be sure to include the supporting data.

5. *Progress notes should be clear and specific.* Do not use vague generalities, such as *good, normal,* or *sufficient.* It is better to say "a 2 x 2 cm area of blood" than "a small amount of blood."

6. *Do not use negative, prejudicial terms* (e.g., *uncooperative, noncompliant, unpleasant*). Instead, describe what the client did that was uncooperative (e.g., "Yelled, 'Go away!' and threw his tray on the floor").

7. *Chart entries should be appropriate and relevant.* You do not need to record everything you know about the client. Recording irrelevant data is a waste of time, and it is sometimes an invasion of privacy.

8. *Progress notes should be complete.* This is essential for communication among caregivers, as well as for legal purposes. For example, if there is no record of turning and skin care, nurses may be found negligent when the client develops a dermal ulcer. Box 7–3 is a guide suggested by Kozier et al. (1991) to help you select essential and complete information about clients.

9. To organize your narrative entry, *include* **D—I—E**. Don't actually label the entry with these letters or words; use them as a memory device.

D-*ata*	What did you observe about the patient (*S-O*)?
I-*ntervention*	What actions did you take? What did you do?
E-*valuation*	What was the patient's response to the actions?
	What did he say or do? How did his condition change?

10. *Be brief.* Do not sacrifice completeness, but *omit unnecessary words,* such as *patient.* It is assumed the entry refers to the patient. Progress notes are usually written in incomplete sentences, but be sure to end each thought with a period. For example, write "300 cc clear emesis," rather than "The patient vomited 300 cc of clear fluid."

How to Chart

1. *Use dark ink.* Most agencies specify black ink. Erasable ink is not acceptable.

2. *Write legibly, or print.* Narcan and Marcaine are different drugs, but they may look very much alike if handwriting is illegible or messy.

3. *Use correct grammar, spelling, and punctuation.*

4. *Use standard symbols, terminology , and abbreviations.* Many agencies have a list of abbreviations and terminology they accept. If not, use only those that are standard and used universally. Other professionals must be able to interpret the terms correctly, especially if the record is ever used as evidence in court. If you are in doubt about an abbreviation, write the term out fully.

5. *Sign each entry with your name and title* (e.g. "Kay Wittman, RN" or "K. Wittman, RN").

6. *Chart entries on consecutive lines. Never skip a line or leave a line blank.* Draw a line through any blank spaces before or after your signature. For example, "Lungs clear to auscultation. Skin warm and dry._____ K. Wittman, RN."

Box 7–3. Essential Charting Information

Essential charting information includes the following:

1. Any behavior changes, for example:
Indications of strong emotions, such as anxiety or fear
Marked changes in mood
A change in level of consciousness, such as stupor
Regression in relationships with family or friends

2. Any changes in physical function, such as:
Loss of balance
Loss of strength
Difficulty hearing or seeing

3. Any physical sign or symptom that:
Is severe, such as severe pain
Tends to recur or persist
Is not normal, such as elevated body temperature
Gets worse, such as gradual weight loss
Indicates a complication, such as inability to void following surgery
Is not relieved by prescribed measures (such as continued failure to defecate or to sleep)
Indicates faulty health habits, such as lice on the scalp
Is a known danger signal, such as a lump in the breast

4. Any nursing interventions provided, such as:
Medications administered
Therapies
Activities of daily living, if agency policy dictates
Teaching clients self-care

5. Visits by a physician or other members of the health team

From Kozier, Erb, and Olivieri,. *Fundamentals of Nursing,* 4th ed. (Redwood City, CA: Addison-Wesley Nursing, 1991), p. 131. Reprinted by permission.

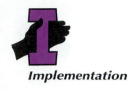

Implementation

7. *Correct errors by drawing a single line through the mistaken entry* and writing the word *error* above it. Initial the error, and then rewrite the entry correctly. These instructions may vary according to agency policy. Never try to erase or obliterate the entry: the incorrect entry should still be visible. Do not insert words above the line or between words.

8. *Be sure the client's name and identification number are on every page.*

Oral Reports

In addition to written records, nurses use oral reports to communicate nursing interventions and client status. When the client's condition is changing rapidly, physicians and other caregivers must be constantly informed. Oral reports are also given when a client is transferred from one unit to another (e.g., from the emergency room to a medical floor), at change of shift, and when family members request reports of the client's condition. A report is given to communicate specific information about what has been observed, done, or considered. It should be concise, but still contain all pertinent information. Remember, a report is a summary, not a detailed accounting.

A **change-of-shift report** is given to the on-coming nurse by the nurse who has been responsible for the patient. The on-duty charge nurse may report to on-coming nursing personnel for all clients on a team or a unit, or a primary nurse may report to the on-coming nurse for her own patients. Reports may be given in a meeting, on walking rounds, or on audiotape. Tape-recorded reports are usually less time-consuming; however, face-to-face reports allow for questions and clarification. A typical change-of-shift report includes the following:

1. *Basic identifying information for each client.* Name, room number, age, medical diagnosis or reason for admission, admission date, and physicians. This will vary depending upon the setting. (e.g., in a long-term care facility, you might omit the admission date).

2. *A description of the client's present condition.* Include only significant measurements. It is not necessary to report that the vital signs are normal, unless this is a change for the client (e.g., "After medication her temperature returned to 98.6°").

3. *Significant changes in the client's condition.* Report both deterioration and improvement in condition (e.g., "At 1400 her blood pressure was 150/94; baseline was under 130/80 until that time"). When reporting changes, organize your report as follows: State what you observed, its meaning (if appropriate), what action was taken, the client's response, and the continuing plan for the on-coming nurse.

Example: "Her respirations are slow and shallow, and she has weak cough effort. I helped her turn and cough hourly. Her lungs are clear, but she still does not deep breathe well. You should continue to have her cough and deep breathe hourly unless you see improvement."

4. *Progress in goal achievement for identified nursing diagnoses* (e.g., "Mrs. Martin has High Risk for Impaired Skin Integrity. We are presently meeting our goal of intact skin").

5. *Results of diagnostic tests or other therapies performed in the last 24 hours* (e.g., "Blood cultures were negative").

6. *Significant emotional responses* (e.g., "She has been crying since she was told she won't be able to go home").

7. *Description of invasive lines, pumps, and other apparatus* (e.g., Foley catheter).

8. *Description of important activities* that occurred on your shift. This should not be a detailed catalog of the patient's day. Report only significant activities (e.g., there is no need to report that all clients showered and ambulated in the hall).

9. *Description of care the on-coming nurse needs to do.* This does not include routine care such as the daily linen change or routine vital signs, unless it is something you were unable to accomplish (e.g., "Her bed still needs to be changed"). Include laboratory and diagnostic tests and preps that the on-coming nurse should do or special observations that she should make (e.g., "She is scheduled for surgery in the morning, and should be NPO after midnight").

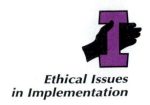

Ethical Issues in Implementation

ETHICAL ISSUES IN IMPLEMENTATION

Items 1 and 2 of the ANA Code of Ethics (Appendix A) emphasize respect for human dignity and the client's right to privacy. Issues of confidentiality and dignity arise frequently in the implementation step. As client advocates, nurses are obligated to protect the client's humanity, and it is during implementation of care that the choice exists for humanization or depersonalization of care.

Item 1 of the ANA Code of Ethics emphasizes *respect for human dignity* (1985). Many of the procedures performed during implementation are invasive or require the client to be exposed or assume awkward positions. Nurses are obliged to respect the client's personhood by providing adequate draping and privacy for such interventions as enemas, catheterizations, and bed baths. These may seem like routine procedures to a busy nurse, but they can be very depersonalizing for the patient. The more skilled you become in technical procedures, the more you should be able to adopt and respect the patient's perspective on what is occurring.

The manner in which you address the patient can also preserve or diminish his dignity. It is easy to fall into the habit of addressing everyone as *dear* or *honey*. Some nurses do this in an effort to express caring; others do it because it is too hard to remember the patients' names. However, patients lose their individuality when they all have the same name—even if it is a "nice" name. This is a particularly disrespectful practice when the patient is older than the nurse. You should not call a patient by his first name unless you know that he prefers it, or you are on a reciprocal first-name basis with him.

Privacy and confidentiality are related to the issue of client dignity. Item 2 of the ANA Code of Ethics treats these subjects as well: "The nurse safeguards the client's right to privacy by judiciously protecting information of a confidential nature" (ANA, 1985).

When you provide good nursing care, patients feel comfortable with you. They may trust you enough to disclose important and personal information (e.g., "This baby does not belong to my husband, but he doesn't know"). Do not chart

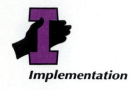

Implementation

such information unless it is important to the care plan, and do not share it with other members of the staff either informally or in reports. Nurses are free to share only information that is pertinent to the patient's health.

The law restricts access to the client's written record. Even if it did not, nurses would have a moral obligation to protect the confidentiality of the record. This means that insurance companies and other agencies have no right to the information in the record without the client's permission; nor does the client's family. Legally, the client must sign an authorization for review, copying, or release of information from the chart. When charts are used for educational or research purposes, the student or researcher is obligated to avoid using the client's name or identifying her in any way.

Widespread use of computer-based record systems increases the risk that the client's privacy will be accidentally or intentionally violated. To help ensure confidentiality, agencies issue passwords to those authorized to use the system. Nurses should be aware of the potential for abuse of computer data systems. Angry employees may break through system security to destroy, change, or distribute data, or computer hackers may break into the system simply for the challenge. To help ensure client privacy, you should not give unauthorized users your password or access to the computer.

SUMMARY

Implementation
- ✓ is action-focused.
- ✓ requires nurses to perform or delegate dependent, independent, and collaborative actions.
- ✓ may use one of four common systems for allocating tasks and authority: functional, team, or primary nursing, or case management.
- ✓ requires nurses to seek help as needed to perform interventions safely and effectively.
- ✓ should preserve confidentiality and client dignity.
- ✓ relates to client readiness and the nurse's cognitive, technical, and inter-personal skills.
- ✓ is completed when the nursing actions have been carried out and re-corded, along with the client's reactions to them. (The client record or chart is a permanent, legal document of the client's health care and status.)
- ✓ is documented in flowsheets and narrative notes, and reported orally at change of shift and when a client is transferred.

Skill-Building Activities

Practice in Critical Thinking: Analyzing Statements

Every day you hear or read many statements. Some statements seem to be correct when you first hear or read them; yet as you think further about them you find that you disagree. In these cases it is especially important to analyze why you agree or disagree.

Begin by considering the statement carefully to make sure you understand what the speaker or author is saying. Next, think about the subject and determine whether you agree with the statement. The following are examples of questions you could consider to help you. Has the author used key words in the same way you use them? Has the author made an assumption with which you do not agree? Has the author made a mistake, like faulty logic or incorrect mathematics? Finally, you should state clearly whether or not you agree, and give reasons for your judgment.

Step 1: Study the statement to make sure you understand what the author is saying.

Step 2: Determine whether or not you agree with the statement.

Step 3: State clearly whether or not you agree, and give reasons for your judgment.

Learning the Skill

1. Analyze the following statement about nursing care delivery systems. Go through the three steps and analyze the statement.

   In primary nursing each patient has one nurse who is accountable for and well informed about his care. Because it provides continuity of care, primary nursing is the preferred model for delivering nursing care.

   Step 1. Study the statement to be sure you understand what the author is saying.

   a. What is meant by primary nursing?

   b. What is meant by continuity of care?

   Step 2. Determine whether or not you agree with the statement.

   a. Has the author left anything out of the argument?

   b. Has the author used any terms incorrectly?

247

c. Has the author used faulty logic?

Step 3. State clearly whether or not you agree, and give reasons for your judgment.

Applying the Skill

1. Analyze the following statement about computer-based records. State clearly whether you agree or not, and state your reasons if you disagree. Try to go through the three steps mentally before writing.

> Computer-based records are a threat to patients' privacy because of the possibility they may be accessed by angry employees or hackers. A great deal of time and expense are involved in teaching nursing staff to use computers for charting and care planning. For these reasons, hospitals should not use computer-based records for charting and care planning.

Step 1. Study the statement to be sure you understand what the author is saying.

a. What is meant by computer-based records?

b. What is meant by patients' privacy?

Step 2. Determine whether or not you agree with the statement.

a. Has the author left anything out of the argument?

b. Has the author used any terms incorrectly?

c. Has the author used faulty logic?

Step 3. State clearly whether or not you agree, and give reasons for your judgment.

2. Analyze the following statement about "charting by exception." In your response, clearly state whether you agree or not, and state your reasons for disagreeing. Try to go through the three steps mentally before writing.

   Charting by exception should not be used because most people believe that if it isn't charted, it wasn't done.

* Adapted from *Critical Thinking Worksheets*, a supplement of *Addison-Wesley Chemistry*, by Wilbraham et al. (Menlo Park, CA: Addison-Wesley Publishing Company, 1990).

(Answer Key, p. 382)

Case Study

Read the following case study. Several of the exercises will refer to it.

Nancy Atwell is a 32-year-old teacher who lives alone. She has been diagnosed as having rheumatoid arthritis for approximately 4 years. This change has made her knees painful and has limited the motion and weight-bearing ability of her knee joints. She has recently been diagnosed as having endometriosis. Medical treatment has been unsuccessful in relieving her pain and dysmenorrhea, and she now enters the hospital to have an abdominal hysterectomy.

On her previous admission for treatment of her arthritis, she was quiet, withdrawn, and extremely concerned for her privacy. Now she seems more outgoing and less overtly concerned about privacy. When questioned, Ms. Atwell states she has had no previous surgical experience, but denies feeling nervous about the operation. She says she is having "quite a bit" of abdominal cramping now.

Her preoperative orders follow:

1. S.S. enema at HS

2. Nembutal 100 mg p.o. at HS

3. NPO after midnight

4. pHisohex shower in A.M.

5. Pre-op med: Demerol 50 mg and Vistaril 25 mg IM at 0600

6. Ibuprofen 500 mg p.o. every 3–4 hours prn for abdominal or joint pain

1. Define and give an example of each of the following types of nursing actions (you do not need to use the case study, but you may if you wish):

Type	Definition	Example
Dependent		
Independent		
Interdependent		

2. What activities may be a threat to Ms. Atwell's privacy and dignity?

3. A nursing diagnosis for Ms. Atwell is "High Risk for Impaired Home Maintenance Management: Inability to manage own care on dismissal r/t single state (no one to help out), pain in knees, and post-op pain and weakness."

   a. What collaborative (interdependent) nursing action might be performed for this nursing diagnosis?

b. What independent nursing action might be performed?

4. Ms. Atwell's nurse is preparing to implement the order for a pHisohex shower. The nurse has the necessary supplies, but she does not know the rationale for giving a pHisohex shower. What should she do?

5. If you were Ms. Atwell's nurse, what would you do to prepare her before you implement the following medical order: Nembutal 100 mg p.o. at H.S.?

6. What is an example of therapeutic communication that might be needed by Ms. Atwell? (One example is given for you.)

   Example: Talking to her to assess for feelings of grief related to her inability to bear children after the hysterectomy.

7. State the guideline for implementing nursing strategies that is demonstrated by the following situations (refer to Box 7–2 on page 223).

   a. It is important for Ms. Bates to be turned frequently, but it causes her a great deal of pain. It is 15 minutes past time to turn her, but she has a visitor—the first one she has had in several weeks. In order to meet Ms. Bates's emotional needs, the nurse decides to wait until the visitor leaves to do the turning.

   Guideline:

b. The physician has ordered Bromocriptine 2.5 mg p.o. The nurse does not know the side effects of this drug, so he looks it up in the Hospital Formulary.

Guideline:

c. The nurse pulls the curtain around the bed and drapes the client's legs and perineum before inserting an indwelling catheter.

Guideline:

d. The nurse asks a colleague to double-check her insulin dosage.

Guideline:

e. The nurse uses sterile technique to insert the urinary catheter.

Guideline:

f. The nurse takes the client's blood pressure before administering an antihypertensive medication.

Guideline:

8. Indicate the type of client record system illustrated by the following statements and examples.

   S—Source-oriented   **P**—Problem-oriented   **C**—Computer-based

   a. ___ Organized according to discipline. Special section for lab reports and so forth.

   b. ___ All disciplines chart on the same progress notes.

   c. ___ Requires a password or code in order to access patients' records.

   d. ___ Information about the client's hypertension is scattered throughout the chart. It is difficult to determine exactly what has been done specifically for the elevated blood pressure.

   e. ___ All health professionals contribute to the problem list and care plan.

   f. ___ Information can be easily retrieved in a variety of forms (e.g., a list of the client's treatments for the day, a list of suggested interventions for his nursing diagnosis).

9. Chart the following information in DAR format (focus charting): Mr. Jarrett says his head hurts. He has his eyes shut tightly; he says the light makes them hurt. The nurse places a cool cloth on his head and closes the door to his room. She gives him Tylenol #3, tabs. i, p.o., at 6 p.m., as ordered. When she reassesses Mr. Jarrett in one hour, he says it still hurts. She plans to disturb him as little as possible and keep the room dark. She wants the evening nurse to call Dr. King if Mr. Jarrett's headache is unrelieved after the second dose of medication.

10. Use Figure 7–9 to chart the following data about Ms. Atwell. Chart in the 1500–2300 column—you are the evening nurse. Much of the normal data can be recorded by making check marks. Everything else should be charted narratively under "Nursing Progress Notes." Notice that this is a two-page form, based on the Roy Adaptation model.

Data

Ms. Atwell seems outgoing and not overtly concerned about privacy. When questioned, she states she has had no previous surgical experience, but denies feeling nervous about the operation. She gets up to go to the bathroom and walks about in the room several times during the evening. She walks erect and with a steady gait.

She eats all of her evening meal. At 9 P.M. (2100) you give her a soapsuds enema; she has a large, unformed stool. You tell her that she cannot have anything to eat or drink after midnight, explaining the rationale for this restriction. She says she understands this. You take this opportunity to do the rest of her preoperative teaching. She states, "I understand."

Your assessment reveals that her oxygenation function is normal. She has +1 edema of her left ankle, which she says is normal for her. Her pedal pulses are strong and equal bilaterally; she has no numbness or tingling in her extremities. Her skin is warm and dry.

She is alert and oriented. She says she is having "quite a bit" of abdominal cramping now. You give her the Ibuprofen at 1800, as ordered, and record it in the medication record (MAR). At 1900, she says, "I feel better now." You assess that she is cooperative (in the "self-concept, interdependence" mode).

254

	DATE	2300-0700	0700-1500	1500-2300
	SIGNATURE			

EXERCISE/REST	Type of activity
	How far? How long?
	Repositioned
	ROM
	Aides (walker, cane, crutches, etc.)
	Sleep
		___Bedrest
		___Reposition
		   q 2 hrs
		___BRP/BSC
		___Chair/WC
		___Walk
		___Sleeping
		___Check q hr
		___Request SR down
		___Tx____hrs
		Patient Response
			___Bedrest
			___Reposition
			   q 2 hrs
			___BRP/BSC
			___Walk
			___Up ad lib
			___Tx ___hrs
			Patient Response
				___Bedrest
				___Reposition
				   q 2 hrs
				___BRP/BSC
				___Walk
				___Up ad lib
				___Tx ___ hrs
				Patient Response

NUTRITION/ FLUID/ELEC	N/V Feeding assistance Tube feedings	___No Problems identified ___Not assessed/sleeping ___NPO	___No Problems identified ___Feed ___Assist Feed ___NPO	___No Problems Identified ___Feed ___Assist Feed ___NPO
ELIMINATION	Stool: freq/char Urine: freq/char Bowel sounds flatus, distention	___No Problems Identified ___Urine ___Abd. status ___Stool ___Incontinent	___No Problems Identified ___Urine ___Abd. status ___Stool ___Incontinent	___No Problems Identified ___Urine ___Abd. status ___Stool ___Incontinent

OXYGENATION	Breathing pattern
	Breath sounds
	Chest tubes
	Sputum
	O_2
	Tissue perfusion
		___Eupneic
		___Lungs clear to
		   auscultation
		___O_2
		___IS c assist
		___Cough/sputum
			___Eupneic
			___Lungs clear to
			   auscultation
			___O_2
			___IS c assist
			___Cough/sputum
				___Eupneic
				___Lungs clear to
				   auscultation
				___O_2
				___IS c assist
				___Cough/sputum

CIRCULATION	Pulse quality/presence
	Heart sounds
	Edema
		___No problems identified
		___Pedal pulses
		___Cap Refill
		___Numbness/tingling
		___Edema
		___TED Hose
		___R/L toes/fingers
		   pink/pale & warm/cool
			___No problems identified
			___Pedal pulses
			___Cap refill
			___Numbness/tingling
			___Edema
			___TED Hose
			___R/L toes/fingers
			   pink/pale & warm/cool
				___No problems identified
				___Pedal pulses
				___Cap refill
				___Numbness/tingling
				___Edema
				___TED Hose
				___R/L toes/fingers
				   pink/pale & warm/cool

TEMP REGUL/ SKIN INTEGRITY	Skin assessment
	Wound/incision
	Rash
	Heparin Lock Site
		___Hep Lock
		___Dressing/incision
		   Normal
		___Warm/dry
		___Cast dry/intact
		___Brace/splint
		___Checked q 2 hr
		   for fit/position
			___Hep Lock
			___Dressing/incision
			   normal
			___Warm/dry
			___Cast dry/intact
			___Brace/splint
			___Checked q 2 hr
			   for fit/position
				___Hep Lock
				___Dressing/incision
				   Normal
				___Warm/dry
				___Cast/dry intact
				___Brace/splint
				___Checked q 2 hr
				   for fit/position

PATIENT DAILY ASSESSMENT
SUMMARY FLOW SHEET
2 NORTH (PILOT)

Figure 7–9. Patient Daily Assessment Summary Flowsheet, 2 North Pilot. Courtesy of Shawnee Medical Center, Merriam, KS.

255

	DATE	2300-0700	0700-1500	1500-2300
	SIGNATURE			
SENSORY/ NEURO	Visual/hearing aid Communication aid Perceptual ability Pain Neuro assessment Level of conscious.	__Alert/oriented __No c/o pain __C/o pain (Location) __See MAR __Dorsi/Plantar flex __Indicates pain relief	__Alert/oriented __No c/o pain __C/o pain (Location) __See MAR __Dorsi/Plantar flex __Indicates pain relief	___Alert/oriented ___No c/o pain ___C/o pain (Location) ___See MAR ___Dorsi/Plantar flex ___Indicates pain relief
ENDOCRINE	Uterine/prostate status Menstrual/lactation Pregnancy Endocrine status	___NA ___No s/s hypo/hyper glycemia ___See Diabetic Record	___NA ___No s/s hypo/hyper glycemia ___See Diabetic Record	___NA ___No s/s hypo/hyper glycemia ___See Diabetic Record
SELF CONCEPT/ INTERDEPENDENCE	Emotional status Coping mechanisms Role of S.O.	___Cooperative ___Freq call lite use/ demands ___Safety assessment min/mod/intense Posey/wrist restraints ___Pt/family emotional support (Mod/intense	___Cooperative ___Freq. call lite use/ demands ___Safety assessment min/mod/intense Posey/wrist restraints ___Pt/family emotional support (mod/intense	___Cooperative ___Freq call lite use/ demands ___Safety assessment min/mod/intense Posey/wrist restraints ___Pt/family emotional support (Mod/intense)
ROLE FUNCTION	Knowledge deficit Learning abilities Discharge planning Adaptive difficulty to new roles	___Nursing cares/ procedures explained ___Special teaching: ___Pt. indicates understanding	___Nursing cares/ procedures explained ___Special teaching: ___Pt. indicates understanding	___Nursing cares/ procedures explained ___Special teaching: ___Pt. indicates understanding

NURSING PROGRESS NOTES

TIME	

Figure 7–9. (concluded)

11. Using the information in Exercise 10, chart in SOAP format all the data that are pertinent for the problem, #2, High Risk for Noncompliance with Pre- and Post-op Instructions r/t lack of knowledge. Your plan for this problem will be to (1) remove water pitcher at 2400 and (2) remind her when she wakes up not to drink anything.

REFERENCES

American Nurses Association. (1973). *Standards of Nursing Practice*. Kansas City, MO.

American Nurses Association. (1985). *American Nurses Association: Code for Nurses*. Kansas City, MO.

American Nurses Association. (1988). *Nursing Case Management*. Kansas City, MO.

Bulechek, G., and McCloskey, J. (1985). *Nursing Interventions: Treatments for Nursing Diagnoses*. Philadelphia: W. B. Saunders.

Burke, L., and Murphy, J. (1988). *Charting by Exception: A Cost-Effective, Quality Approach*. New York: John Wiley and Sons.

Feutz, S. (1989). *Nursing and the Law*. 3rd ed. Eau Claire, WI: Professional Education Systems.

Gordon, M. (1987). *Nursing Diagnosis: Process and Application*. 2nd ed. New York: McGraw-Hill.

Groah, L., and Reed, E. (1983). Your responsibility in documenting care. *Association of Operating Room Nurses Journal, 37* (May): 1174, 1176–77, 1180–85.

Guzzetta, C. (1987). Nursing diagnoses in nursing education: Effect on the profession. Part 1. *Heart and Lung. 16* (November): 629–635.

Kozier, B., Erb, G., and Olivieri, J. (1991). *Fundamentals of Nursing: Concepts, Process and Practice*. 4th ed. Redwood City, CA: Addison-Wesley.

Lampe, S. (1985). Focus charting: Streamlining documentation. *Nursing Management, 16* (7): 43–46.

Roy, C. (1980). The Roy adaptation model. In Riehl, J. P., and Roy, C., eds., *Conceptual Models for Nursing Practice*. 2nd ed. New York: Appleton-Century-Crofts.

CHAPTER 8

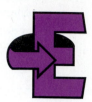

EVALUATION

OBJECTIVES

Upon completing this chapter, you should be able to do the following:
- Define evaluation as it relates to (1) the nursing process and (2) quality assurance.
- State the importance and purpose of evaluation in (1) the nursing process and (2) quality assurance.
- Describe the process of evaluating client progress toward goal achievement.
- Given predicted outcomes and client data, write two-part evaluative statements.
- Describe a process for modifying the nursing care plan.
- Describe a process for nursing quality assurance.
- Differentiate between criteria and standards.
- Explain how quality-assurance evaluation supports the moral principles of beneficence and nonmaleficence.

INTRODUCTION

In the course of their work, nurses make frequent and varied evaluations. Because the client is the nurse's primary concern, the most important evaluations involve the following:

1. The client's progress toward health goals

2. The value of the nursing care plan in helping the client to achieve his goals

3. The overall quality of care given to defined groups of clients

This chapter first examines the universal characteristics of evaluation and then discusses evaluation as a step of the nursing process (see Figure 8–1). Finally, it explains the process of quality assurance.

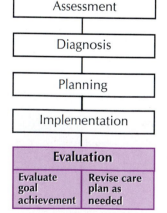

Figure 8-1. The Evaluation Step in the Nursing Process

UNIVERSAL CHARACTERISTICS OF EVALUATION

Before examining evaluation as it is used in the nursing process, it may be helpful to analyze a more universal definition of the term. In general, **formal evaluation** is a deliberate, systematic process in which a judgment is made about the *quality, value, or worth* of something by comparing it to *previously identified criteria or standards*. Almost anything can be the subject of evaluation (e.g., a painting, a highway system, a teaching method, or a person's character). Furthermore, various aspects or properties of a thing can be evaluated. If you are evaluating a painting, for instance, you can assess the artist's use of color or the extent to which the painting elicits emotion. If you were evaluating teaching methods, you might measure the teacher's ability to hold student interest, promote student learning, or minimize student stress. The important thing to remember is that you must decide *in advance* what properties you are going consider and how you will measure those properties.

Standards and Criteria

Although *standards* and *criteria* are sometimes used interchangeably, most texts differentiate between these terms. A **standard** is established by authority, custom, or consensus as a model of what should be done. In nursing, standards describe quality nursing care and are used for comparison when evaluating job performance. Nursing standards should be based on scientific and ethical knowledge and research, as well as on currently accepted nursing practice. Some standards, like those written for routines of care on a nursing unit, are specific enough to serve as criteria. Others are broad and abstract, as in the ANA's *Standards of Nursing Practice* (1973). The following example compares standards from each of these sources. Note the difference in specificity.

> **Example:**
>
> | *Broad:* | *Specific:* |
> | --- | --- |
> | (*ANA Standard I*) | (*Standard for a Nursing Unit*) |
> | The collection of data about the health status of the client/patient is systematic and continuous. The data are accessible, communicated, and recorded. | Temperature will be taken q4h. (Assess q2h if membranes ruptured.) Temp. will be assessed qh if > 99.6. |

When standards are broad, more specific criteria must be developed to guide the collection of data for evaluation. **Criteria** are measurable or observable qualities that describe specific skills, knowledge, behaviors, attitudes, and so on. Two criteria that could be used to evaluate ANA Standard I follow:

1. Vital signs are taken and recorded on the flowsheet every hour.
2. Flowsheets are kept on a clipboard at the foot of the bed while in use and transferred to the chart daily by 0700.

Because they are concrete and specific, criteria serve as guides for collecting evaluation data, as well as for making judgments about such data. The predicted outcomes you learned to write in Chapter 6 are examples of criteria. The preceding standard for the nursing unit could also be used as a criterion for evaluating because it describes specific, observable behaviors.

Criteria should be both valid and reliable. A criterion is **valid** if it actually measures what it is intended to measure. For example, the white-blood-cell count is often used to "measure" the presence of infection. However, it would not be valid if used alone, because the white count is not elevated in all infections; in addition, the white count is sometimes elevated when there is no infection. More valid indicators might be a blood culture or a bacterial count of a body fluid.

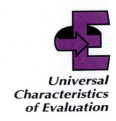

Universal Characteristics of Evaluation

Distinctive Characteristics of Evaluation:
° Determination of quality or value
° Use of predetermined criteria or standards

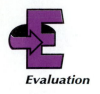

Evaluation

A **reliable** criterion yields the same results every time it is used, no matter who uses it (e.g., determining a patient's age by asking his friends is less reliable than asking the patient or checking his birth certificate). Box 8–1 presents a comparison of standards and criteria.

Types of Evaluation

Evaluation is often classified into three types: (1) structure, (2) process, and (3) outcome. Each type of evaluation requires different criteria and methods, and each has a different focus. In a health-care agency, the structure in which care is given, the caregiving processes, and the outcomes produced are interrelated.

Structure evaluation focuses on the setting in which care is given. It answers the question, What effect does the setting have on the quality of care? Structure evaluation examines the organization of the system for delivering care, looking at such factors as administrative and financial procedures, communication and staff-development processes, staffing patterns, qualifications of personnel, physical facilities, and availability of supplies and equipment.

Process evaluation focuses on the activities of the caregiver. It is concerned with actual performance in relation to the client's needs, and answers questions like the following:

In what manner is the care given?
Is care relevant to the client's needs?
Is care appropriate, complete, and timely?
What is the level of the caregiver's skills? The quality of the caregiver's performance?

Your nursing instructor probably uses a process-oriented tool to evaluate your clinical performance.

Outcome evaluation focuses on the client's health status and satisfaction with the results of care. Outcomes are evaluated by comparing clients' changes or responses to their health goals. Outcome evaluation answers the following questions:

Box 8–1. Comparison of Standards and Criteria

	Standards	**Criteria**
Similarities	Describe what is acceptable or desired	Describe what is acceptable or desired
	Serve as basis for comparison	Serve as basis for comparison
Differences	Describe nursing care	Describe expected nurse or client behaviors
	May be broad or specific	Specific, observable, measurable
Example	ANA standards	Predicted outcomes on patient care plan

To what degree were the client's health goals achieved?

To what degree, and in what way, did the interventions contribute to goal achievement?

Determining the relationship between nursing interventions and goal achievement is one example of outcome evaluation.

Aspect of Care	Focus	Criterion Examples
Structure	Setting	Exit signs are clearly visible.
Process	Caregiver activities	Initial interview is completed within 8 hours after admission of client.
Outcome	Patient responses	B/P < 140/90 at all times.

EVALUATION IN THE NURSING PROCESS

In the context of the nursing process, **evaluation** is a planned, ongoing, deliberate activity in which the client, family, nurse, and other health-care professionals determine (1) the client's progress toward goal achievement and (2) the effectiveness of the nursing care plan. Recall the two universal characteristics of evaluation:

Determination of quality or value

Use of preselected criteria or standards

The nurse and client determine the *quality* of the client's health by using as *predetermined criteria* the predicted responses identified in the planning step. They determine the *value* of the nursing care plan by using as *standards* the excellent application of each step of the nursing process.

Universal Definition	Nursing Process Definition
Determination of quality or value	**1.** of the client's health. **2.** of the nursing care plan.
Use of predetermined criteria or standards:	Criteria/standards are: **1.** the predicted outcomes identified in the planning step. **2.** Use of the nursing process according to guidelines such as those in the "Guidelines for Writing Nursing Orders" in Chapter 6.

Evaluation is an ongoing process that begins with the initial baseline assessment and continues during each contact with the client. Frequency of evaluation depends on frequency of contact, which is determined by the client's status or the condition being evaluated. When a patient has just returned from surgery, the nurse may evaluate for signs of change in status

Evaluation

Evaluation is a planned, on-going, deliberate activity in which the nurse, client, significant others, and other health-care professionals determine

1. the extent of client goal achievement, and
2. the effectiveness of the nursing care plan.

---

every 15 minutes. The following day, the nurse may evaluate the client only every 4 hours. As the client's condition improves and she approaches dismissal, evaluation gradually becomes less frequent.

Critical Thinking in Evaluation

Critical thinking is an integral part of the evaluation step. You will use it to apply knowledge, identify relevant facts, analyze data, and test hypotheses. When developing the criteria for evaluation, you will apply knowledge of physiology, psychology, and other fields to the specific client situation in order to know what outcomes can reasonably be expected. When collecting evaluation data, you will use critical thinking to determine the significant data for the goal being evaluated. Critical thinking continues as you analyze the data to judge the congruence between predicted and actual outcomes. In a sense, you hypothesized during the planning step that a particular nursing intervention would produce a desired client outcome; in the evaluation step you test that hypothesis.

Relationship to Other Steps

Effective evaluation depends upon the effectiveness of the steps that precede it. Assessment data must be accurate and complete so that the predicted outcomes written in the planning step will be appropriate for the client. The predicted outcomes (planning) must be stated in concrete, behavioral terms if they are to be useful for evaluating actual client outcomes. Finally, without the implementation step, there would be nothing to evaluate.

Evaluation overlaps with assessment. During evaluation, the nurse collects data (assessment), but for the purpose of evaluating (evaluation) rather than diagnosing. The *act* of data collection is the same; the differences are in (1) when it is collected and (2) how it is used. In the assessment step the nurse uses data to make nursing diagnoses; in the evaluation step, it is used to assess the effect of nursing care on the diagnoses.

	Assessment Data	*Evaluation Data*
When Collected	In assessment step Before care is given	In evaluation step After care is given
Purpose/Use	Diagnosis of client status	Evaluation of change in client status

Although it is the fifth and final step in the nursing process, evaluation does not end the process; the information it provides is used to begin another cycle. After implementing the care plan, the nurse compares client responses to goals and then uses this information in reviewing the care plan and each step of the nursing process.

Evaluation of Client Progress

In the context of the nursing process, outcome evaluation focuses primarily on the client's progress toward achieving health goals. The nurse compares the **actual outcomes** (client responses) to the **predicted outcomes** identified during the planning step and makes a judgment about whether or not the goals have been met. Evaluation data is collected by observing the client's behavior and responses, examining care plans and client records, and talking to the client, family, friends, and other health team members.

Evaluation of client outcomes may be ongoing or intermittent. **Ongoing evaluation** is done while, or immediately after, implementing an intervention to enable you to make on-the-spot modification. **Intermittent** evaluation, performed at specified times, shows the amount of progress toward goal achievement and enables you to correct any inadequacies in the client's care and modify the care plan as needed. Evaluation continues until the client's health goals are achieved or until he is discharged from the agency.

Terminal evaluation indicates the client's condition at the time of discharge. It includes understanding of follow-up care and status of goal achievement, especially with regard to self-care abilities. Most agencies have a special Discharge Record (see Figure 7–5) for the terminal evaluation, as well as for instructions regarding medications, treatments, and follow-up care. As you work with the client throughout her stay, you should prepare her for eventual discharge by gradually promoting more self-care and talking about the time when she will be leaving.

Responsibility for Evaluation

Professional standards of practice (American Nurses Association, 1973) identify evaluation as a mutual nurse-client activity. Family and other team members provide data and participate, but the nurse is responsible for initiating and recording the evaluation.

By performing organized, systematic evaluation of client outcomes, nurses demonstrate caring and responsibility. Examining outcomes shows that nurses care not only about planning and delivering care, but also about its effect upon those whose lives they touch. Without evaluation, nurses would not know whether the care they give actually meets the client's needs.

Evaluation enables the nurse to improve care. It promotes efficiency by eliminating unsuccessful interventions and allowing the nurse to focus on actions that are more effective. Only by evaluating the client's progress in relation to the plan of care can the nurse know whether to continue, change, or terminate the plan.

Finally, by linking nursing interventions to improvements in client status, evaluation can demonstrate to employers and consumers that nurses play an important role in achieving client health.

Procedure for Evaluating Client Progress

For each of the client's nursing diagnoses you will (1) review the stated goals or predicted outcomes, (2) collect data about the client's responses to nursing interventions, (3) compare actual outcomes to predicted outcomes and draw a conclusion about whether the goals have been met, (4) record the evaluative statement, and (5) relate the nursing orders to the client outcomes. The following discussion provides a step-by-step guide for evaluating client progress.

Review Predicted Outcomes   The predicted outcomes, identified in the planning stage, describe how the client is expected to look, feel, or be, or what he will be able to do if the nursing interventions are effective. A nursing diagnosis may have only one predicted outcome, but usually there are several. You may

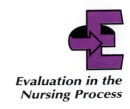

Evaluation in the Nursing Process

Standard VII.
The client's/patient's progress or lack of progress toward goal achievement is determined by the client/patient and the nurse.

Standard VIII.
The client's/patient's progress or lack of progress toward goal achievement directs reassessment reordering of priorities, new goal setting, and revision of the plan of nursing care (ANA, 1973).

Evaluation

find it helpful to make a working list of the predicted outcomes before collecting evaluation data. Table 8–1 illustrates this and the following step in the evaluation process.

Collect Evaluation Data Collect data about the client's responses to the nursing interventions. Use the nursing diagnosis and its list of predicted outcomes to guide your ongoing focus assessment. In the example in Table 8–1, in order to get the data under "Actual Outcomes" during interactions with Sam Rizzo, the nurse focused on his facial expression and muscle tension and listened for statements reflecting his level of anxiety and his knowledge of routines and treatments.

The professional nurse responsible for the care plan is also responsible for evaluating the client's response to care. The client is the best source of information about subjective symptoms such as pain, nausea, or anxiety. Family input is often helpful as well, especially in ambulatory or home health settings where you are not present to observe client responses. To help make their data useful, you need to provide detailed guidelines (e.g., when to make observations, what to look for, how to get the data, how to describe what they experience or observe).

The nature of the goal determines the type of information you will collect. Goals can be classified as cognitive, psychomotor, or affective, or as pertaining to body appearance and functioning. For cognitive goals you might ask the client to repeat information or apply new knowledge (e.g., choose low-fat foods from a menu). For psychomotor goals you could ask the client to demonstrate a skill, such as drawing up insulin. For affective goals, you might talk to the client and observe her behavior for cues to changes in values, attitudes, or beliefs. You can obtain data about body appearance and functioning by interviewing, observing,

Table 8–1. Evaluation Example: Sam Rizzo

Nursing Diagnosis: Moderate Anxiety r/t unfamiliar environment and dyspnea

Compare Predicted Outcomes . . .	to Actual Outcomes (Data) . . .	Conclusion
Broad goal: Will experience reduced anxiety, as evidenced by		
1. verbalization of feeling less anxious.	When dyspneic, states "What should I do? Can you help me?"	Goal not met
2. relaxed facial muscles.	Face relaxed except during episodes of dyspnea.	Goal partially met
3. absence of skeletal muscle tension.	No skeletal muscle tension, except during episodes of dyspnea.	Goal partially met
4. verbalizes understanding of hospital routines and treatments.	States, "I feel better since you explained about the fire drill. I thought there was a real fire."	Goal met
	States, "I understand about the hospital routines and the breathing treatments. Those things really aren't causing any anxiety."	

and examining the client, as well as from secondary sources such as laboratory results. Some examples of data-collection methods for the different types of goals appear in Table 8–2.

Compare Actual and Predicted Outcomes, and Draw a Conclusion

Comparing data to preestablished criteria is a necessary component of evaluation: without this step, evaluation has not occurred. If the nursing process has been effective up to this point, it is relatively simple to determine if a goal has been met. Is the client's response (actual outcome) what you wanted it to be (predicted outcome)? Is it at least the best you can expect given the time and circumstances? Include the client in decisions about the level of goal achievement. Go over the predicted outcomes with the client, and ask him if he believes they have been achieved. Three possible conclusions about outcome achievement are possible:

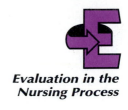
1. Goal met   The desired client response occurred, and

The actual outcome is congruent with the predicted outcome.

2. Goal partially met   Some, but not all, predicted outcomes were achieved, or

The predicted outcome is achieved only part of the time.

3. Goal not met   The desired client response did not occur by the target time, or

The actual outcome does not match the predicted outcome.

Note that these conclusions refer to specific predicted outcomes, not to achievement of the broad general goal (which is not necessarily written on the care plan). *Outcome achieved* might be more accurate than *goal met,* but you are not likely to see that terminology in actual practice. The term *goal met* is more concise and easier to say and write; therefore, it is the term most used. Table 8–1 shows how actual outcomes would be compared to predicted outcomes in order to draw conclusions about Sam Rizzo's goal achievement.

Table 8–2. Evaluation Data-Collection Methods

Type of Goal	Predicted Outcome	Example of Data Collection Activity
Cognitive	By the end of the week, names foods to avoid on a low-fat diet.	Using a chart of the Four Basic Food Groups, ask the client to tell you which foods to avoid.
Psychomotor	Within 24 hours after delivery, positions baby correctly at breast.	Observe the mother breastfeeding the infant.
Affective	After orientation to routines and procedures, states he is feeling less anxiety.	Listen for spontaneous statements about anxiety, or ask, "How are you feeling?"
Body function and appearance	Heart rate < 100 at all times.	Auscultate apical heart rate.

Evaluation

Write the Evaluative Statement   An evaluative statement consists of two parts: (1) the judgment about whether the goal was met ("Conclusion" in Table 8–1) and (2) data to support the judgment ("Actual Outcomes" in Table 8–1). Following are the evaluative statements that would be written for Sam Rizzo, using the data and conclusions in Table 8–1.

Predicted Outcome	*Evaluative Statement*
1. Verbalization of feeling less anxious	2/14. Goal not met. When dyspneic, states, "What should I do? Can you help me?" No statements of feeling less anxious.
2. Relaxed facial muscles	2/14. Goal partially met. Face relaxed except during episodes of dyspnea.
3. Absence of skeletal muscle tension	2/14. Goal partially met. No skeletal muscle tension, except during episodes of dyspnea.
4. Verbalizes understanding of hospital routines and treatments	2/14. Goal met. States, "I feel better since you explained about the fire drill. I thought there was a real fire." Also states, "I understand about the hospital routines and the breathing treatments. Those things really aren't causing any anxiety."

Some care plans have a special column for the evaluative statement; in other systems you may record the evaluative statement in the progress notes. In still other systems you may record the evaluation data but not the conclusion about goal achievement.

Relate Nursing Interventions to Outcomes   It is important to establish whether or not the patient outcomes were actually caused by the nursing actions. You cannot automatically assume that a nursing intervention was the reason a goal was or was not met. A number of variables can have an impact on goal achievement, for example:

> Actions and treatments performed by other health-care professionals
> Influence of family members and significant others
> Client's attitudes, desire, and motivation
> Client's failure to give accurate or sufficient information during data collection
> Client's prior experiences and knowledge

Nurses cannot control all the variables that might influence the outcome of care; therefore, in determining the effect of a nursing action, you should try to identify other factors that might have promoted or interfered with its effectiveness.

The preceding steps should tell you whether or not the care plan has been effective in achieving goals and resolving or preventing the client's problems. The final step—whether or not the goals were met—is to review the nursing care plan and each of the nursing process steps in its development. This step should always follow the step comparing interventions to outcomes. However, because it uses a different type of evaluative process than just explained, the final step is considered separately in the next section.

Evaluation of the Nursing Care Plan

Changes in the client's condition and the status of her goal achievement (from the outcome evaluation) determine whether, but not how, the care plan should be revised. After finishing the outcome evaluation, you should examine the nursing care plan to see if it needs modification. You will probably modify the care plan if (1) the client's condition changes or (2) if the health goals were not met. You should obtain client input for modifying the plan, just as you did when developing it.

Some agencies use a pink or yellow highlighter to mark through discontinued sections of the care plan. Others have a status column in which to write the date of any revisions. These methods do not obliterate the original plans; thus they can be photocopied or used for reference as needed.

The nursing care plan is evaluated primarily by process evaluation while the client is still receiving care, so that modifications can benefit the client. Data is obtained from client examination, interviews and records, or from staff conferences. In evaluating a care plan, you need to (1) draw conclusions about the status of client problems, and (2) review each step of the nursing process, evaluating the quality of the diagnoses, goals, and nursing orders, and also review the manner in which each step was performed.

Draw Conclusions About Problem Status

Decisions about care plan modifications depend in part upon whether client goals were met, not met, or partially met. The various alternatives for each of these situations are considered in the following discussion.

The fact that goals have been met usually indicates that nursing interventions are no longer needed for a particular problem. However, you will sometimes need to continue or modify a care plan, even though goals were met. You will draw one of the following conclusions about the client's problem when outcome evaluation indicates that a **goal has been met.**

1. *Problem Resolved.* When the problem stated in the actual or potential nursing diagnosis has been resolved, nursing care is no longer needed for that problem. You can conclude that the problem has been resolved if all the predicted outcomes for that problem have been achieved. If this is the case, document that the goals were met, and discontinue the nursing diagnosis. In Mr. Rizzo's case (Table 8–1), the Anxiety problem can be considered resolved when Goals 1, 2, and 3 have been met.

2. *Potential Problem Prevented; Risk Factors Remain.* When the potential problem stated in the nursing diagnosis has not occurred, but the risk factors are still present, nursing care is still required for continued goal achievement. You will probably continue with the same nursing diagnosis, goals, and nursing orders. For example, suppose that Tamara Jordan's nursing diagnosis is High Risk for Puerperal Infection r/t membranes having ruptured several days before delivery of her baby. The goal is that she will not develop puerperal infection. When the nurse evaluates her progress on day 2 postpartum, Tamara's temperature is normal and she has no other signs of infection—all goals for this problem are being met. However, this problem could still develop, so the nurse keeps it in the care plan and continues to assess for it.

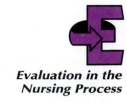

Evaluation in the Nursing Process

Process for Evaluating Client Outcomes

1. Review the predicted outcomes on the client's care plan.
2. After implementing the nursing order, collect data relevant to the expected outcomes.
3. Compare actual outcomes (data) to predicted outcomes (goals), and draw one of the following conclusions: goal met, goal partially met, or goal not met.
4. Record the two-part evaluative statement: Goal status + supporting data.
5. Relate nursing actions to goal achievement.
6. Review and modify care plan as needed, depending on goal achievement and changes in client's condition.

Evaluation

3. *Possible Problem Ruled Out.* In this case you should discontinue the problem, goals, and nursing orders.

4. *Actual Problem Still Exists.* Even though the goal was met, the problem may still exist, particularly if the goal was only one of several written for the problem. The Anxiety diagnosis in Table 8–1 illustrates this point. One of Mr. Rizzo's goals was met: he verbalized understanding of hospital routines and treatments. However, the other goals were either not met or only partially met, so his diagnosis of Anxiety still exists. The nursing orders related to explaining routines and treatments can probably be discontinued, but the other nursing interventions for Anxiety should be continued or modified to make them more effective.

5. *All Problems Resolved; No New Problems.* When all goals have been met and no new problems have developed, the client is discharged from nursing care. In an acute-care setting this is not likely to occur before dismissal from the institution.

It is important to identify variables that have contributed to goal achievement, so that you can reinforce positive behaviors and use them in promoting continued and future goal achievement. For example, if your evaluation shows that a child eats better for his mother, you could arrange his mealtimes so that his mother feeds him when she is there.

You may have some, but not enough, evidence that the goal has been met; or perhaps the goal is being met at one time and not another. One of Mr. Rizzo's goals, for instance, is absence of muscle tension. He does achieve this outcome at times, but not when he is dyspneic. You will conclude one of the following when evaluation indicates that a **goal has been partially met.**

1. *The problem has been reduced; care plan needs revisions.* As in Mr. Rizzo's case, you may conclude that the problem has been reduced but that nursing interventions are still needed. Since the goal is not being fully met, the care plan may need to be modified.

2. *The problem has been reduced; continue with the same plan, but allow more time.* After examining the care plan, you may wish to continue with the same plan but give the client more time to achieve the goal. To decide, you must assess why the goal has not been fully met.

Even when goals have not been met, you cannot automatically conclude that the care plan needs revision. Recall that client, family, and other variables also influence the success of the plan; therefore, you must reexamine the entire care plan and each step of the nursing process. You may conclude one of the following when a **goal has not been met:**

1. The problem still exists. Continue with the same plan.
2. The problem still exists. Revise the plan.

Review All Steps of the Nursing Process

As you can see, whether or not goals have been met, there are a number of decisions to make about continuing, modifying, or terminating nursing care for each problem. Before making specific modifications, you must first determine why the plan was not effective. This requires that you review the entire care plan and the nursing process steps involved in its development. This section provides a checklist of questions and actions for use in your review of each step of the nursing process.

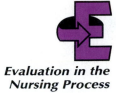

Evaluation in the Nursing Process

Assessment Step   Examine the initial and ongoing assessment data in the client's chart (e.g., data base, progress notes). Errors or omissions in data influence subsequent steps of the nursing process and may require changes in every section of the care plan.

Example: Wasumita Singh answers the nurses in brief phrases; she does not initiate conversation. Her nurses initially believed her communication problem was caused by her difficulty with English. When evaluating her progress, the nurse concludes that her Impaired Verbal Communication problem still exists. However, on reviewing Ms. Singh's chart, she finds new data: a psychiatric consultation note indicating that Ms. Singh is deeply depressed. The nurse realizes now that Ms. Singh's communication problem is more than simply a language barrier.

You may find that new data have become available since the client's initial assessment, or perhaps the client's condition has changed. For example, Ms. Ray's care plan states that she can ambulate "with help of one." However, she has become progressively weaker and now cannot bear weight at all; thus the nursing order is no longer appropriate.

The following checklist will help you to review the assessment step. Ask yourself each of the questions. If you answer no, proceed to the next question. If you answer yes to a question, take the suggested actions, and then move to the next question.

EVALUATION CHECKLIST—ASSESSMENT STEP

Questions to Ask	*Actions to Take*
1. Were the assessment data incomplete or inaccurate?	☐ Yes. Reassess the client. Record the new data. Change care plan as indicated.
2. Are there data that still need to be validated?	☐ Yes. Validate with client (by interview and physical examination), significant others, or other professionals. Record validation (or failure to validate). Change care plan as indicated.
3. Have new data become available that require changes in the plan (e.g., a different problem etiology, new goals, new nursing orders)?	☐ Yes. Record the data in the progress notes. Change care plan as indicated.
4. Has the client's condition changed?	☐ Yes. Record data about client's present status. Change care plan as indicated.

Move to a review of the diagnosis step.

Evaluation

Diagnosis Step If your examination of the assessment step results in a revision of the data base, you may need to revise or add new nursing diagnoses. Even if data were complete and accurate, you must still analyze the diagnostic process and each of the diagnostic statements. The nursing diagnosis could be incorrect because of errors in the diagnostic process, or the diagnostic statement may have been poorly written. Perhaps the nurse who wrote the statement had a clear idea of the client's problem, but was unable to communicate the idea when writing the diagnostic statement. Other nurses might therefore have focused their interventions inappropriately.

Use the following list of questions to help you review the diagnosis step. Take the suggested actions as needed.

EVALUATION CHECKLIST—DIAGNOSIS STEP

Questions to Ask

1. Is the diagnosis irrelevant or unrelated to the data base?

2. Is the diagnosis inadequately supported by the data?

3. Has the problem status changed (actual, possible, potential)?

4. Is the diagnosis stated unclearly?

5. Does the etiology incorrectly reflect the factors contributing to the problem?

6. Is the problem one that cannot be treated primarily by independent actions?

7. Is the diagnosis broad and general (rather than individualized for *this* patient)?

8. Has the nursing diagnosis been resolved?

Proceed to a review of client goals.

Actions to Take

☐ Yes. Revise the diagnosis.

☐ Yes. Collect more data. Support or revise diagnosis.

☐ Yes. Relabel the problem.

☐ Yes. Revise the diagnostic statement.

☐ Yes. Revise the etiology.

☐ Yes. Label as collaborative and consult appropriate health-care professional.

☐ Yes. Revise diagnosis. Revise goals and nursing orders as suggested by the new nursing diagnosis.

☐ Yes. Delete diagnosis and related goals and nursing orders.

Planning Step If you have made additions to the data or changed the nursing diagnosis, you will need to revise the goals and nursing orders. However, if the data and the diagnostic statement are satisfactory as initially written, the reason for lack of goal achievement may lie in the goals themselves. Perhaps the goals were unrealistic, or perhaps the best nursing strategies were not chosen. The following questions will help you decide whether your goals should be revised.

EVALUATION CHECKLIST—GOALS

Questions to Ask	*Actions to Take*
1. Have nursing diagnoses been added or revised?	☐ Yes. Write new goals.
2. Is the goal unrealistic in terms of patient abilities and agency resources?	☐ Yes. Revise goal.
3. Was insufficient time allowed for goal achievement?	☐ Yes. Revise time frame.
4. Are there aspects of the client's problem that the goals do not address?	☐ Yes. Write additional goals.
5. Do the predicted outcomes, as written, fail to demonstrate resolution of the problem specified in the nursing diagnosis?	☐ Yes. Revise goals.
6. Have client priorities changed? Has the focus of care changed?	☐ Yes. Revise goals.
7. Were they the nurse's goals instead of the client's?	☐ Yes. Get client input. Write goals valued by the client.

Proceed to review of nursing orders.

EVALUATION CHECKLIST—NURSING ORDERS

Questions to Ask	*Actions to Take*
1. Have nursing diagnoses or goals been added or revised in previous review steps?	☐ Yes. Write new nursing orders.
2. Do the nursing orders seem unrelated to the stated client goals?	☐ Yes. Revise or develop new nursing orders.
3. Is the rationale insufficient to justify the use of the nursing order?	☐ Yes. Revise or develop new nursing orders.
4. Are the nursing orders unclear or vague, so that other staff may have had questions about how to implement them?	☐ Yes. Revise nursing orders. Add details to make more specific and/or individualized to the client.
5. Do the nursing orders lack instructions for timing of the strategies?	☐ Yes. Revise nursing orders. Add times.
6. Was the order clearly ineffective?	☐ Yes. Delete it.
7. Are the orders unrealistic in terms of staff and other resources?	☐ Yes. Revise orders or obtain resources.
8. Have new resources become available that might enable you to change the goals or nursing orders?	☐ Yes. Write new goals or nursing orders reflecting the new capabilities.
9. Do the nursing orders fail to address all aspects of the client's goals?	☐ Yes. Add new nursing orders.

Proceed to review of implementation step.

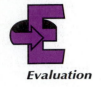

Evaluation

Implementation Step   If all sections of the nursing care plan appear to be satisfactory, perhaps the lack of goal achievement is due to the manner in which the plan was implemented. To find out what went wrong in the implementation step, consult the progress notes, the client, significant others, and other caregivers. Use the following checklist as a guide.

EVALUATION CHECKLIST—IMPLEMENTATION

Questions to Ask	*Actions to Take*
1. Did the nurse fail to get client input at each step in developing and implementing the plan?	☐ Yes. Obtain client input, revise plan and implementation as needed.
2. Were the nursing interventions unacceptable to the client?	☐ Yes. Consult client; change nursing orders or implementation approach.
3. Did the nurse fail to prepare the client for implementation of the nursing order (e.g., fail to explain what client should expect or do)?	☐ Yes. Continue plan. Prepare client before implementing. Reevaluate.
4. Did the nurse lack the knowledge or skill to perform techniques and procedures correctly?	☐ Yes. Continue same plan. Have someone else implement or help the nurse to acquire the knowledge or skills. If neither of these is possible, delete nursing order.
5. Did client and/or family fail to comply with the therapeutic regimen? Were strategies performed incorrectly?	☐ Yes. Reassess motivation, knowledge, and resources. Add goals and nursing orders aimed at teaching, motivating, and supporting client in carrying out the regimen. Set time for reevaluation.
6. Did other personnel fail to carry out nursing orders? Why?	☐ Yes. Implement the nursing order or ensure that others will do so. Set time for reevaluation.
7. Was the plan of care implemented in a manner that failed to communicate caring?	☐ Yes. This is a problem that must be addressed by staff development and personal development.

After making the necessary modifications to the care plan, implement the new plan, and begin the nursing process cycle again.

Evaluation Errors

Probably the most common evaluation error is failure to perform systematic evaluation of patient outcomes. Many nurses are more action-oriented than analytic and reflective, so it is easy in the press of a busy day to make a plan and act; you may have to make determined efforts to find time to observe and record the client's responses to the actions. Remember that quality care is not guaranteed simply because you have implemented the nursing orders. Only when you evaluate client outcomes can you be assured that the care has met the client's needs.

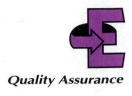
Usually the nurse does, in fact, observe the client's response, but she may not document it or consciously use it in an evaluation process that would enable her to modify interventions. You must be sure to document the evaluative statements in the client's record so that other nurses will be able to judge the effectiveness of your interventions. Otherwise, they might continue with approaches that you have already discovered to be ineffective.

Another error may occur when a nurse uses irrelevant data to judge the level of goal achievement. You should consider only data that is clearly related to the predicted outcome. Box 8–2 provides examples of both relevant and irrelevant data related to Mr. Rizzo's Anxiety problem from Table 8–1.

Errors are also possible in judging the congruence between actual and predicted client outcomes; actual outcomes may be measured inaccurately, or data may be incomplete. In the example of Table 8–1, if the nurse observed Sam Rizzo only during periods when he was not dyspneic, she might erroneously conclude that his anxiety was relieved.

QUALITY ASSURANCE

In addition to evaluating goal achievement for individual clients, nurses are also involved in evaluating and modifying the overall quality of care given to groups of clients. Table 8–3 compares quality assurance and nursing process evaluation.

A **quality-assurance** program is an ongoing, systematic process designed to evaluate and promote excellence in health care given to groups of clients. Quality assurance frequently refers to evaluation of the level of care provided in an agency, but it may be as limited in scope as an evaluation of the performance of one nurse or as broad as the evaluation of the overall quality of care in an entire country.

Quality assurance evaluation is done both because it benefits professions and because consumers and government agencies mandate it. As health costs rise, increasingly sophisticated consumers demand accountability from professionals. The public wants to know that it receives maximum quality for the high price it pays.

Box 8–2. Relevant and Irrelevant Data: Sam Rizzo	
Relevant data	When dyspneic, states "What should I do? Can you help me?" Face relaxed; no skeletal muscle tension, except during episodes of dyspnea. States, "I feel better since you explained about the fire drill. I thought there was a real fire." States, "I understand about the hospital routines and the breathing treatments. Those things really aren't causing any anxiety."
Irrelevant data	Temperature 98.6°. Watching television except when wife is here.

Evaluation

Background

Quality assurance is not a new concept. Florence Nightingale (1858) developed standards for patient care, which she supported with evidence gathered from hospital wards. Evaluation of health care has changed in the past twenty years in response to consumer pressures and government concerns about cost containment and quality control. Since the United States government mandated professional review of health-care services in 1972, it has been increasingly required by other private and government agencies. The 1972 Joint Commission for Accreditation of Hospitals standards were an impetus for institutions, as well as the nursing profession, to place more emphasis on evaluating the quality of nursing care. Since that time, regulatory agencies such as the Joint Commission for Accreditation of Healthcare Organizations and state boards of nursing have required documentation that nursing care is being given according to nursing standards. Nursing quality assurance is now a major part of the overall evaluation of care in an institution. Nurses are involved in developing standards to describe quality nursing care in their setting and in conducting quality-assurance evaluations.

In 1982 a system of peer review organizations (PROs), managed on a statewide basis, replaced the earlier professional standards review organizations (PSROs) (Werner, 1985). Hospitals receiving federal funds must now conduct utilization reviews through PROs. The PROs use **peer review**, which means that the members of the profession delivering the care develop and implement the process for evaluating that care. This has been a further impetus for nurses to become involved in developing standards that describe good nursing care.

Nursing Quality Assurance

Quality assurance enables nursing to demonstrate accountability to society for the quality of its services. Consumers, administrators, and bureaucrats do not always clearly perceive the relationship between quality nursing care and improved patient outcomes; professional survival requires that nurses demonstrate this link.

Table 8–3. Comparison of Quality Assurance and Nursing Process Evaluation

	Nursing Quality Assurance	The Nursing Process
Scope of evaluation	Groups of clients	Individual clients
Subject of evaluation	Overall quality of care	1. Progress toward achieving client goals
		2. Review of nursing care plan
Type of evaluation	Structure, process, outcome	1. Outcome evaluation of patient progress
		2. Process evaluation of nursing care plan
Responsibility for evaluation	Chief nurse in the institution	Nurse caring for client

In an effort to control health-care costs, Medicare began in 1983 to use a prospective payment system (PPS), in which hospitals are reimbursed on the basis of the client's diagnosis rather than on the number of days the client stays in the hospital. This method provides strong incentive for early discharge and has raised both professional and consumer concerns about quality. Since the advent of the PPS, there has been a great deal of pressure on home-health and extended-care agencies to accommodate those discharged from acute-care settings. Clients frequently complain of being discharged from hospitals before they feel ready to leave, of bed shortages in nursing care facilities, and of abuses in home health care. Unfortunately, while resources for treating clients in hospitals are becoming more limited, sufficient alternative treatment settings are not yet available. Providing adequate care is difficult under these circumstances, and nurses are challenged to provide a satisfactory level of care. Monitoring and promoting quality of care is an important nursing function.

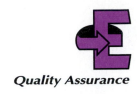

Quality Assurance

Types of Quality-Assurance Evaluations

Quality assurance requires evaluation of three essential components of care: structure, process, and outcome, which were defined in the first part of this chapter; this section explains how they relate to nursing quality assurance. Nurses were traditionally evaluated by supervisors on characteristics such as dependability, communication, and clinical skills. However, such process evaluation does not consider whether the nursing care was effective in improving the client's health. On the other hand, outcome evaluation by itself does not take into account that variables other than the nursing care may affect the client's health. Quality assurance requires consideration of the interaction of these three components.

Quality assurance usually involves a **nursing audit**, in which client records are reviewed for data about nursing competence. A committee establishes standards of care (e.g., for safety measures, documentation, preoperative teaching), and a number of charts are randomly selected and reviewed to compare nursing interventions against these standards.

Structure Evaluation

Structural standards describe desirable environmental and organizational characteristics that indirectly influence care. Pertinent data includes information about policies, procedures, fiscal resources, facilities, equipment, and the number and qualifications of personnel. The data is obtained by direct observation of the physical facilities and examination of written records such as policies and financial records. Criteria that might be written for structure evaluation include (1) "Call light is within reach," (2) "Narcotics are kept in double-locked cabinet," (3) "Policies for medication errors are written and easily accessible." Although adequate staff and resources do not insure quality care, they are certainly important factors.

Process Evaluation

In nursing quality assurance, process evaluation concentrates on the activities of the nurse. Process standards focus on the manner in which the nurse uses the nursing process. They describe what the nurse should do for the client or what constitutes proper performance of a procedure. The ANA *Standards of Nursing Practice* (1973) are an example of process standards. Some examples of specific, observable criteria for evaluating process standards follow:

Evaluation

Checks client's identification band before giving medication.

Performs and records chest assessment, including auscultation, once per shift.

Explains procedures (e.g., catheterization) prior to implementation.

Data for concurrent process evaluation is obtained by observing nursing performance, by interviewing the client, and by auditing the client's records while he is still in the institution. Process questions that might be asked concurrently are (1) Does the nurse administer medications safely? and (2) Is privacy provided during treatments and procedures?

A positive relationship should exist between the quality of the nurse's practice and the outcomes for the patient. This is an important premise of the nursing profession and an important focus for nursing research. Of course, the patient's health may become worse instead of better no matter how expertly the nurse performs, but overall, good nursing care should improve patient outcomes.

Process evaluation after the client is discharged involves an audit of client records to obtain evidence of the nurse's application of the nursing process. This emphasizes the need for careful documentation of nursing care and client responses (see Chapter 7). Retrospective process evaluation may also use postdischarge questionnaires or telephone interviews as sources of data. Examples of process questions that might be answered retrospectively follow:

Were medications given on time?

How soon after admission was the client's nursing history complete?

Is the nursing care plan complete?

Do the nursing progress notes provide evidence that the care plan was implemented?

Outcome Evaluation

Outcome evaluation focuses on demonstrable changes in the client's health status that occur as a result of nursing care. Evaluation criteria are written in terms of client responses or health states—just as they are for evaluation of an individual client's progress (e.g., "Verbalizes feelings about Caesarean birth"; "Skin over bony prominences is intact and free from redness"). Additionally, the criterion states what percent of clients are expected to have this outcome when nursing care is satisfactory.

Example: Skin over bony prominences is intact and free from redness.
Expected compliance: 100%

Taken alone, this means that you would expect that with good care, no clients in the institution will develop redness over a bony prominence. If used alone, however, outcome evaluation fails to consider the effect of variables other than nursing care; some clients' nutritional and mobility status may be so compromised that no amount of care can prevent redness over bony prominences. A process evaluation for such a client might show that a good care plan was written and that the client received hourly turning and skin care—indicating that the nursing care was adequate even though the outcome was poor. A structure evaluation might also show that the nursing unit was chronically understaffed, which would validate a process evaluation that reveals that the client often went for more than 2 hours without being repositioned—providing the reason for the poor processes and poor outcome.

Client responses are the data used for outcome evaluation. Data is obtained from nursing audits, as well as client interviews and questionnaires. Judgments made after the client is discharged can be used to determine whether the nursing care plan was effective. Of course, the information comes too late to improve outcomes for that particular client, but it can contribute to improved care for future clients.

It is not always easy to demonstrate the relationship between nursing care and client outcomes. Medical, or disease-related, outcomes are easy to observe. For instance, a temperature of 98.6° and a white-blood-cell count of 8,000 provide good evidence that there is no infection, and it is easy to attribute these results to the effects of the antibiotic that was given. The nursing perspective is more holistic, so it is sometimes difficult even to define the outcomes desired. Emotional, social, or spiritual responses, for instance, are hard to write in measurable terms. It is also difficult to measure the degree to which the outcome was caused by the nursing care, since many variables contribute to improvement (or deterioration) in the client's health (e.g., the nature of the client's illness, medical interventions, quality of nursing care, availability of resources, client motivation, and family participation).

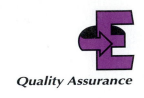

Quality Assurance

A Procedure for Quality-Assurance Evaluation

The quality-assurance process is similar to the nursing process; it involves data collection, comparison of data to criteria, identification of problems, generation and implementation of solutions, and reevaluation. It is different in that it focuses on nurses and institutions rather than patients, does not rely as heavily on outcome evaluation, and is concerned with groups of clients rather than individuals. The following steps are included in the quality-assurance models of most organizations:

1. *Decide the topic to be evaluated.* The topic might be the care for a group of clients with a particular medical diagnosis, care for all clients in a hospital, or record keeping on a nursing unit.

2. *Identify standards of care.* Determine whether structure, process, or outcome standards are appropriate. Recall that standards are broad guidelines and are not measurable or useful in data collection. Therefore, this step is sometimes omitted, and only the criteria are actually written.

3. *Establish criteria* for measuring the standards of care. Process and outcome criteria are specific, observable characteristics that describe the desired behaviors of the nurse or client.

4. *Determine expected compliance or performance levels.* A performance level is the percent of times you would expect the criterion to be met. This may vary from 0% to 100%, depending on how the criterion is stated. For example, you might expect that 95% of the time, an admission data base would be completed within 4 hours after the client was admitted.

5. *Collect data related to the criteria.* Data may be obtained from client interviews, chart audits, direct observation of nursing activities, questionnaires, or special evaluation tools, depending on the criterion you are evaluating.

Evaluation

6. *Analyze the data.* Identify discrepancies between the data and the criteria. Determine reasons for the discrepancies, using information about structures, processes, and outcomes. Identify problems. In the example in Item 4, if fewer than 95% of the admission data bases were completed in the specified time, it would be important to find out why this is happening.

7. *Generate solutions for correcting discrepancies and solving problems.* For instance, more in-service education may be needed for nurses, or perhaps the staffing pattern should be changed, or a new data-collection form used.

8. *Implement the solutions.* The purpose of evaluation is to maintain the quality of care being delivered. Once problems have been identified, action must be taken to see that they do not recur.

9. *Reevaluate* to determine if the solutions were effective.

ETHICAL CONSIDERATIONS IN EVALUATION

The moral principle of **beneficence** holds that we ought to do good things for other people, that is, benefit them. A nurse who holds the hand of a dying patient honors this principle. The principle of **nonmaleficence** holds that we should not harm others. For example, a nurse upholds this principle when she withholds morphine from a client whose respirations are already depressed. You can think of these principles as being on a continuum, with the duty to do no harm taking precedence over the other duties:

Nonmaleficence ⟶ Beneficence

Do no harm → Try to prevent harm → Remove harmful things → Do good

Some simple examples to help you understand this continuum follow:

Nonmaleficence	Do no harm	Do not push a stranger into the lake.
	Try to prevent harm	If a stranger starts to fall into the lake, try to grab him and keep him from falling in.
	Remove harmful things	If you see that a person is about to stumble over a rock, which will cause him to fall in the lake, warn him or remove the rock.
Beneficence	Do good	If you happen upon the scene after a stranger has fallen into the lake, jump in and rescue him.

It is easy to see how the first situation is a stronger duty than the last one.

Nurses are morally obligated under the principles of beneficence and nonmaleficence to seek to benefit patients and not harm them. Quality assurance and evaluation of client progress fulfill this obligation by enabling nurses to improve the quality of care they deliver. Quality assurance not only contributes to improved nursing care, it can produce changes in the total health-care system and improve communication and collaboration between health-care disciplines.

The ANA code of ethics (1985) in Appendix A includes at least four items that imply that evaluating care is a nursing responsibility:

Item 4. The nurse assumes responsibility and accountability for individual nursing judgments and actions.

Item 8. The nurse participates in the profession's efforts to establish, implement, and improve standards of nursing.

Item 9. The nurse participates in the profession's efforts to establish and maintain conditions of employment conducive to high-quality nursing care.

Item 11. The nurse collaborates with members of the health professions and other citizens in promoting community and national efforts to meet the health needs of the public.

Summary

SUMMARY

Evaluation
✓ is a deliberate, systematic process in which the quality, value, or worth of something is determined by comparing it to previously identified criteria or standards.
✓ in nursing, is a planned, ongoing, deliberate activity in which the nurse, client, significant others, and other health-care professionals determine the client's progress toward goal achievement and the effectiveness of the nursing care plan.
✓ considers *structure* (focusing on the setting in which care is given), *process* (focusing on nursing activities), and *outcomes* (focusing on the changes in client health status that result from nursing care).
✓ does not end the nursing process, because the information it provides is used to begin another cycle.
✓ involves five steps: (1) *review* of the stated client goals or predicted outcomes, (2) *collection* of data about the client's responses to nursing interventions, (3) *comparison* of actual client outcomes to the predicted outcomes and drawing a conclusion about whether the goals have been met, (4) *recording* of evaluative statements, and (5) *relating* the nursing orders to the client outcomes.
✓ requires the nurse to consider all variables that may have influenced goal achievement and to modify the care plan as needed.

Quality-assurance evaluation
✓ is an ongoing, systematic process designed to evaluate and promote excellence in health care.
✓ is usually concerned with the care given to groups of clients.
✓ frequently refers to evaluation of the level of care provided in an agency, but it may be as limited in scope as an evaluation of the performance of one nurse or as broad as the evaluation of the overall quality of care in an entire country.
✓ commonly uses the methods of retrospective chart audit and peer review.

Skill-Building Activities

The word *synthesis* means putting things together to form something new. Chemists synthesize new compounds for use as medicines by thoughtfully combining various kinds of reactants and determining what the products are. We can also put ideas together to develop new ideas. Concepts, data, ideas, and methods from one source are linked with those from other sources. We call this process *synthesizing ideas*. It is an important skill because it allows us to come up with new ideas to deal with the different situations we encounter in everyday life.

Nurses synthesize when they use concepts and ideas from nursing theories and related knowledge to bring patient data together into meaningful relationships. First, cues are clustered by identifying relationships between them. Knowledge of physiological and psychological norms is combined with knowledge of nursing theories and other concepts to explain the clustered data. Further synthesis is done as the information is formed into a meaningful whole: the nursing diagnosis.

Learning the Skill

To synthesize an idea, you start with ideas that you believe are connected—ideas that might help you with a problem you are trying to understand. Suppose you are interested in gardening and you want to figure out how to fertilize your plants to grow the largest possible crop of tomatoes. You might be able to solve this problem by putting ideas about plants and fertilizers together. Here is some information you can use.

Tomatoes grow from the flowers on tomato plants.

Larger vines have more room for flowers.

Fertilizer that is high in nitrogen encourages plants to grow large, leafy vines, but it does not encourage the growth of flowers.

Fertilizer that is low in nitrogen encourages plants to grow lots of flowers.

Notice that these statements do not indicate how fertilizer affects tomato crops. That means that you must combine these ideas to synthesize a new statement about the effect of fertilizers on tomato crops.

1. How does the number of tomatoes on a vine relate to the number of flowers?

2. How does the size of the vine relate to the number of flowers?

3. How can you fertilize to grow large vines?

4. Does fertilizing for large vines solve the problem of growing lots of tomatoes?

5. How should you fertilize to grow lots of tomatoes?

As you worked your way through these questions, you were practicing the skill of synthesizing an idea. By answering Question 5, you synthesized a new idea by combining the four original ideas you were given.

Applying the Skill

Max Dupree is 75 years old. He has a medical diagnosis of peripheral arterial disease, characterized by decreased circulation in both his lower legs. Mr. Dupree has atherosclerosis and arteriosclerosis, which have caused his arteries and arterioles to become stiff and resistant, as well as smaller in radius. He is a heavy smoker. Even if you are not familiar with the nursing care of a patient with peripheral arterial disease, you should be able to synthesize a *potential* nursing diagnosis (problem + etiology) for Mr. Dupree, based on the following facts.

> All body cells need oxygen and nutrients, and are sensitive to any reduction in their supply.
>
> Oxygen and nutrients are carried to the tissues in the arterial blood.
>
> Vessel resistance (including vessel size) is one of the most important factors in determining arterial blood flow.
>
> The physiological effects of decreased peripheral circulation depend on the degree to which *reduced blood flow* exceeds *tissue demands* for oxygen and nutrients. If tissue needs are high, then even a small reduction in flow can create symptoms.
>
> Metabolic rate is a measure of the rate at which energy is being expended. An increased metabolic rate causes an increase in oxygen use.
>
> Physical exercise greatly increases the metabolic rate.
>
> Metabolic activity in muscles that lack oxygen results in hypoxia and a buildup of metabolites, producing muscle spasms.

(*Note:* Do not write a diagnosis of Altered Peripheral Tissue Perfusion, since independent nursing interventions for that diagnosis are limited in this case. Additionally, if you use this diagnosis, the etiology will either consist of pathophysiology or a medical diagnosis, neither of which can be addressed by nursing orders.)

1. First, use synthesis to determine a potential problem for Mr. Dupree.

    a. What is the connection between the radius of the arteries/arterioles and the amount of blood flow to the tissues?

b. What is the connection between decreased blood flow and the amount of oxygen that reaches the tissues?

c. Knowing Mr. Dupree's diagnosis, and using the facts in (*a*) and (*b*), what can you say about the probable state of oxygenation of the muscle tissues in Mr. Dupree's lower legs?

d. What is the connection between hypoxia, muscle spasms, and pain?

e. How does the balance (imbalance) between reduced blood flow and tissue demands affect the severity of symptoms or the likelihood that the patient will have symptoms?

f. Taking (*d*) and (*e*) into account, you could say that Mr. Dupree will probably have Pain **if**

g. Therefore, you could diagnose the problem: High Risk for Pain in Lower Legs. Given that Mr. Dupree has a constant state of reduced blood flow to his legs, he will probably have pain whenever his legs experience an increased need for oxygen.

2. Now use synthesis to determine an etiology for Mr. Dupree's potential problem of Pain.

   a. What determines the likelihood that a symptom will be produced by a reduction in peripheral blood flow?

   b. What is the connection between metabolic rate and oxygen use?

   c. What is the connection between exercise and metabolic rate?

   d. Combine the ideas in (*a*) and (*b*). What is the connection between exercise and the demands of the skeletal muscle tissues for oxygen (especially in Mr. Dupree's legs)?

   e. Combine the ideas in (*a*) and (*d*). Under what circumstances is Mr. Dupree most likely to experience the problem (symptom) of Pain?

f. Therefore, for Mr. Dupree, the etiology of High Risk for Pain in Lower Legs is exercise. Your diagnosis is: High Risk for Pain in Lower Legs r/t exercise. You do not have enough information to determine how much exercise it will take to produce pain, nor how severe the pain would be.

Reviewing What You Have Learned

In your own words, explain what synthesizing an idea means.

* Adapted from *Critical Thinking Worksheets*, a supplement of *Addison-Wesley Chemistry*, by Wilbraham et al. (Menlo Park, CA: Addison-Wesley Publishing Company, 1990).

Applying the Nursing Process

(Answer Key, p. 385)

1. Place a check mark (✔) beside the criteria that are specific, measurable, or observable.

    a. ___ The nurse gives safe care.

    b. ___ Medications are recorded at the time they are given.

    c. ___ Every patient will have an arm band with name and hospital number.

    d. ___ Temperature will be less than 100.1° during entire stay.

    e. ___ Each unit will have an adequate number of wheelchairs.

    f. ___ Data collection is systematic.

2. Match the data source to the letter of the type of evaluation for which it would be used.

   a. Structure

   b. Process

   c. Outcome

   1. ____ Charts

   2. ____ Procedure manuals

   3. ____ Verbal data from the client

   4. ____ Observation of the client (e.g., VS)

   5. ____ Observation of nursing activities

   6. ____ Staff orientation plans

   7. ____ Most performance-evaluation forms

   8. ____ System for measuring client acuity

3. Match the criterion (or question) to the letter of the type of evaluation for which it would be used.

   a. Structure

   b. Process

   c. Outcome

   1. ____ Client will state he is free from pain.

   2. ____ The nurse washes her hands before drawing up the medication.

   3. ____ How many wheelchairs are kept on the unit?

   4. ____ Client's B/P will be < 130/90.

   5. ____ All direct caregivers are registered nurses.

   6. ____ Bed is in low position with wheels locked.

   7. ____ Are all monitors in working order?

4. Your client has a nursing diagnosis of Altered Oral Mucous Membranes r/t prolonged NPO and mouth breathing. Some of the nursing orders follow:

   1. Instruct client to rinse mouth as needed with a solution of 25% acetic acid and water.

   2. Reinforce importance of oral hygiene after meals and as needed.

   3. Remind client to breathe through nose as much as possible.

   4. Lubricate lips with mineral oil.

   a. Write at least two outcome criteria you could use to determine whether this problem has been resolved.

b. State how you would obtain the data needed to determine if each criterion has been met (e.g., interview the patient, etc.)

Case Study

Refer to the following case study for Exercises 5 and 6.

Ms. Nancy Atwell is a 32-year-old unmarried teacher who has been diagnosed as having rheumatoid arthritis for approximately 4 years. This change has made her knees painful and has limited the motion and weight-bearing ability of the knee joints themselves. She has recently been diagnosed as having endometriosis, and now enters the hospital to have a hysterectomy. On her previous admission for treatment of her arthritis, she had been quiet, withdrawn, and extremely concerned for her privacy. Now she seems more outgoing and less overtly concerned about privacy. When questioned, Ms. Atwell states that she has had no previous surgical experience, but denies feeling nervous about the operation. Her preoperative orders follow:

1. S.S. enema at HS
2. Nembutal 100 mg p.o. at HS
3. NPO after midnight
4. pHisohex shower in A.M.
5. Pre-op med: Demerol 50 mg and Vistaril 25 mg IM at 0600.

5. The nurse identified for Ms. Atwell a diagnosis of "High Risk for Anxiety r/t lack of knowledge of effects and procedure of hysterectomy." Her goal is to find out whether Ms. Atwell is anxious and if she is, to relieve her anxiety. (The first answer is provided for you).

   a. Give an example of a verbal cue that would indicate achievement of this objective.

   Ms. Atwell states, "I'm confident everything will go all right. I certainly don't have any experience with this kind of thing, but I know you will tell me what I need to know. I feel pretty relaxed, actually."

   b. Give an example of a nonverbal cue that would indicate achievement of this objective.

   c. Give an example of a verbal cue that would indicate the objective has not been achieved.

   d. Give an example of a nonverbal cue that would indicate the objective has not been achieved.

6. The following nursing diagnoses and goals appear on Ms. Atwell's care plan. Using the new data charted by the nurse after implementing care for each diagnosis, write an evaluative statement for each diagnosis.

Nursing Diagnosis	Goal	New Data (Progress Notes)
High Risk for Anxiety r/t lack of knowledge of effects & procedure of hysterectomy	Will state not anxious about effects of surgery. Will show no physical signs of anxiety.	Pre-op teaching done. States understanding of surgical procedure. Says she expects to have some post-op pain, but is sure she can manage with meds. No facial tension, hands folded loosely in lap while talking.

Evaluative statement for care plan:

Nursing Diagnosis	Goal	New Data (Progress Notes)
High Risk for Grief r/t loss of childbearing ability 2° hysterectomy	Will express her feelings about sterility/desire for children, prior to discharge.	During pre-op teaching, ct. was told she would not have menstrual periods after her hysterectomy and would not be able to become pregnant. She stated "Periods are a nuisance anyway," but did not comment further.

Evaluative statement for care plan:

Nursing Diagnosis	Goal	New Data (Progress Notes)
High Risk for Noncompliance with NPO order r/t lack of understanding of importance	Will state reasons for remaining NPO for O.R. after pre-op teaching. Will remain NPO after midnight.	9 P.M.—Pre-op teaching done. States relationship of NPO to anesthesia, aspiration, etc. this evening. 11:50 P.M.—Water pitcher removed; NPO sign up. 2:30 A.M.—Ct. up to bathroom, drinking water from cupped hands. Stated she forgot about drinking restriction and would not drink any more.
Evaluative statement for care plan:		

7. For the three nursing diagnoses in exercise 6, draw a line through parts of the care plan that could be discontinued after evaluation.

8. Circle the correct word(s).

   a. A (retrospective audit) (nursing audit) is the application of objective criteria to evaluate a client's record after discharge from the hospital.

   b. Evaluation of the quality of care (is) (is not) a new concept.

   c. As the nurse is helping a client to ambulate, the client becomes pale and short of breath. The nurse did not expect this reaction, and quickly helps the client back to bed. This demonstrates that evaluating is a/an (terminal) (ongoing) process.

   d. A goal on the care plan reads, "Client will be able to ambulate to bathroom by May 1, without pallor or shortness of breath." This goal is an example of a (criterion) (standard).

9. The nursing diagnosis is "High Risk for Impaired Skin Integrity: Dermal Ulcer r/t inability to move about in bed and poor nutritional status." The goal is, "Skin integrity will be maintained." The nurse notes that the client's skin is intact, with no redness over bony prominences, and concludes that the goal has been met. Circle the letter of the correct action. The nurse should

   a. decide the problem no longer exists, document that the goal was met, and discontinue the nursing care planned to meet that goal.

   b. decide that the problem still exists even though the goal was met, and continue the same nursing interventions.

REFERENCES

American Nurses Association. (1973). *Standards of Nursing Practice*. Kansas City, MO.

American Nurses Association. (1985). *Code for Nurses with Interpretative Statements*. Kansas City, MO.

Joint Commission on the Accreditation of Hospitals. (1973). *Joint Commission on the Accreditation of Hospitals: Procedure for Retrospective Patient Care Audit in Hospitals, Nursing Edition*. Chicago.

Nightingale, F. (1858) *Notes on Matters Affecting the Health, Efficiency, and Hospital Administration of the British Army*. London: Harrison and Sons.

Werner, J. (1985). PSROs and hospital accreditation. In McCloskey, J., and Grace, H., eds., *Current Issues in Nursing*. 2nd ed. Boston, MA: Blackwell Scientific Publications.

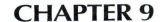

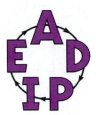

CHAPTER 9

CREATING A PATIENT-CARE PLAN

OBJECTIVES

Upon completing this chapter, you should be able to do the following:

- Describe the content of a comprehensive patient-care plan.
- Compare and contrast standardized and individually written care plans.
- Explain how model care plans, standards of care, protocols, and policies are used in creating a patient-care plan.
- List guidelines for writing patient-care plans.
- Explain how a well-written care plan supports two conventional ethical principles of nursing.
- Develop a complete plan of care for a client using either inductive or deductive diagnostic reasoning and a nursing framework.
- Describe the steps necessary in using the nursing process to develop a comprehensive patient-care plan.

INTRODUCTION

Chapters 3 through 8 presented the five steps of the nursing process and illustrated how each step is applied, using nursing models as frameworks for collecting, organizing, and analyzing data. The nursing process steps are summarized for you in Figure 9–1.

This chapter describes and provides examples of each section of a comprehensive care plan. It next presents a step-by-step Care-Planning Guide, which summarizes how the entire nursing process is used to develop a care plan for a client. Finally, the Nikki Winters case (begun in Chapter 3) is used to demonstrate how to create a comprehensive care plan by combining standard (preprinted) and individually written care plans.

THE PATIENT-CARE PLAN

A care plan is a written guide for goal-oriented nursing action. A **comprehensive care plan** is made up of several different documents that (1) address the patient's nursing diagnoses and collaborative problems; (2) describe any routine care needed to meet basic needs (e.g., bathing, elimination); and (3) specify nursing responsibilities in carrying out the medical plan of care (e.g., preparing the patient for a laboratory test, keeping the patient NPO before surgery). A

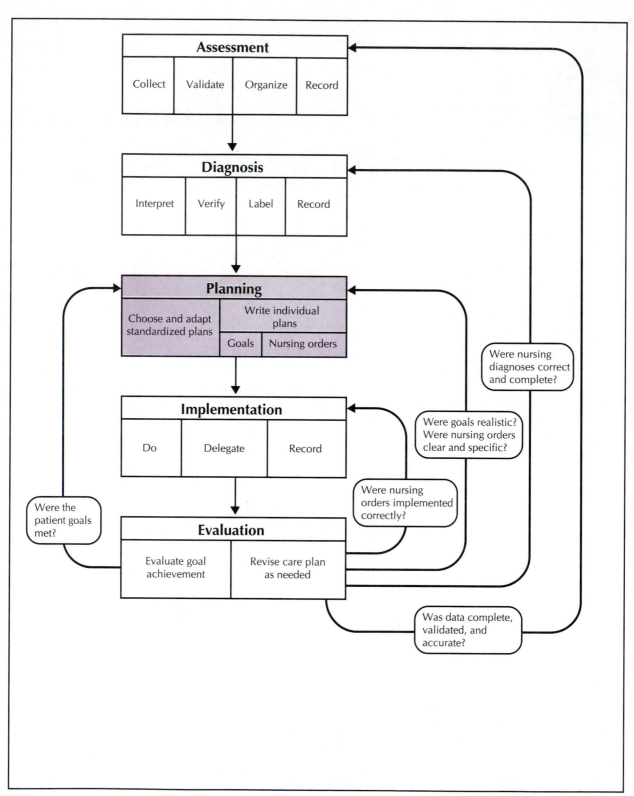

Figure 9-1. The Five Steps of the Nursing Process

complete plan of care integrates dependent, interdependent, and independent nursing functions into a meaningful whole, providing a central source of patient information.

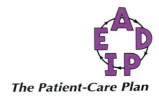

The Patient-Care Plan

The **nursing care plan** is the section of the comprehensive care plan that prescribes the independent nursing actions for the patient's nursing diagnoses and collaborative problems. Some nurses also use the term *care plan* to mean the goals and nursing orders written for a *single* nursing diagnosis, as in, "Ms. Sifuentes needs a *care plan* for Impaired Skin Integrity related to total immobility," and "What is your *plan of care* for Mr. Debicki's Anxiety?" A comprehensive care plan usually contains several of these single-problem care plans.

The professional nurse who obtained the data base should initiate the care plan as soon as possible after the patient is admitted to the agency. As a nurse, you will have the primary responsibility for planning care, but you should involve the patient and support people to the extent of their ability, as in all steps of the nursing process.

Benefits of a Written Plan

A formal, written care plan has a number of benefits for the client, the nurse, and the profession. A written care plan, first of all, **provides direction for individualizing care**. A care plan is organized according to each client's nursing diagnoses and health problems. Even if a standardized plan is used to address routine care, it must be individualized. A written plan identifies the client's unique needs and preferences for nurses who do not know him well. Even for those who do know him well, an individualized plan is a reminder that clients are people—not gallbladders, kidneys, or fractured hips.

A written care plan also **provides continuity of care**. It is important—sometimes crucial—that all caregivers use the same approach with a particular patient. For example, Jed Goldstein is being treated on an adolescent mental health unit. The staff has been trying to modify his manipulative behavior. Val Benitez, RN, has been floated to the mental health unit from the intensive care unit. She does not know Jed, but she reads an order on the nursing care plan: "Do not respond to negative talk about staff on other shifts." Later, Jed begins to complain about the night nurse. Val's usual response with ICU patients is to remain neutral but encourage them to express their feelings. Instead, she remembers the nursing order and changes the subject. Val is not an experienced psychiatric nurse; without the care plan, her nurturing instincts and past experience would have prompted her to respond differently. This would not have been therapeutic for Jed, and would have undermined the work of the nurses on the other shifts.

Over a 24-hour period, at least two or three different nurses care for a patient. During the course of his hospitalization, many different nurses, including part-time, per diem, and float nurses, will interact with him. This means that some of them will not be familiar with his unique reactions to illness. A written plan is, therefore, a valuable reference. The written plan is used as a reference at change-of-shift reports, nursing rounds, and patient-care conferences; it is also sent with the patient if he is transferred within the facility or to another facility.

A written plan **facilitates coordination of the client's care**. In addition to nursing interventions, clients receive care from a number of departments in an agency: laboratory tests, X rays, physical therapy, and so on. The comprehensive

Benefits of a Written Care Plan
- Individualized, goal-oriented care
- Continuity of care
- Coordinated care
- Efficient use of human and material resources
- Direction for documenting progress notes
- Guide for staffing assignments
- Third-party reimbursement
- Adequate discharge planning

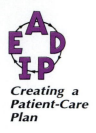

care plan is the one source of information that incorporates every aspect of a client's care. Nurses are responsible for coordinating the client's care to provide maximum comfort and conservation of his energy.

A written plan **promotes efficient functioning of the nursing team**. Written, individualized instructions assure that time will not be wasted with ineffective approaches (as in the Jed Goldstein example above) and that efforts will not be duplicated. Furthermore, a written plan transmits information more accurately than is possible in oral reports alone, and it is always available as a resource to the entire health team.

A written plan **provides direction for documentation**. The nursing care plan specifically outlines nursing observations and interventions, including client and family teaching. It provides a convenient reference for organizing the nursing progress notes and for assuring they are complete. Let's continue with the example of Jed Goldstein. Near the end of her shift, Val Benitez sat down to chart. She had talked to several patients that day. One patient had become physically ill and had to be transferred to a medical unit, and another had tried to run away. It was difficult to organize her thoughts, especially since this was her first day with these patients. As she scanned Jed's care plan, the nursing order, "Do not respond to negative talk about staff" reminded her that she should chart Jed's attempted manipulation and her own intervention.

Written care plans **provide a guide for staff assignments**. Clients with complex needs can be assigned to personnel with the necessary skills, or a client may be assigned to one nurse, with some aspects of his care delegated to someone else. The number of clients assigned to a nurse depends upon the complexity of their needs, which can easily be determined from their care plans. For example, after reviewing the care plans to determine the level of care needed by the patients on her unit, the charge nurse assigned Bryan, an LPN, to care for a caseload of six patients. He will give total care for these patients, except for the following:

1. The nursing assistant will make beds for the clients who can be out of bed.
2. A registered nurse will maintain the primary IVs and give the IV push medications.

Written care plans are **used as documentation for third-party reimbursement**. Medical insurance companies examine the client's record to determine which charges they will pay. As proof of care given, a precise, well-documented care plan facilitates hospital and client reimbursement for nursing and other services.

And finally, a written plan **helps to assure adequate discharge planning**. To assure adequate care, it has become increasingly important to include written discharge plans in the client's permanent record. (Discharge planning was introduced in Chapter 6 and will be discussed in this chapter as well.)

Systems for Storing Care Plans

Care plans must be easily accessible to all members of the health-care team, and stored so that the nurse does not have to wait while someone else is using the records. They may be kept at the bedside or in the patient's medical record, or all the care plans for a unit may be stored together in a central location (e.g., computer, Kardex, or notebook).

A **Kardex** is a holder for care plans written on specially designed 6 x 11-inch cards. Each Kardex holds several care plans. The Kardex care plan should become part of the client's medical record when it becomes inactive, although this does not happen in all agencies.

Some institutions keep the care plans for a group of patients in a **notebook** in a central location. This is similar to the Kardex system, except that the care plan cards are 8½ × 11 inches and punched to fit in a notebook binder.

In agencies that use problem-oriented medical records (POMR), the nursing care plan is documented in a special format and kept in the patient's **chart**. In this system, the patient's problems, goals, and nursing orders are recorded in the progress notes. All team members contribute to the plan, addressing one or more of the problems on the list. With this system, the nursing care plan is scattered throughout the progress notes, but it is accessible to all those involved in the patient's care.

Computers are also being used to create and store nursing care plans. The computer can generate both standardized and individualized care plans (see Figure 9–12 for an example of a computer-generated care plan). The nurse can access the patient's stored care plan from a centrally located terminal at the nurses' station or from terminals in patient rooms.

With this system, the nurse chooses the appropriate nursing diagnoses from a menu suggested by the computer. The computer then lists possible goals and interventions for those diagnoses. The nurse chooses those appropriate for the patient and types in any additional goals or interventions not listed in the menu. The nurse can read the plan on the computer screen or print out an updated working copy each day. Computerized care plans are easy to review and update, and since they do not rely on human memory, they are likely to be thorough and accurate. Charting is also more thorough and accurate. While the nurse is charting, the computer reads the specific interventions on the care plan and prompts the nurse to document the patient's responses to each intervention.

One disadvantage is that most nurses are not yet computer-literate. It takes time and effort to learn to use each new system, but it pays off in more efficient use of the nurse's time. For this reason, more and more agencies are using computerized record systems. In this era of information explosion, computer literacy is becoming another essential nursing skill.

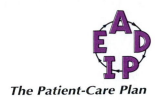

The Patient-Care Plan

Content of the Comprehensive Care Plan

A comprehensive patient-care plan covers all aspects of the patient's care. Any nurse, even one who does not know the patient, should be able to find in the care plan the instructions needed to provide competent care. Regardless of whether it is preplanned (standardized) or written from scratch, every comprehensive care plan should include (1) a brief patient profile, (2) instructions for meeting basic care needs, (3) nursing responsibilities for the medical plan, and (4) the care plan for the patient's identified nursing diagnoses and collaborative problems (the nursing care plan). Many care plans also include special sections for discharge and teaching plans. Figure 9–2 illustrates the various components of a comprehensive care plan.

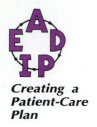

Creating a Patient-Care Plan

Client Profile

The client profile includes the client's name, age, admitting diagnosis, support people, and other pertinent personal or demographic data. This should be a brief summary, available at a glance, to give a quick overview of the client. On the computer care plan (see Figure 9–12), the profile data appears at the top of each page. The notebook Kardex (Figure 9–3) shows Nikki Winters's profile data, taken from Figure 3–3 in Chapter 3. This profile data is grouped in a section at the bottom of the Kardex. Notice that even if the nurse is not acquainted with Ms. Winters, she can quickly find out how to reach Mr. Winters in case of an emergency. She can also see the date and type of surgery, as well as the physician to call if she needs medical orders.

Instructions for Meeting Basic Needs

Regardless of the client's nursing diagnoses, the nurse must know what routine assistance is needed for hygiene, nutrition, elimination, and other basic needs. Most comprehensive care plans have a separate section for these instructions, often on a Kardex or basic care flowsheet, where they can be found quickly and conveniently. From Figure 9–3, the nurse can quickly determine that Ms. Winters cannot have a drink of water (she is NPO), that she needs a bedbath, that her siderails should be up, and that she is not to be out of bed. Because instructions for meeting basic needs change rapidly as the client's condition changes, this section of the care plan is usually marked with pencil so it can be easily altered.

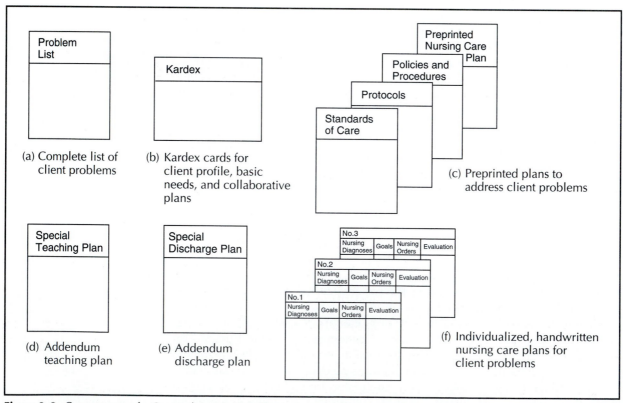

Figure 9–2. Components of a Comprehensive Care Plan

SHAWNEE MISSION MEDICAL CENTER

Date ord.	Radiology	Date Sch	DONE	Date ord.	Laboratory	Date Sch	DONE	Date ord.	Special Procedures	Date Sch	DONE
4/6/91	Chest X-ray	4/6	4/6	4/6/91	Hgb, Hct	4/6	4/6	4/6	C+S Urine	4/7	
				"	Serum Electrolytes	4/6	4/6				
				"	BUN	"	"				
				"	Blood Glucose	"	"				
				"	Cholesterol	"	"				
				4/7	Hgb, Hct	4/8					

Daily Tests

Ancillary Consults

Daily Weight

Diet: NPO p̄ midnight

Food Allergies: NKA

Hold:

Bowel/Bladder			Physical Therapy	Date	Treatments
☒ Foley	IN 4/6				
	OUT 4/8				
☒ Cath care Bid					
☐ Incontinent					
☐ Colostomy					
☐ Ileostomy					
☐ Urostomy					

Feeding/Fluids

☒ Self
☐ Assist
☐ Feeder
☐ Force
☐ Restrict

Activities

☒ Bedrest
☐ BRP
☐ Dangle
☐ Chair
☐ Commode
☐ Up ad Lib
☐ Turn
☐ Ambulate

Communication

	meal	Ext	IV
7-3	NPO		
3-11			
11-7			

☒ I&O
☒ IV LR
☒ Other PCA-M.S.

Transportation
per w/C

Hygiene
☒ Bedbath
☐ Assist
☐ Self Bath
☐ Shower
☐ Tub
☐ Vanity
☐ Oral Care

Cardio-Pulmonary | 4/7 | Incentive Spirometer q̄ 4h

Safety Measures

☒ Siderails
☐ Restraints
☐ Other

Drug Allergies: None Known

Isolation: In Out

Religious Rites: None | Code Blue: Yes

Emergency Instructions:
Relatives: John Winters
Phone: 631-1098

Clergy: None
Religion: None

Surgery & Dates:

Consults & Dates

Diagnosis: Endometriosis, dysmenorrhea | TAH and BSO 4/6/91

Room	Name	Adm Date	Age	Physician
416	WINTERS, NIKKI	4/6/91	37	Faye Humboldt, M.D.

Figure 9–3. Kardex Care Plan: Client Profile, Basic Needs, Medical Plan. Courtesy of Shawnee Mission Medical Center, Merriam, KS.

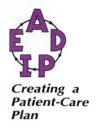

**Creating a
Patient-Care
Plan**

In addition to the routine care marked on the form, you may need to write individualized nursing diagnoses for clients who have special basic needs requirements, for example, those with Bathing/Hygiene Self-Care Deficit, Urinary Incontinence, or Altered Nutrition. These would be written in the nursing care plan section (Figure 9–4).

Aspects of the Medical Plan to Be Implemented by the Nurse

A comprehensive care plan includes nursing activities necessary for carrying out medical orders, for example, dressing changes and IV therapy. It also includes a section for scheduling prescribed diagnostic tests and treatments to be carried out by other departments (e.g., physical therapy). In Figure 9–12 this type of information is listed under "Active Doctor's Orders" and "Active Ancillary Orders." In Figure 9–3 it appears mainly in the top section of the form.

It is better to have a separate section for these activities, but you may also see them included as a part of the nursing care plan for a nursing diagnosis or collaborative problem; for example, in the section for "Laboratory" in Figure 9–3, a physician-ordered "C & S urine." However, if you were creating a student care plan, you might not have a Kardex form to work with. For Ms. Winters, you might wish to write a collaborative problem: "Potential Complication of Indwelling Catheter: Urinary Tract Infection related to vehicle for transmission of pathogens." The medical order for a culture and sensitivity of the urine would then be incorporated into the nursing interventions for that problem.

Date	Nursing Diagnosis	Predicted Outcomes	Nursing Orders	Rationale	Evaluation
7/15/92	Decisional Conflict r/t value conflicts regarding termination of treatment AMB tearfulness. Statements of inability to decide.	1. By 7/16 will discuss feelings about the situation with nurse and significant other. 2. etc.	1. Spend at least 15 minutes sitting with client during each visit. 2. Listen without making judgements. 3. etc.	1. Demonstrates support and caring. 2. Demonstrates acceptance of client's value and worth unconditionally. 3. etc.	7/16 Goal #1 Goal met. Discussed feelings of guilt with wife.

Figure 9–4. Sample Format for Nursing Care Plan

Example:

Medical order (in bold print) included in student care plan:

Problem	Nursing Orders
Potential Complication of Indwelling Catheter: Urinary Tract Infection	1. Teach pt. signs of urinary tract infection before dismissal. 2. **Discontinue Foley cath on Day 2 post-op. Collect specimen for C & S** before discontinuing.

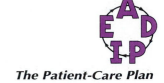

The Patient-Care Plan

Nursing Diagnoses and Collaborative Problems

The **nursing care plan**, a part of the comprehensive patient care plan, includes a list of all the client's actual and potential health problems, as well as the goals and nursing orders for those problems. This part of the care plan **reflects the independent component of nursing practice, and is the part that best demonstrates the nurse's clinical expertise.** The nursing care plan may be preplanned and preprinted, or it may be individually written from scratch. For predictable, routine problems, the goals and nursing orders are often available in preplanned, printed standards of care, standardized care plans, protocols, and agency policies and procedures. A special plan of care is handwritten for unusual problems or ones that need special attention.

Regardless of whether nursing orders are handwritten or chosen from a preprinted plan, the nursing care plan must be individualized to fit the unique needs of each patient. The problem list you develop for the patient (Chapters 4 and 5) will help to individualize care because each patient will have a different set of problems and etiologies.

Standards of Care According to Carpenito (1991) **standards of care** are "detailed guidelines that represent the predicted care indicated in a specific situation" (p. 17) such as the following:

A medical diagnosis (e.g., preeclampsia, abdominal hysterectomy)
A defined situation (e.g., postpartum, relinquishing infant)
A treatment or diagnostic test (e.g., artificial ventilation, colonoscopy)
A selected nursing diagnosis label (e.g., Anticipatory Grieving)
A collaborative problem (e.g., Potential Complication of Thrombophlebitis: Pulmonary Embolus

Standards of care are preplanned, preprinted directions for care, developed by nurses for groups of clients rather than individuals. The standards identify the nursing diagnoses and collaborative problems that occur in a defined situation. They describe achievable rather than ideal nursing care for those problems, taking into account the particular circumstances and client population of the institution. Standards define the interventions for which nurses are held accountable. They do not contain medical orders.

Standards of care are not necessarily placed in the client's care plan or medical record, but are reference documents, stored as permanent hospital records. They are either filed on the unit or in the computer for easy reference. If they are not actually kept as a part of the client's care plan, then the problem list (see Figure 9–5) should indicate which standards of care apply to the patient.

STORMONT VAIL REGIONAL MED CTR   04/06/91   16:17
TOPEKA   KS 66604

Patient: WINTERS, NIKKI
Location: 551 A   Sex:F   Age:37Y   Birthdate:1/25/54   Ht: 5Ft 2In   Wt.:128 Lbs
Account #: 8-37838-1 MRN: 299333 Vst#: 00279 3

PROBLEM LIST

	Type of Plan	Start	Stop	Identified by
1. CHRONIC ABDOMINAL PAIN 2° ENDOMETRIOSIS	Individual NCP	4/6/91	4/7/91	S. Ibarra, RN
2. ACUTE ABDOMINAL PAIN 2° SURGICAL INCISION	Standards of Care for Abd. Hysterectomy	4/6/91		S. Ibarra, RN
3. POTENTIAL COMPLICATION OF HYSTERECTOMY: HEMORRHAGE URINARY RETENTION THROMBOPHLEBITIS TRAUMA TO URETER, BLADDER OR RECTUM INCISION INFECTION	Standards of Care for Abd. Hysterectomy	4/6/91		S. Ibarra, RN
4. POTENTIAL COMPLICATION OF INTRAVENOUS THERAPY: INFLAMMATION PHLEBITIS INFILTRATION	2-South Procedure for IV Therapy	4/6/91		S. Ibarra, RN
5. POTENTIAL COMPLICATION OF FOLEY CATHETER: URINARY TRACT INFECTION RETENTION AFTER REMOVAL	Standards of Care for Abd. Hysterectomy	4/6/91		S. Ibarra, RN
6. HIGH RISK FOR COLONIC CONSTIPATION R/T INADEQUATE FLUID AND FIBER INTAKE, LACK OF EXERCISE, POSTOPERATIVE EFFECTS OF GENERAL ANESTHETIC, MORPHINE SULFATE PCA, AND TEMPORARY IMPAIRED MOBILITY	Model Care Plan for Constipation	4/6/91		S. Ibarra, RN
7. ALTERED HEALTH MAINTENANCE POSSIBLY R/T LACK OF KNOWLEDGE ABOUT CARDIAC DISEASE RISK FACTORS AND OTHER HEALTH-SEEKING BEHAVIORS	Individualized NCP	4/6/91		S. Ibarra, RN
8. POSSIBLE LOW SELF-ESTEEM R/T COMPLEX FACTORS AND POSSIBLY R/T THREATS TO SEXUAL IDENTITY 2° ENDOMETRIOSIS SYMPTOMS AND HYSTERECTOMY	Individualized NCP	4/6/91		S. Ibarra, RN

Figure 9–5. Initial Problem List for Nikki Winters

Depending on the institution, standards of care may or may not be organized according to problems or nursing diagnoses. Figure 9–6 is an example of standards of care organized according to common problems; Figure 9–7 is an example of standards of care that list only the nursing interventions, without identifying the problems to which they apply.

For some clients, all necessary nursing care may be contained in the standards of care; others will need additional interventions. These can be added as printed model care plans or developed by the nurse and handwritten on a blank care plan form.

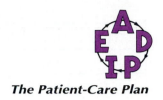

The Patient-Care Plan

Model (Standardized) Care Plans Do not confuse *standardized care plans* with *standards of care*. To avoid confusion, some nurses prefer to call them *model care plans*. Although they have some similarities, there are important differences between standards of care and model care plans:

1. Model care plans are kept with the client's active care plan (in the Kardex or computer). When no longer active, they become a part of her permanent medical record. This is not usually true of standards of care.

2. Model care plans provide more detailed instructions than standards of care. They contain deviations (either additions or deletions) from the standards for the agency.

3. Model care plans take the usual nursing process format:

   Problem → Goals → Nursing orders → Evaluation.

   This is usually not true of standards of care.

4. Model care plans allow you to add addendum care plans. They usually include checklists, blank lines, or empty spaces to allow you to individualize goals and nursing orders. This is not usually true for standards of care.

Model care plans are similar to standards of care in that they are preplanned, preprinted guides for nursing interventions for specific nursing diagnoses, or for all the nursing diagnoses associated with a particular situation or medical condition. They are developed by nurses, and while they are not standards of care, following them ensures that acceptable standards of care are provided. Refer to Figure 9–8 for a computer-generated model care plan for a single problem, High Risk for Colonic Constipation.

Many commercial books of model care plans are available. They can be used as guides when developing your care plans, but remember that they do not address the client's individualized needs, and they can cause you to focus on predictable problems and miss cues to important special problems the client is experiencing. If you use a model care plan as a student, do the following:

1. Consult your instructor to be sure you are using a reliable source.

2. First perform a nursing assessment and make your own list of all the client's actual and potential problems. You can then consult the model care plan to be sure your list is complete.

3. Using client input, establish specific, individualized goals before consulting the model care plan. Consulting the model first may inhibit your creativity.

STANDARDS OF CARE: ABDOMINAL HYSTERECTOMY (Postoperative Care)

Problem	Nursing Interventions
Potential Complication of Hysterectomy: Hemorrhage/Shock	1. VS on admission; then q15min x 4, q30min x 2, q4h x 24 hrs; then b.i.d. and prn. Include pulse rate and volume. 2. Check abdominal dressing on VS schedule. 3. Urine output on VS schedule. 4. On VS schedule, assess for restlessness, decreased level of consciousness, skin pallor or cyanosis.
Potential Complication of Hysterectomy and Indwelling Catheter: **a.** Trauma to Ureter, Bladder **b.** Urinary Tract Infection **c.** Urine Retention	1. On VS schedule, observe for cloudy or bloody urine. 2. Observe and teach patient to report flank/back pain. 3. After catheter removed, monitor for retention. If no void in 6 hrs, straight cath. On second cath, insert indwelling catheter (per protocol). 4. Monitor for symptoms of frequency, burning on urination. Teach patients s/s of UTI.
Potential Complication of Hysterectomy: Thrombophlebitis	1. Monitor q8h for leg pain, swelling, or superficial redness. 2. Check Homan's sign q8h. 3. If symptoms noted, institute bedrest, notify physician, instruct patient not to massage legs. 4. Teach patient importance of adequate fluids and ambulation. 5. Do not gatch bed or place pillows under knees.
Potential Complication of Hysterectomy: Incision Infection	1. Monitor q8h for redness, edema or drainage. 2. Teach patient to wash hands before touching incision. 3. Clean around drainage tubes q8h and prn.
High Risk for Altered Respiratory Function r/t decreased ciliary action and decreased mobility 2° anesthesia, pain, and narcotic analgesics	1. Auscultate lungs on VS schedule. 2. Assist patient to turn, cough, and deep breathe hourly x 24; then q2h x 24. 3. Explain importance to patient. 4. Encourage fluids to extent of medical orders.
Acute Pain r/t abdominal incision	1. Provide pad and teach to splint incision when TCDB or moving. 2. Teach need to ask for prn analgesic; teach to request before pain becomes too severe. 3. Ask to rate pain on 1–10 scale before and after medication. Evaluate results within 30 min after giving IM analgesics (1 hr. for p.o.). 4. Monitor comfort level at least q2h. 5. Assess B/P and resp. before giving narcotics.
High Risk for Self-Concept Disturbance r/t perceived threats to sexual identity 2° surgery of reproductive system	1. Encourage to express feelings about surgery and its effects. 2. Teach usual physiological effects of hysterectomy. 3. Assess amount of support given by significant other.

Figure 9–6. Example of Problem-Oriented Standards of Care

STANDARDS OF CARE: Patient with Thrombophlebitis

Goal:
1. To monitor for early signs and symptoms of compromised respiratory status.
2. To report any abnormal signs and/or symptoms promptly to the medical staff.
3. To initiate appropriate nursing actions when signs and/or symptoms of compromised respiratory status occur.
4. To institute protocol for emergency intervention should the client develop cardiopulmonary dysfunction.

SUPPORTIVE DATA: The purpose of these standards of care is to prevent, monitor, report, and record the client's response to a diagnosis of thrombophlebitis. Thrombophlebitis places the client at risk for pulmonary embolism. The hemodynamic consequences of embolic obstruction to pulmonary blood flow involve increased pulmonary vascular resistance, increased right ventricular workload, decreased cardiac output, and development of shock and pulmonary arrest.

CLINICAL MANIFESTATIONS: Nursing assessments performed q3–4h should monitor for the following signs/symptoms:

- Dyspnea (generally consistently present)
- Sudden substernal pain
- Rapid/weak pulse
- Syncope
- Anxiety
- Fever
- Cough/hemoptysis
- Accelerated respiratory rate
- Pleuritic type chest pain
- Cyanosis

PREVENTIVE NURSING MEASURES:

- Encourage increased fluid intake to prevent dehydration.
- Maintain anticoagulant intravenous therapy as prescribed (See Protocol for Anticoagulant Administration).
- Maintain prescribed bedrest.
- Prevent venous stasis from improperly fitting elastic stockings; Check q3–4h.
- Encourage dorsiflexion exercises of the lower extremities while on bedrest.

INDIVIDUALIZED PLANS/ADDITIONAL NURSING/MEDICAL ORDERS

Do not massage lower extremities.

Intake and output q8h.

Initiated by: *S. Ibarra, RN*   Date: *4-9-91*

Figure 9–7. Example of Non-Problem-Oriented Standards of Care

Diagnosis: **(HIGH RISK FOR) COLONIC CONSTIPATION**

Etiology/
Risk Factors:
- ✔ DECREASED ACTIVITY
- ✔ INADEQUATE DIETARY FIBER
- ✔ DECREASED FLUID INTAKE
- __ IMMOBILITY
- __ CHRONIC LAXATIVE USE
- __ CHRONIC ENEMA USE
- __ EMOTIONAL DISTURBANCES
- __ NEGLECT OF URGE TO DEFECATE
- __ EMBARRASSMENT OVER DEFECATING IN HOSPITAL ENVIRONMENT
- __ RELUCTANCE TO USE BEDPAN
- ✔ NARCOTIC ANALGESICS
- ✔ EFFECTS OF ANESTHESIA
- ✔ SEDENTARY LIFESTYLE, LACK OF EXERCISE
- __ METABOLIC CONDITIONS (E.G., HYPERCALCEMIA)

Predicted
Outcomes:
- ABDOMEN SOFT, NOT DISTENDED *at all times*
- BOWEL SOUNDS AUSCULTATED IN ALL 4 QUADRANTS BY *4-9*
- PASSES SOFT, FORMED STOOL BY *4-10*
- NAMES AND CHOOSES HIGH FIBER FOODS BY *4-10*
- VERBALIZES INTENT TO DRINK ADEQUATE FLUIDS AFTER DISMISSAL *-by 4-10*
- VERBALIZES PRESENCE OF OPTIMAL PATTERN OF BOWEL MOVEMENTS *-by 4-10*
- RESUMES USUAL PATTERN OF BOWEL MOVEMENTS *c̄ no constipation*

Nursing
Orders:
- ~~DETERMINE USUAL BOWEL HABITS~~ *done. S.I.*
- ABDOMINAL ASSESSMENT q *shift* INCLUDE BOWEL SOUNDS, DISTENTION
- MONITOR AND RECORD B.M., INCLUDING FREQUENCY AND CONSISTENCY
- DOCUMENT PASSAGE OF FLATUS
- ASSESS EACH SHIFT FOR SIGNS AND SYMPTOMS OF CONSTIPATION: HEADACHE, ABDOMINAL DISTENTION, CRAMPING, RECTAL PRESSURE, ABDOMINAL FULL-NESS, PALPABLE MASS
- IF NO B.M. IN *4* DAYS, CHECK FOR IMPACTION. OBTAIN ORDER FOR ENEMA, DIGITAL REMOVAL OF STOOL
- ~~TEACH TO REQUEST PAIN MEDICATION PRIOR TO DEFECATION TO DECREASE PAIN OF PASSING STOOL~~
- PROVIDE PRIVACY DURING BOWEL ELIMINATION
- ~~PLACE IN HIGH FOWLER'S POSITION FOR B.M. UNLESS CONTRAINDICATED~~ *Up to B.R*
- TEACH PATIENT ABOUT MEDICATIONS THAT CAUSE CONSTIPATION
- ENCOURAGE TO DRINK WARM LIQUIDS
- ENCOURAGE ACTIVITY AS ORDERED AND AS TOLERATED *See post-op M.D. orders*
- ~~MONITOR SERUM CALCIUM LEVELS~~
- INSTRUCT IN ISOMETRIC ABDOMINAL STRENGTHENING EXERCISES
- DIETARY CONSULT FOR INCREASING FIBER IN DIET
- REQUEST ORDER FOR STOOL SOFTENERS AND BULK FORMING LAXATIVES
- INSTRUCT PATIENT IN MEASURES TO PREVENT CONSTIPATION AFTER DISCHARGE:
    - EAT HIGH-FIBER, BULK-FORMING FOODS (E.G., BRAN, WHOLE GRAINS, RAW FRUITS)
    - INCREASED PHYSICAL ACTIVITY
    - INCREASED FLUID INTAKE (2500 CC/DAY UNLESS CONTRAINDICATED)
    - DEFECATE WHEN URGE IS FELT; DO NOT POSTPONE

S. Ibarra, RNC

Figure 9–8. Model Nursing Care Plan for a Single Nursing Diagnosis

4. Write as many of your own nursing orders as you can. Refer to the model to be sure you have not omitted any important interventions.

5. Be sure the nursing interventions in the model are appropriate for your client and possible to implement in your institution. Delete any that do not apply.

6. Individualize the goals and nursing orders to fit your client.

Example:

Standardized Nursing Order	*Individualized Nursing Order*
Force fluids as ordered or as tolerated by patient.	Force fluids to 2400 cc per 24 hours:

Individualized Nursing Order details:

Force fluids to 2400 cc per 24 hours:

7–3: Offer 200cc water or apple juice hourly.

3–11: Offer 200cc water or apple juice hourly while awake.

11–7: Offer water or juice when awakening patient for VS or meds.

Pt. prefers ice in his water or juice.

Protocols Protocols are preplanned and preprinted. Like standards of care and model care plans, they can cover the common actions required for a particular medical diagnosis, defined situation, treatment, or diagnostic test. For example, there may be a protocol for admitting a patient to the intensive care unit, or a protocol covering the administration of magnesium sulfate to a preeclampsia patient. Protocols are different, though, because they may include both medical orders and nursing orders. Figure 9–9 is a protocol for administering anticoagulants. When a protocol is used, it can be added to the nursing care plan and become a part of the patient's permanent record. An alternative is to keep all protocols in the hospital's file of permanent records and write "See protocol" on the care plan, as in Figure 9–13.

Policies and Procedures When a situation occurs frequently, an institution is likely to develop a policy to govern how it is to be handled. A hospital may have a policy that specifies the number of visitors a patient may have; a policy may also be similar to a protocol and specify, for example, what is to be done in the case of cardiac arrest. As with protocols and standing orders, the nurse must recognize the situation and then use judgment in implementing the policy. Hospital policies must be interpreted to meet patient needs.

Example: While on a business trip, Fred Gonzalez was in an automobile accident. He has been hospitalized in serious condition for several days. It is 8:55 P.M., and Mr. Gonzalez's wife has just arrived on the unit for her first visit. Even though hospital policy requires that visitors leave at 9 P.M., the nurse decides that implementing the policy would not meet Mr. Gonzalez's needs.

If a policy covers a situation pertinent to the patient-care plan, it is usually simply noted on the care plan (e.g., "Make Social Service referral per Unit Policy"). Hospital policies and procedures are institution records, not patient records, so they are not actually placed in the care plan.

The Patient-Care Plan

PROTOCOL FOR ANTICOAGULANT THERAPY: Care of the patient receiving intravenous Heparin Sodium.

GOAL: **1.** To administer Heparin Sodium correctly via the intravenous route as prescribed.

               2. To initiate appropriate nursing actions if hemorrhagic side effects of Heparin Sodium administration occur.

SUPPORTIVE DATA: The purpose of this protocol is to safely administer Heparin Sodium to clients requiring anticoagulant therapy. Administration is done according to the medical prescription based on clotting profiles. Continuous pump infusion is the preferred method for administration of Heparin Sodium. Evidence suggests a lower incidence of hemorrhagic complications.

SPECIAL PRECAUTIONS: Heparin is contraindicated in hemorrhagic blood dyscrasias, aneurysms, trauma, alcoholism, recent surgery, severe hepatic or renal disease, recent cerebrovascular hemorrhage, infections, and ulcerative wounds.

PHARMACODYNAMICS: Heparin Sodium interferes with clotting mechanisms along the clotting cascade. It primarily acts as an antagonist to thrombin and prevents conversion of fibrinogen to fibrin. It is used for short-term therapy, and its action is prompt and predictable. The partial thromboplastin time (PTT) should be monitored closely.

PREADMINISTRATION:

               1. Assess the client's general skin condition to establish a baseline for future assessment of ecchymotic areas.

               2. Report the PTT results to the physician.

               3. Explain the procedure to the client.

ADMINISTRATION:

               1. Perform venipuncture as prescribed (See Policy and Procedure Manual)

               2. Administer Heparin solution via volume-control pump.

               3. Monitor vital signs preadministration, q4h and as client needs/responses indicate.

               4. Assess q4h for

                    a. bleeding gums

                    b. ecchymotic areas

                    c. signs of pain

               5. Monitor PTT & platelet count as prescribed & keep physician informed.

               6. Assess IV site q3–4h.

               7. Check IV tubing for kinks/leaks q3–4h.

               8. Monitor Heparin infusion for prescribed infusion amount q2h.

ANTIDOTE: Protamine Sulfate (order from pharmacy and keep on unit).

DOCUMENTATION: Record procedure and client's tolerance/response.

Figure 9–9. Protocol for Anticoagulant Therapy

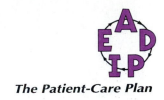

The Patient-Care Plan

Format for Nursing Care Plans Care-plan forms differ from agency to agency. However, the format for this section of the plan usually consists of at least three columns: nursing diagnoses, patient goals, and nursing orders. Some agencies add a column for assessment data (the *A.M.B.* part of the nursing diagnosis), and some add a column for evaluating patient responses to the nursing interventions. Planning usually progresses horizontally across the page: Nursing Diagnosis → Patient Goals → Nursing Orders → Evaluation. Figure 9–4 shows a typical format. In this format, you could write the assessment data in the same column as the nursing diagnosis if you use the *A.M.B.* format. A few agencies add a column for a **rationale**, which consists of principles or scientific reasons for selecting a specific nursing action. It may also explain why the action is expected to achieve the goal. Professional functioning requires an understanding of the rationale underlying the nursing orders, even when the rationale is not written on the care plan.

If care plans are to be useful in the clinical setting, they must be concise and easy to use. Still, the format chosen should include adequate space to write individualized nursing orders, even when preprinted plans are used.

Student Care Plans Care plans in practice settings are designed primarily for nurses to use in delivering care. Student care plans are designed, in addition, to provide a learning experience. Student care plans are commonly assigned for these purposes:

1. To help the student learn and apply the nursing process.

2. To provide a guide for giving nursing care to meet the client's needs while in the clinical setting.

3. To help the student learn about the client's pathophysiology or psychopathology and the associated nursing care.

Therefore, you will probably be required to handwrite your student care plans without incorporating any preprinted plans. You may be expected to develop a list of all your patient's actual and high-risk (potential) nursing diagnoses and collaborative problems, not just the unusual ones, and to develop detailed nursing interventions for them. Your instructors may also ask you to provide an in-depth rationale for your nursing interventions, and perhaps to cite literature to support your rationale.

Special Teaching Plans

In response to health-care trends such as shorter hospital stays and emphasis on wellness, teaching has become an important part of the nursing role. At the same time, nurses are caring for more and sicker patients, and find they have less time for teaching. Careful planning is therefore essential. To assure that teaching is emphasized, many institutional care plans include a special section for teaching needs. Teaching needs may also be addressed in standards of care, in model care plans, or by individually written nursing diagnoses. It is usually better to include teaching interventions as a part of the nursing orders for every nursing diagnosis, rather than write a single Knowledge Deficit problem to cover all the patient's various learning needs (see the *Nursing Diagnosis Guide* at the end of the text).

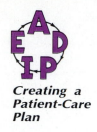

Creating a Patient-Care Plan

When a patient has complex learning needs (e.g., a newly diagnosed diabetic, a new mother without a support system), a Knowledge Deficit problem *may* be appropriate. For such patients you may wish to develop a special teaching plan to ensure efficient use of your time and maximize the patient's learning. Figure 9–10 is an example of a section of an individualized teaching plan.

Addendum Discharge Plans

All clients need some degree of discharge planning, but a separate, formal discharge plan may not always be needed. Often, you can include discharge assessments and teaching in the nursing orders for other nursing diagnoses. For example, in Figure 9–8 (the model care plan for Constipation), one of the nursing orders is to teach Ms. Winters measures to prevent constipation after discharge. Such routine discharge planning is called **standard discharge planning** and is the responsibility of the nurse caring for the client and family (Carpenito, 1991, p. 26). Many institutions have a standardized, preprinted discharge plan, like the one in Figure 9–11.

A separate discharge plan is required for clients with special needs; for example, those who are to be placed in a nursing home or other continuing-care agency, those with newly diagnosed long-term diseases such as diabetes, those with complex self-care needs, those who lack financial or social support, and so forth. Such **addendum discharge plans** require collaborative action and usually involve a discharge-planning coordinator other than the staff nurse (Carpenito, 1991, pp. 26–27).

CARE-PLANNING GUIDE

Now that you are familiar with the various documents that make up a comprehensive care plan, you should be able to follow the steps of the nursing process and make a care plan for an actual patient. The guide in Box 9–1 compresses all the steps of the nursing process into a concise but detailed reference to use in planning care. The care plan developed for Nikki Winters in this chapter follows this guide.

Each chapter in this book included a detailed guide for carrying out a particular step of the nursing process. For example, Box 4–3 (in Chapter 4) is a list of steps to follow in the diagnostic process. If you need to review any of the steps in the following Care-Planning Guide, refer to the appropriate chapter in this book, where the step is expanded for you. In addition to proceeding step-by-step through the Care-Planning Guide, you should refer to Box 9–2 when writing care plans.

Nursing Diagnosis: High Risk for Altered Health Maintenance r/t lack of knowledge of insulin therapy				
Met	Learning Objective	Content	Teaching Strategy	Learning Strategy
	1st Session Client will describe the basic patho-physiology of diabetes mellitus (cognitive).	Location and function of pancreas How cells use glucose Function of insulin Effects of insulin deficiency (elevated blood sugar, mobiliza-tion of fats and proteins, ketones, etc.)	Explain. Transparency of the pancreas.	Read pamphlet, "Your Pancreas."

	2nd Session
	Ct. will demonstrate ability to draw up correct amount of insulin (psychomotor).
		Syringe markings
		
		Sterile technique
		
		Preparation
			Point out on enlarged drawing; then actual syringe.
			
			Demonstrate and discuss.
			
			Demonstrate and discuss:
			  How to mix insulin.
			  Read label carefully, be sure syringe and label concentrations match.
			  Clean top of bottle with alcohol.
			  Withdraw correct amount.
				Practice with syringe and vial of sterile water.

Figure 9–10. Sample Teaching Plan (Partial): Diabetes Mellitus

RESEARCH MEDICAL CENTER
RESEARCH BELTON HOSPITAL
DISCHARGE PLAN

1. Does this patient require referrals prior to discharge?
   Yes _____ No _____
   If yes, check the criteria identified for making referrals. Indicate person contacted and date referred.

   A. SOCIAL SERVICES #4264 - RBH #1276
   Notified _____ on _____
   Over 65 years with:
   ___ Loss of continence, bowel/bladder
   ___ Loss of independent ambulation
   ___ Admission/Discharge nursing home
   ___ Need for Home Health
   ___ Disoriented/Confused
   ___ Under 65 with one or more significant problems affecting discharge/home care

   B. FOOD SERVICE #4125 or send req - RBH #1277
   Notified _____ on _____
   ___ Involuntary weight loss (greater than 10 lbs. in 6 mos.)
   ___ Appearance of malnourishment
   ___ Food Allergy
   ___ Special diet/religious food needs

   C. INFECTION CONTROL #4039 - RBH Notify Shift Coordinator
   Notified _____ on _____
   ___ Temperature elevation above 38.8
   ___ WBC greater than 10,000
   ___ Isolation ordered
   ___ Draining ulcerations or lesions
   ___ HIV positive/orders for HIV
   ___ Hepatitis B known positive
   ___ Rash present

   D. SKIN CARE
   ___ Score of 5 *'s on Admission Profile
   ___ Initiate Skin Care Protocols
   ___ Score of 10 *'s on Admission Profile
   ___ Notify 276-3991 for consult

   E. OTHER: _____
   Notified _____ on _____

2. What teaching needs do you identify for this patient?
   _____
   _____
   _____

3. Care plan reviewed with patient/family? Y N
   (If unable to review with patient/family, indicate reason)
   _____
   _____

   _____
   Signature of RN

   FOR SKILLED UNIT ONLY

   A. List patient's main goal.
   _____
   _____

   B. List Date Notified
   ___ ___ Physical Therapy
   ___ ___ Occupational Therapy
   ___ ___ Speech Therapy
   ___ ___ Activities Therapy
   ___ ___ Chaplaincy Service
   ___ ___ Pharmacist
   ___ ___ Respiratory Therapy

   C. ___ Patient and/or family informed that patient's own clothing may be worn; laundering will be done by patient's family.

   D. ___ Care plan reviewed at 14 days with patient/family
   Date _____ Signature _____

Figure 9–11. Discharge Plan. Courtesy of Research Medical Center, Kansas City, MO.

Box 9–1. Care-Planning Guide

1. **Collect data.**
   a. Interview, physical exam.
   b. Validate data.
   c. Organize according to framework.
2. **Analyze and synthesize data.**
   a. Group related cues according to framework.
   b. Form new cue clusters as needed.
   c. Identify deviations from normal.
3. **List all problems (working list).**
   a. Human responses that need to be changed.
   b. Medical, nursing, collaborative.
   c. Actual, high risk, possible
4. **Make formal list of labeled problems.**
   a. Label nursing diagnoses (Problem + Etiology)
      (1) Problem: Compare pt. data to defining characteristics, definitions, and risk factors.
      (2) Etiology: Related factors (risk, causal, contributing factors).
   b. Label Collaborative Problems (Potential complications of . . .).
5. **Determine which problems can be addressed by**
   a. standards of care.
   b. model care plans.
   c. protocols.
   d. policies/procedures (e.g., note on formal problem list: High Risk for Pulmonary Embolus—See Standards of Care).
6. **Individualize model care plans, protocols, and so forth, as needed.**
7. **Transcribe medical, collaborative, ADLs, and basic care needs to Kardex.**
8. **Develop individualized care plan for remaining nursing diagnoses and collaborative problems.**
   a. Develop individualized goals.
      (1) State desired client responses.
      (2) Opposite of problem response.
      (3) Measurable/realistic.
   b. Choose nursing orders.
      (1) Address etiology: reduce/remove related factors.
      (2) Address problem: relieve symptoms.
      (3) Address goal: how to bring about desired behaviors.
      (4) Health promotion, prevention, treatment, observation.
      (5) Physical care, teaching, counseling, environment management, referrals, emotional support, activities of daily living.
      (6) For complex orders, refer to policies and protocols (See "Unit Procedure for IV Therapy").
   c. Include any special, complex teaching or discharge plans.
9. **Implement care plan (do or delegate; record in chart).**
10. **Evaluate results of care.**
    a. Compare patient progress to original goals.
    b. Revise care plan as needed.
       (1) Collect more data, if needed.
       (2) Revise, discontinue, or continue problem.
       (3) Change goals if unachievable.
       (4) Revise, discontinue, or keep nursing orders.

Box 9–2. Guidelines for Writing Comprehensive Care Plans

1. **Include each of these components:**
   a. Client profile
   b. Basic needs
   c. Aspects of medical plan
   d. Nursing diagnoses and collaborative problems
   e. Special or complex teaching or discharge needs

2. **Date and sign the initial plan and any revisions.** The date is important for evaluation; the signature demonstrates nursing accountability.

3. **List or number the nursing diagnoses in order of priority.** Priorities can be changed as the client's needs change.

4. **List the nursing orders for each problem in order of priority** or in the order in which they should be done. For instance, you would assess the client's level of knowledge before you teach him to log-roll.

5. **Write the plan in clear, concise terms.** Use standard medical abbreviations and symbols. Use key words rather than complete sentences. Leave out unnecessary words, like *client* and *the* (e.g., write "Turn & reposition q2h" rather than "Turn and reposition the client every two hours").

6. **Write legibly, in ink.** When the plan cannot be erased, accountability is emphasized and more importance is placed on what is being written. If a nursing diagnosis is resolved, write "Discontinued" and a date beside it, highlight it, or date a special "Inactive" column. Goals and nursing orders can be discontinued similarly.

7. **For detailed treatments and procedures, refer to other sources** (e.g., standards of care) instead of writing all the steps on the care plan. You might write, "See unit procedure book for diabetic teaching," or you might attach a standard nursing care plan for a problem (e.g., "See standard care plan for Ineffective Breastfeeding"). This saves time, and focuses the written part of the care plan on the unique needs of the client.

8. **Be sure the plan is holistic.** It should consider the client's physiological, psychological, sociocultural, and spiritual needs.

9. **Be sure the plan is individualized** and addresses the client's unique needs. Include the client's choices about how and when care is given. For example, "Prefers evening shower."

10. **Include the collaborative and coordination aspects of the client's care.** You may write nursing orders to consult a social worker or physical therapist, or you may simply coordinate tests and treatments. The medical plan should be incorporated into the nursing care plan so that the two plans do not conflict.

11. **Include discharge plans** (e.g., arrangements for follow-up by a social worker or community health nurse).

CREATING A COMPREHENSIVE CARE PLAN

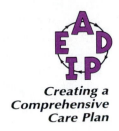

Creating a Comprehensive Care Plan

Read the following case study, which describes the course of Nikki Winters's hospitalization. Then follow the steps of the care-planning guide (Box 9–1) and the guidelines in Box 9–2 to develop a comprehensive plan for Ms. Winters.

Case Study: Nikki Winters

Framework: NANDA Unitary Person.
Medical Diagnosis: Hysterectomy, Endometriosis

Day 1 (Admission and Surgery)

Nikki Winters was admitted for a scheduled abdominal hysterectomy. She had been treated unsuccessfully for endometriosis, which was causing dysmenorrhea, painful intercourse, and heavy menstrual bleeding associated with cramping and back pain. Her hemoglobin remained low in spite of iron therapy. Ms. Winters's complete assessment data appears in Figure 3–3 in Chapter 3, so it is repeated here only in part.

Admission medical orders included NPO for surgery, heating pad for abdominal cramping or backache, IV of 1000 cc Lactated Ringers to be started at 0600 and run at 125 cc/hour, and Foley catheter to dependent drainage.

Ms. Winters had a routine surgery and uneventful recovery period. She returned to her room at 1600, still drowsy from the anesthetic. Her vital signs were within her normal baseline limits. At 2000 she was helped to sit on the side of the bed for 10 minutes. Her incisional pain was well controlled with morphine given by a patient-controlled analgesic (PCA) pump. Her abdominal dressing remained dry and intact throughout the night.

Day 2 (Day 1 Post-op)

By evening of the first postoperative day, Ms. Winters was able to walk around the room without help. She continued to use her PCA pump to control her pain. She began taking clear liquids and experienced no nausea.

Day 3 (Day 2 Post-op)

Ms. Winters's dressing was removed. The incision edges were well approximated, with minimal pink drainage. She had only slight pink, serous drainage on her vaginal pads. Her Foley catheter was removed, and she voided 4 hours later. She began taking a soft diet. She was making good progress and looking forward to going home.

During the evening, however, Ms. Winters's right thigh became sore. It was painful when she moved about. The nurse examined it and noted that it was swollen, pink, and warm to the touch when compared to the left leg. Ms. Winters's vital signs were BP 124/82, P-88, R-20, and temperature 100.4°. Sheryl notified the physician, who ordered Doppler ultrasound studies, confirming a deep vein thrombosis. He also ordered a Lee-White Clotting Time test and intravenous Heparin ("Heparin drip"). Ms. Winters was placed on complete bedrest, and a hot, moist pack was applied to her right thigh.

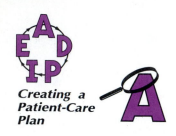

Creating a Patient-Care Plan

Assessment

Step 1: Collect Data

To collect Ms. Winters's admission data, her nurse, Sheryl Ibarra, used a data-collection form (Figure 3–3 in Chapter 3) based on the Unitary Person Framework adopted by NANDA in 1984. Sheryl compared the interview and physical examination data in order to validate her findings. Table 4–4 in Chapter 4 summarizes all the admission data collected in each of the Human Response Patterns. Sheryl summarized the data in this way so that she would have a worksheet to use during data analysis.

Diagnosis

Step 2: Analyze and Synthesize Data

Sheryl circled all the cues that seemed significant or that were outside the norm (see Box 4–1). For example, in the Knowing pattern, Sheryl circled that Ms. Winters is a smoker and that her father died of a heart attack, because both of these pieces of information may increase Ms. Winters's risk for heart problems.

She then thought about how the abnormal cues in one group might be related to cues in another group—inductively forming new cue clusters (refer to Table 4–4). For instance, in the Relating pattern, Ms. Winters reported that she has had infrequent sexual intercourse during the past six months because of pain, and says, "That won't be a problem after surgery." In the Knowing pattern, she reported having dysmenorrhea for the past six months; this relates to and validates the Relating data. In the Feeling pattern, Sheryl noted data about abdominal cramping and back pain that are aggravated by intercourse. All these pieces of information seemed related, so Sheryl inductively grouped them together into a new cue cluster (Cluster 1). This cue cluster represents a problem that is essentially physiological and fits best in the Feeling pattern.

Notice in Cluster 3 that Sheryl found cues in the Knowing, Moving, and Exchanging patterns that, taken together, indicate that Ms. Winters may need to pay more attention to health-promotion and disease-prevention activities—a problem of Health Maintenance in the Moving pattern. Each piece of data alone (e.g., that she smokes, doesn't eat a well-balanced diet, exercise, get regular checkups, or do breast self-exams) might not be significant; but when Sheryl considered them together their importance became clear. All the new cue clusters are listed in Table 4–4 in Chapter 4. Notice that the same piece of data may appear in more than one new cluster (e.g., "heavy bleeding past six months" is in both Clusters 1 and 2). Examine Table 4–4 carefully, to see if you can follow the reasoning for each of the cue clusters. If you need to review the NANDA Human Response Patterns, see Table 3–5 in Chapter 3.

Step 3: Make a Working Problem List

Recall that a nursing diagnosis is a judgment about the client's responses to health problems or life processes. In this step Sheryl made a judgment about the most likely explanation for each cue cluster. She then decided whether it represented an actual, high-risk, or possible problem; she also concluded whether the problem was medical, collaborative, or a nursing diagnosis.

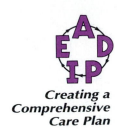

For Cluster 1, the most likely explanation was that the unsatisfactory sexual relationship was caused by Ms. Winters's disease symptoms. Surgical removal of her uterus would be expected to stop her pain and bleeding, allowing her to resume satisfactory sexual intercourse. This is a medical problem that will be solved without nursing intervention; therefore, Sheryl did not include it in her care plan.

For Cluster 2, a likely explanation was that Ms. Winters might lack knowledge about cardiac disease risk factors and other health-seeking behaviors, such as breast self-exam, balanced diet, and exercise. Her financial resources seemed adequate, and Ms. Winters had complied with past therapies for her endometriosis, so Sheryl concluded that the problem was probably caused by lack of knowledge rather than lack of motivation or resources. This cue cluster represents an actual problem of Altered Health Maintenance, which Sheryl identified as a nursing diagnosis because she can intervene independently.

Cluster 3 represents a Pain problem, caused by Ms. Winters's endometriosis. Since there are some independent nursing interventions for this problem, Sheryl decided to include it on the care plan as an actual nursing diagnosis. However, she realized it would only apply prior to surgery; after surgery the problem would change.

The cues in Cluster 4 all seemed related somehow to Ms. Winters's self-concept. Sheryl thought Ms. Winters might not have good self-esteem, but she really did not have enough data to draw that conclusion. She hypothesized that her endometriosis symptoms and the hysterectomy might create a threat to her sexual identity. She also realized that low self-esteem usually develops over a long period of time and that many factors contribute to it. She would need more data before deciding if this were an actual problem, so she concluded that the cue cluster represented a possible nursing diagnosis of Low Self-Esteem.

Sheryl concluded that Cluster 5 represented the medical problem of anemia, for which Ms. Winters was already receiving iron pills. Further, the bleeding would stop after surgery, so the problem required no nursing intervention and was not included in the care plan.

Cluster 6 contained cues for a nursing diagnosis of Colonic Constipation. However, since Ms. Winters had no symptoms of constipation, Sheryl concluded this was a potential rather than an actual problem.

In addition to the problems identified from the cue clusters, Sheryl identified the potential collaborative problems that existed for Ms. Winters because of her impending surgery and medical therapies. The following is Sheryl's working problem list, before it was put into standard NANDA terminology:

Working Problem List

Cue Cluster	Probable Explanation
1	Symptoms of medical problem. No formal statement needed.
2	Actual Altered Health Maintenance. Possibly caused by lack of knowledge about cardiac disease risk factors and other health-seeking behaviors (such as breast self-exam, balanced diet, and regular exercise program). Nursing diagnosis.

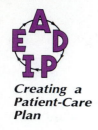

Creating a Patient-Care Plan

3	Moderate, chronic Pain (abdominal cramps and backache). Caused by disease process (endometriosis). Nursing diagnosis.
4	Possible Low Self-Esteem. Caused by complex factors and possibly by threats to her sexual identity brought on by endometriosis symptoms and impending hysterectomy. Nursing diagnosis.
5	Medical problem (anemia). Currently being treated. Requires no nursing interventions. Do not include in care plan.
6	High Risk for Constipation. Caused by inadequate fluid and fiber intake and lack of exercise. Will probably be aggravated by postoperative effects of anesthesia, narcotic analgesics, and temporary decreased mobility. Nursing diagnosis.

Collaborative Problems

Potential Complications of Hysterectomy: Hemorrhage; urinary retention; thrombophlebitis; trauma to ureter, bladder, or rectum; incision infection.

Potential Complications of Intravenous Therapy: Inflammation, phlebitis, infiltration.

Potential Complication of Foley Catheter: Urinary tract infection, retention after removal.

Strengths

Communicates adequately. Stable family situation. Adequate finances. Adequate social network. Essentially healthy history—no major illnesses. Understands about surgery and therapeutic effects. No perceptual or sensory difficulties. Able to solve problems and make decisions. Motivated to comply with therapies.

Step 4: Make Formal List of Labeled Problems

Sheryl referred to her list of NANDA diagnostic labels (see inside front cover for list of diagnostic labels organized by Human Response Patterns) to make the formal list of nursing diagnoses and collaborative problems for Ms. Winters's care plan. For the nursing diagnoses, Sheryl compared the data to the defining characteristics in her nursing diagnosis handbook to be sure she had chosen the correct NANDA label. After verifying the diagnoses with Ms. Winters, she wrote them on the care plan in order of priority (see Figure 9–5). Note that this is the *initial* problem list, written on the day Ms. Winters was admitted to the hospital.

Planning

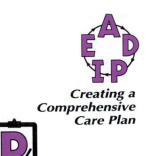

Creating a Comprehensive Care Plan

Step 5: Determine Which Problems Can Be Addressed by Standards of Care, Standardized Care Plans, Protocols, Policies, and Procedures.

After developing the formal problem list, Sheryl needed to decide how each of the problems was to be addressed (i.e., with preplanned interventions or individualized plans). For each problem, she asked the following series of questions.

1. *Are there standards of care for clients with this medical diagnosis or situation?* Sheryl's unit, 2-South, has standards of care for abdominal hysterectomy patients (Figure 9–6). Sheryl concluded that these standards describe all the care necessary for Problems 2, 3, and 5 (incision pain and the potential complications of surgery and catheterization). Since no special plan was necessary, she simply listed these three problems on the formal problem list (Figure 9–5) and wrote beside them, "Standards of Care for Abd. Hysterectomy."

   Even though Pain can be a nursing diagnosis, the medical order for PCA morphine would be the major factor in controlling Ms. Winters's postoperative pain; also, the standards of care contain the independent nursing interventions for Pain (e.g., "Teach to splint incision . . ."). For this reason, a handwritten, individualized plan was not needed for this problem.

2. *Is there a model nursing care plan for the client's medical diagnosis or condition?* In Ms. Winters's case, because there were standards of care for abdominal hysterectomy patients, and because her needs did not exceed the standards, Sheryl did not look for a model care plan for this medical diagnosis.

3. *For the **collaborative problems** not completely covered by the standards of care, do any of the following exist to direct your interventions?*

   Physician's orders (you may need to call to obtain these)
   Standing orders
   Protocols
   Policies and procedures

   Ms. Winters's only collaborative problem not addressed by standards of care was Problem 4, Potential Complications of IV Therapy. The physician's orders specified the type of IV fluid and the prescribed rate of flow. Sheryl noted this information on a Kardex form (Figure 9–3). The 2-South *Policies and Procedures* notebook contains a section on "Intravenous Therapy," which specifies how often IV tubing is to be changed, what focus assessments to make, and so forth. Sheryl noted this source on the formal problem list (Figure 9–5) beside Problem 4.

   If there are collaborative problems that are not covered by any of the above documents, they must be written on the care plan, and individualized goals and nursing orders must be developed for them.

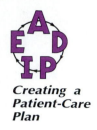

**Creating a
Patient-Care
Plan**

4. For the **nursing diagnoses** not covered by the standards of care, determine the following:

   a. Which nursing diagnoses really need individualized nursing care plans? Remember that an individualized plan is needed only if the care is not completely covered by standards of care, protocols, or other routine nursing care. Sheryl determined that Problems 1, 6, 7, and 8 needed care beyond that specified in the standards of care and unit procedures.

   b. Is there a preprinted model care plan for the nursing diagnosis? Recall that model care plans may exist for a medical diagnosis or for a single nursing diagnosis. Sheryl used a preprinted plan (Figure 9–8) for Problem 6, High Risk for Colonic Constipation.

   You may not use the procedure in Step 5 for beginning student care plans, but you will certainly use it when you develop working care plans as a professional nurse. While you are learning to write care plans, your instructors may ask you to make a complete list of the client's nursing diagnoses and collaborative problems, and to write your own goals and nursing orders for each problem—even the ones that are routine. You will usually not have the option of using standards of care, standing orders, protocols, and model care plans.

Step 6: Individualize Standardized Documents as Needed

Besides the handwritten care plans for the three nursing diagnoses, Sheryl planned to use the following documents to direct Ms. Winters's care:

   2-South "Standards of Care for Abdominal Hysterectomy"
   2-South "Procedure for Intravenous Therapy"
   2-South "Model Care Plan for Colonic Constipation"

The "Standards of Care" and the "Procedure for Intravenous Therapy" were in the 2-South files and required no alterations for Ms. Winters. Because they are a part of the permanent agency records and reflect the care given to all patients with those therapies, Sheryl did not add copies to Ms. Winters's permanent care plan record. Sheryl individualized the Model Care Plan for Colonic Constipation (Figure 9–8), and noted it on the Problem List (Figure 9–5). She then signed and placed the modified plan with the rest of Ms. Winters's comprehensive care plan.

Step 7: Transcribe Medical, Collaborative, ADLs, and Basic Care Needs to Special Sections of the Kardex

Because 2-South uses computerized care plans, Sheryl typed the medical orders into the computer. Each day she can obtain a list of orders in effect for that day (see Figure 9–12, "Active Doctor's Orders"). Instructions for Ms. Winters's diet, activity, hygiene needs, intravenous therapy, and so on, are also found on page 2 of the care plan; some appear under "Active Ancillary Orders." (Note: page 1 of Ms. Winters's care plan is her Problem List, Figure 9–5.)

Step 8: Develop Individualized Care Plan for Remaining Nursing Diagnoses and Collaborative Problems

Sheryl needed to develop goals and nursing orders for Chronic Pain $2°$ endometriosis, Altered Health Maintenance, and Possible Low Self-Esteem. Since there was no model care plan for these, Sheryl developed the goals and nursing orders based on her own nursing knowledge and information about Ms. Winters and typed them into the computer (see Figure 9–12, pages 3 and 4).

STORMONT VAIL REGIONAL MED CTR   04/06/91   16:17
TOPEKA, KS 66604

Patient: WINTERS, NIKKI
Location:551A   Sex:F   Age:37 Y   Birthdate:1/25/54   Ht:5Ft 2In   Wt:128 Lbs
Account #:8-37838-1 MRN:299333 Vst#:00279 3   Admitted date:04/06/91
Discharge Date: / /   Admitting Diagnosis: Endometriosis
Surgical Procedure: TOTAL ABDOMINAL HYSTERECTOMY
Drug Allergies: Penicillin   Admitting Dr.:Humboldt, F.
Food Allergies: None   Consult Dr. 1:
Other Allergies: None   Consult Dr. 2:
Religion: None   Consult Dr. 3:
Marital Status: MARRIED   Pri Care Phy: Humboldt, F.
Diabetic? N   Pregnant? N   Smoker? Y   Infectious? N   Fasting? N
Hygiene? Bed Bath 4/7/91

ACTIVE DOCTOR'S ORDERS

	Start	Stop	Entered by
ACTIVITY			
AD LIB	4/6/91	4/7/91	RRT
INTAKE & OUTPUT			
ROUTINE	4/6/91		RRT
I.V. THERAPY/FLUIDS			
PERIPHERAL - LR @125CC/HOUR			
START 4/7/91 AT 0600.	4/7/91		RRT
VITAL SIGNS/NEURO/CIRCULATION			
ROUTINE	4/6/91		RRT
K-PAD PRN ABD. CRAMPS OR BACKACHE	4/6/91	4/7/91	RRT

ACTIVE ANCILLARY ORDERS

	Ord#	Freq	Priority	Order Dt Sts	Entered by
DIETARY					
NPO AFTER MIDNIGHT	5	1 TIME	ROUT	4/6/91 Ordered	RRT
DIAGNOSTIC RADIOLOGY					
CHEST PA & LAT 71020	4	1 TIME	ROUT	4/6/91 Ordered	RRT

NURSING CARE PLAN

Prob.
No.

	Start	Stop	Status
1. Nursing Diagnosis:CHRONIC MODERATE ABDOMINAL PAIN	4/6/91	4/7/91	IN PROGRESS
Related to: 2° ENDOMETRIOSIS	4/6/91		
Desired Outcomes: REPORTS REASONABLE COMFORT	4/6/91		IN PROGRESS
REPORTS PAIN IS < 4 on A SCALE OF 1-10	4/6/91		IN PROGRESS
PAIN DOES NOT INTERFERE WITH SLEEP	4/6/91		IN PROGRESS

Figure 9–12. Initial Care Plan for Nikki Winters. Adapted courtesy of Stormont Vail Regional Medical Center, Topeka, KS.

STORMONT VAIL REGIONAL MED CTR   04/06/91   16:17
TOPEKA, KS 66604

Patient: WINTERS, NIKKI
Location: 551A   Sex:F   Age:37 Y   Birthdate:1/25/54   Ht:5Ft 2In   Wt:128 Lbs
Account #: 8-37838-1 MRN: 299333 Vst#: 00279 3

NURSING CARE PLAN

		Start	Stop	Status
Nursing Orders:	ASSESS INTENSITY OF PAIN (SCALE 1-10) EVERY 4 HR	4/6/91		IN PROGRESS
	ASSESS NONVERBAL CUES FOR PAIN EVERY 4 HR	4/6/91		IN PROGRESS
	INSTRUCT TO REQUEST MED BEFORE PAIN SEVERE	4/6/91		IN PROGRESS
	K-PAD AT BEDSIDE; INSTRUCT IN USE	4/6/91	4/7/91	IN PROGRESS
	TEACH RELAXATION TECHNIQUES-MUSCLE RELAXATION	4/6/91		IN PROGRESS
7. Nursing Diagnosis:	ALTERED HEALTH MAINTENANCE	4/6/91		IN PROGRESS
Related to:	POSSIBLY R/T LACK OF KNOWLEDGE ABOUT CARDIAC DISEASE RISK FACTORS AND OTHER HEALTH-SEEKING BEHAVIORS	4/6/91		
Desired Outcomes:	VERBALIZES INTENT TO DO BSE AFTER DISCHARGE	4/6/91		IN PROGRESS
	ACKNOWLEDGES EFFECTS OF SMOKING ON HEART BY DISCHARGE	4/6/91		IN PROGRESS
	AGREES TO STOP SMOKING WHILE IN HOSPITAL	4/6/91		IN PROGRESS
	VERBALIZES IMPORTANCE OF REGULAR EXERCISE	4/6/91		IN PROGRESS
	VERBALIZES INTENT TO HAVE REGULAR CHECK-UPS	4/6/91		IN PROGRESS
Nursing Orders:	GIVE LITERATURE ON BSE	4/10/91		
	DEMONSTRATE BREAST SELF-EXAM	4/10/91		
	GIVE PAMPHLET AND REFER TO SMOKING CLINIC	4/10/91		
	DISCUSS NEED FOR EXERCISE; BENEFITS OF WALKING	4/10/91		
	IDENTIFY FACTORS INTERFERING WITH EXERCISING	4/6/91		IN PROGRESS
	IDENTIFY FACTORS INTERFERING WITH BSE	4/6/91		IN PROGRESS
	IDENTIFY FACTORS CONTRIBUTING TO SMOKING	4/6/91		IN PROGRESS
	PROVIDE NONJUDGMENTAL ENVIRONMENT TO PROMOTE DISCUSSION OF HEALTH HABITS	4/6/91		IN PROGRESS
8. Nursing Diagnosis:	POSSIBLE LOW SELF-ESTEEM	4/6/91		IN PROGRESS
Related to:	COMPLEX FACTORS	4/6/91		IN PROGRESS
	POSSIBLY R/T THREATS TO SEXUAL IDENTITY 2° ENDOMETRIOSIS SYMPTOMS AND HYSTERECTOMY			
Desired Outcomes:	CONFIRM OR RULE OUT LOW SELF-ESTEEM BY DISCHARGE	4/6/91		IN PROGRESS
Nursing Orders:	PROVIDE NONJUDGMENTAL ENVIRONMENT FOR DISCUSSION	4/6/91		IN PROGRESS
	EXPLORE RECENT CHANGES THAT MAY BE CAUSING LOW SELF-ESTEEM (PAINFUL INTERCOURSE, BLEEDING, HYSTERECTOMY)	4/6/91		IN PROGRESS
	HELP TO EXPLORE AND IDENTIFY STRENGTHS	4/6/91		IN PROGRESS

Figure 9–12. (continued)

```
┌─────────────────────────────────────────────────────────────────────────────────┐
│                    DAILY CARE ACTIVITY SHEET                         PAGE 4       │
│  STORMONT VAIL REGIONAL MED CTR                        04/06/91    16:17          │
│  TOPEKA, KS 66604                                                                 │
│  Patient: WINTERS, NIKKI                                                          │
│  Location:551A      Sex:F    Age:37 Y    Birthdate:1/25/54    Ht:5Ft 2In   Wt:128 Lbs │
│  Account #:8-37838-1 MRN:299333 Vst#:00279 3                                      │
│                      NURSING CARE PLAN                                            │
│                                               Start   Stop   Status              │
│       ASSESS FOR NEGATIVE FEELINGS ABOUT SELF   4/6/91        IN PROGRESS         │
│       ASSESS FOR EXPRESSIONS OF SHAME/GUILT     4/6/91        IN PROGRESS         │
│       OBSERVE FOR DIFFICULTY IN MAKING DECISIONS 4/6/91       IN PROGRESS         │
│       OBSERVE FOR HYPERSENSITIVITY TO CRITICISM 4/6/91        IN PROGRESS         │
│       IDENTIFY HUSBAND'S FEELINGS ABOUT         4/6/91        IN PROGRESS         │
│          HYSTERECTOMY, TO DETERMINE IF CLIENT'S                                   │
│          FEARS ARE REALISTIC                                                      │
└─────────────────────────────────────────────────────────────────────────────────┘
```

Figure 9–12. (concluded)

Implementation

Step 9: Implement the Care Plan (Do or Delegate)

Most of Ms. Winters's care plan was scheduled to be put into effect after her surgery. During the morning of her admission, Sheryl performed the preoperative teaching, as outlined in the standards of care. She also talked with Mr. Winters to assess his feelings about his wife's surgery. The following are Sheryl's nursing progress notes for the morning.

4/6/91

0630   Ibuprofen 500 mg given p.o. for c/o abd. cramping. Pt. using K-pad; demonstrated and taught use._____S. Ibarra, R.N.

0730   States abd. cramps now "about 2" on a 1–10 scale. Goals for pain control are being met. Preoperative teaching done per unit standards, including need to be NPO. Verbalizes understanding; returned demonstration of T.C.D.B. _____S. Ibarra, R.N.

0930   Discussed with Mr. Winters his feelings about his wife's surgery. He verbalized understanding of the procedure, expected results, and effects. States that he, too, has been frustrated with their sexual relationship, but that he expects "everything will be o.k." after the surgery. He says he does not have any "especially negative feeling" about hysterectomy—that any changes will be "for the better." _____S. Ibarra, R.N.

Implementation during the rest of the day consisted of routine care given according to the Standards of Care for Abdominal Hysterectomy and the 2-South Procedure for IV Therapy. Ms. Winters was drowsy and in pain after surgery, so the individualized problems were not addressed. The same was true on her first post-op day (Day 2 in the case study). On Day 3, the nurses began to address the individualized nursing diagnoses on the care plan. The diagnosis of Low Self-Esteem was confirmed and found to be a long-standing problem for Ms. Winters. This was also the day that Ms. Winters developed thrombophlebitis.

319

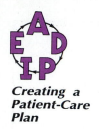

Creating a Patient-Care Plan

Evaluation

Step 10: Evaluate Results of Care

During evaluation, the nurse compares patient progress to the predicted outcomes and revises the care plan if necessary. The computerized nursing care plan used on 2-South does not have a column for evaluative statements. It does have "Start/Stop" columns and a column for "Status." Therefore, when the nurses make a judgment about goal achievement, the supporting patient data must be charted in the nursing progress notes. Sheryl did this when she charted Ms. Winters's pain relief after receiving Ibuprofen. On the first day, Sheryl evaluated care for the following problems:

Problem 1: Chronic Moderate Abdominal Pain 2° Endometriosis. Sheryl concluded that two of the desired outcomes had been met: (1) reports reasonable comfort and (2) reports pain is < 4 on a scale of 1–10. She concluded that the Ibuprofen and K-pad had been effective interventions, since they were the only ones that had been tried. In the evening after surgery, this problem was no longer appropriate; it was discontinued, and a new problem was added to the care plan: "Acute Abdominal Pain 2° surgical incision."

Problem 2: Acute Abdominal Pain 2° surgical incision. Ms. Winters obtained adequate pain relief from the PCA morphine during the night. This was a newly added nursing diagnosis and did not require revision.

Problems 3, 4, and 5: No symptoms of complications were observed; the care plan for these problems was not changed.

Problems 6 and 7: These problems could not be evaluated, as no care was given for them.

Problem 8: Possible Low Self-Esteem r/t complex factors and possibly r/t threats to sexual identity. Sheryl had obtained some further information from Ms. Winters's husband about this diagnosis, but not enough to confirm or rule out the problem. Therefore, she concluded the goal had not been met and that the care plan should continue. She did, however, delete the nursing order to "identify husband's feelings about hysterectomy." She did not want nurses on other shifts to repeat this activity, since she had already talked to Mr. Winters. She simply entered the date in the "Stop" column on the computer screen, as shown below:

	START	STOP
ASSESS FOR EXPRESSIONS OF SHAME/GUILT	4/6/91	IN PROGRESS
OBSERVE FOR DIFFICULTY IN MAKING DECISIONS	4/6/91	IN PROGRESS
OBSERVE FOR HYPERSENSITIVITY TO CRITICISM	4/6/91	IN PROGRESS
IDENTIFY HUSBAND'S FEELINGS ABOUT HYSTERECTOMY, TO DETERMINE IF CLIENT'S FEARS ARE REALISTIC	4/6/91	**4/6/91**

STORMONT VAIL REGIONAL MED CTR   04/09/91   16:17
TOPEKA   KS 66604

Patient: WINTERS, NIKKI
Location:551A   Sex:F   Age:37 Y   Birthdate:1/25/54   Ht:5Ft 2In   Wt:128 Lbs
Account #:8-37838-1 MRN:299333 Vst#:00279 3

PROBLEM LIST

Prob. No.		Type of Plan	Start	Stop	Identified by
2.	ACUTE ABDOMINAL PAIN 2° SURGICAL INCISION	Standards of Care for Abd. Hyst.	4/6/91		S. Ibarra, RN

3.	POTENTIAL COMPLICATION OF HYSTERECTOMY:
	   HEMORRHAGE
	   URINARY RETENTION
	   INCISION INFECTION
		Standards of Care
		for Abd. Hyst.
			4/6/91		S. Ibarra, RN

4.	POTENTIAL COMPLICATION OF
	   INTRAVENOUS THERAPY:
	   INFLAMMATION, PHLEBITIS, INFILTRATION
		2-South Procedure
		for IV Therapy
			4/6/91		S. Ibarra, RN

5.	POTENTIAL COMPLICATION OF
	   FOLEY CATHETER:
	   URINARY TRACT INFECTION
	   RETENTION AFTER REMOVAL
		Standards of Care
		for Abd. Hyst.
			4/6/91		S. Ibarra, RN

6.	HIGH RISK FOR COLONIC CONSTIPATION R/T
	   INADEQUATE FLUID AND FIBER INTAKE,
	   LACK OF EXERCISE, MORPHINE SULFATE
	   PCA, AND TEMPORARY IMPAIRED MOBILITY
		Model Care Plan
		for Constipation
			4/6/91		S. Ibarra, RN

7.	ALTERED HEALTH MAINTENANCE POSSIBLY R/T
	   LACK OF KNOWLEDGE ABOUT CARDIAC
	   DISEASE RISK FACTORS AND OTHER
	   HEALTH-SEEKING BEHAVIORS
		Individualized NCP	4/6/91		S. Ibarra, RN

8.	LOW SELF-ESTEEM R/T
	   COMPLEX FACTORS AND THREATS TO
	   SEXUAL IDENTITY 2° ENDOMETRIOSIS
	   SYMPTOMS AND HYSTERECTOMY
		Individualized NCP	4/6/91		S. Ibarra, RN

9.	POTENTIAL COMPLICATION OF
	   THROMBOPHLEBITIS:
	   PULMONARY EMBOLUS
		Standards of Care
		for
		Thrombophlebitis
			4/8/91		S. Ibarra, RN

10.	MODERATE CRAMPING PAIN IN RIGHT LEG R/T INFLAMMATORY PROCESS	Model Care Plan for Pain	4/8/91		S. Ibarra, RN

11.	POTENTIAL COMPLICATIONS OF HEPARIN
	   THERAPY:
	   SPONTANEOUS BLEEDING
	   THROMBOCYTOPENIA
		2-S Protocol for
		Anticoagulant
		Therapy
			4/8/91		S. Ibarra, RN

Figure 9–13. Revised Care Plan for Nikki Winters. Adapted courtesy of Stormont Vail Regional Medical Center, Topeka, KS.

STORMONT VAIL REG MED CTR   04/09/91   16:17
TOPEKA   KS 66604

Patient: WINTERS, NIKKI
Location:551A   Sex:F Age:37 Y   Birthdate:1/25/54   Ht:5Ft 2In   Wt:128 Lbs
Account #:8-37838-1 MRN:299333 Vst#:00279 3

NURSING CARE PLAN

	Start	Stop	Status
Nursing Diagnosis: ALTERED HEALTH MAINTENANCE	4/6/91		IN PROGRESS
Related to: R/T LACK OF KNOWLEDGE ABOUT CARDIAC DISEASE			
RISK FACTORS AND OTHER HEALTH BEHAVIORS			
Desired Outcomes: VERBALIZES INTENT TO DO BSE AFTER DISCHARGE	4/6/91		IN PROGRESS
ACKNOWLEDGES EFFECTS OF SMOKING ON HEART	4/6/91		IN PROGRESS
BY DISCHARGE			
AGREES TO STOP SMOKING WHILE IN HOSPITAL	4/6/91		IN PROGRESS
VERBALIZES IMPORTANCE OF REGULAR EXERCISE	4/6/91	4/9/91	GOAL MET
VERBALIZES INTENT TO HAVE REGULAR CHECK-UPS	4/6/91	4/9/91	GOAL MET
Nursing Orders: GIVE LITERATURE ON BSE	4/10/91		
DEMONSTRATE BREAST SELF-EXAM	4/10/91		
GIVE PAMPHLET AND REFER TO SMOKING CLINIC	4/10/91		
DISCUSS NEED FOR EXERCISE; BENEFITS OF	4/10/91		
WALKING			
IDENTIFY FACTORS INTERFERING WITH EXERCISING	4/6/91	4/9/91	DONE
IDENTIFY FACTORS INTERFERING WITH BSE	4/6/91		IN PROGRESS
IDENTIFY FACTORS CONTRIBUTING TO SMOKING	4/6/91		IN PROGRESS
PROVIDE NONJUDGMENTAL ENVIRONMENT TO PROMOTE	4/6/91		IN PROGRESS
DISCUSSION OF HEALTH HABITS			
Nursing Diagnosis: LOW SELF-ESTEEM	4/6/91		IN PROGRESS
Related to: COMPLEX FACTORS			IN PROGRESS
THREATS TO SEXUAL IDENTITY			IN PROGRESS
2° ENDOMETRIOSIS SYMPTOMS AND HYSTERECTOMY			
Desired Outcomes: WILL IDENTIFY AND ACKNOWLEDGE SOME	4/8/91		IN PROGRESS
STRENGTHS BY DISMISSAL			
PARTICIPATES IN DECISIONS ABOUT PLAN OF CARE	4/8/91		IN PROGRESS
EXPRESSES AN INTEREST IN OBTAINING	4/8/91		IN PROGRESS
COUNSELING BY DISMISSAL			
Nursing Orders: PROVIDE NONJUDGMENTAL ENVIRONMENT FOR	4/6/91		IN PROGRESS
DISCUSSION			
HELP TO EXPLORE AND IDENTIFY STRENGTHS	4/6/91		IN PROGRESS
ASSESS FOR NEGATIVE FEELINGS ABOUT SELF	4/6/91		IN PROGRESS
ASSESS FOR EXPRESSIONS OF SHAME/GUILT	4/6/91		IN PROGRESS
OBSERVE FOR DIFFICULTY IN MAKING DECISIONS	4/6/91		IN PROGRESS
OBSERVE FOR HYPERSENSITIVITY TO CRITICISM	4/6/91		IN PROGRESS
HELP TO OBTAIN NAMES OF COUNSELORS	4/9/91		IN PROGRESS

Figure 9–13. (concluded)

Nursing Diagnosis: PAIN *in left leg*			
Etiology	Client Outcomes	*Nursing Actions	Teaching Plan

__Fractures
__Muscle spasms
__Arthritis
__Vascular occlusion
__Vasospasm
✔Phlebitis
__Vasodilation
✔Inflammation
__Trauma
__Surgical wound
__Procedures (specify):
_____
__Immobility
__Pressure
__Medications
__Chemical irritants
__Stress
 	
Defining Characteristics
 	
✔Reports pain
__Guarded position
__Facial mask of
  pain
__Crying/moaning
__Restlessness
__Anxiety/fear
__Elevated BP
__Elevated Pulse
__Elevated Resp.
__Diaphoresis
__Dilated pupils
__Pallor
__Nausea/vomiting
__Muscle tension
__Altered sleep
  pattern
	✔Pt. will convey
	  relief of pain.
	__Pt. will state
	  methods to reduce
	  pain.
	__Pt. will convey
	  ability to tolerate
	  pain.
	✔Pt. will discuss the
	  proper use of pain
	  medication.
		__Assess factors that
		  decrease pain
		  tolerance.
		__Acknowledge the
		  presence of pain.
		__Identify factors that
		  increase or decrease
		  pain.
		✔Explain causes of pain
		  x 1 and prn.
		✔Encourage pt. to
		  discuss pain experi-
		  ence *prn.*
		✔Provide patient emo-
		  tional support *during
		  pain and prn.*
		✔Teach relaxation
		  techniques *initially and
		  reinforce prn.*
		✔Maintain warm, moist
		  compresses as pre-
		  scribed *continuously.*
		__Maintain cold packs as
		  prescribed.
		__Medicate prior to
		  activity.
		✔Medicate prior to
		  severe pain.
		__Assess V.S. prior to
		  adm. of analgesics.
		✔Evaluate effect of pain
		  relief measures *20-30
		  min p̄ administration.*
		__Offer assurance of
		  other relief measures.
		*Identify frequency of
		  nursing action/s.
			__Explain expecta-
			  tions regarding
			  pain.
			✔Develop a plan
			  with pt. for pain
			  control.
			__Teach specific
			  pain-reduction
			  techniques (i.e.,
			  splinting, turning).
			✔Teach side effects
			  of analgesics to
			  report.

Plan Initiated by: *S. Ibarra RN* _____ Date: _4-8-91_____

Plan/Outcomes Evaluated by: _____ Date: _____

Plan/Outcomes Evaluated by: _____ Date: _____

Figure 9–14. Model Care Plan: Pain

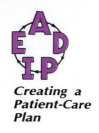

On Day 2, no changes were made in the care plan. On Day 3, Ms. Winters developed thrombophlebitis. As a result of this, Sheryl added three new problems to the care plan:

Problem 9: Potential Complication of Thrombophlebitis: Pulmonary Embolus

Problem 10: Moderate Cramping Pain in Right Leg r/t inflammatory process

Problem 11: Potential Complications of Heparin Therapy: Spontaneous Bleeding, Thrombocytopenia

Figure 9–13 shows Ms. Winters's problem list and care plan on 4/8/91, after it was modified. Care for Problem 9 was covered completely by the 2-South "Standards of Care for Thrombophlebitis" (Figure 9–7). For Problem 10, Sheryl individualized a 2-South model care plan for Pain (Figure 9–14). Problem 11 was covered by the "Protocol for Anticoagulant Therapy" (Figure 9–9). Sheryl added the three problems to the master problem list and then reviewed the remainder of the care plan.

Notice, also, that Sheryl removed thrombophlebitis as a potential complication of hysterectomy in Problem 3 because it had become an actual problem.

Sheryl concluded that Ms. Winters's Acute Abdominal Pain 2° Surgical Incision was being adequately controlled, since she was using the PCA pump infrequently and rating the pain as less than 3 on the 1–10 scale. There was no special action needed for this problem other than the routine standards of care.

For the Altered Health Maintenance nursing diagnosis, no nursing orders had yet been implemented, so Sheryl continued this plan unchanged.

Because of newly acquired data, she changed the Low Self-Esteem diagnosis from "possible" to "actual." She wrote new goals appropriate for the actual problem, discontinued some of the data-collection orders, and kept the orders aimed at promoting self-esteem.

For the nursing diagnosis, High Risk for Colonic Constipation, Sheryl modified the etiology to reflect Ms. Winters's current status by removing the reference to the general anesthetic. She had auscultated bowel sounds, and Ms. Winters was passing flatus, so she modified some of the desired outcomes accordingly. She also decided to decrease the frequency of abdominal assessments.

WELLNESS IN THE ACUTE-CARE SETTING

Even in an acute-care setting, nurses do not focus entirely on problems and illness needs. You can increase your wellness focus by being sure to identify client strengths and to use those strengths in working to relieve the client's problems. One of Ms. Winters's strengths is that she is able to communicate adequately. Realizing this, her nurse planned to use discussion, pamphlets, and diagrams as nursing interventions. Because Ms. Winters has a stable family situation and finances, Sheryl decided that a special discharge plan was not needed.

Clients have health-promotion and illness-prevention needs beyond their admitting medical diagnoses. During the admission assessment the nurse noticed that Ms. Winters was omitting some practices that contribute to good health:

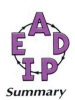

regular exercise, eating balanced meals, and performing breast self-exams. Because Ms. Winters has an essentially healthy history with no major illnesses (a strength), she is not at immediate risk for cardiac or breast problems. However, these cues are important enough to merit a diagnosis of Altered Health Maintenance. Notice, though, that the problem is only seventh in priority because the nurses must focus on Ms. Winters's more basic and immediate needs—pain and potential complications of hysterectomy and thrombophlebitis. This illustrates the difficulty of addressing wellness needs in an acute-care setting. They have been identified and plans made to give Ms. Winters some information, but on postoperative Day 3, this has not yet been done. Still, if the nurses can manage to carry out the plan before dismissal, Ms. Winters may follow through on her own to improve her health-style.

ETHICAL CONSIDERATIONS

Some would say that because nursing affects people when they are most vulnerable, everything a nurse does has a moral aspect. Following this line of reasoning, the act of creating patient-care plans has a moral dimension.

Conventional ethical principles are those that are widely held, expressed in practice, and enforced by sanctions. Among the basic conventional principles held by nurses are the following:

1. Nurses have an obligation to be competent in their work.
2. The good of the patient should be the nurse's primary concern.

A nurse who is careless and uncaring violates both principles. Other nurses on the unit may sanction her by avoiding her or perhaps even by reporting her behavior to a supervisor. These ethical principles suggest that nurses have a moral duty to promote client healing. A well-written nursing care plan aids healing by assuring that the client's needs are communicated and met. When all caregivers understand her needs and preferences, the client is reassured and less anxious and can conserve her energies for healing.

Although not a conventional principle of nursing, the moral principle of **justice** (in the sense of fairness) is also supported by good planning. In this era of cost-containment, limited health-care resources, and staffing shortages, it is important not to misuse human and material resources. A written care plan makes the most efficient use of the nurse's time, assuring that efforts will not be duplicated or time wasted in ineffective interventions.

SUMMARY

A comprehensive care plan
✓ is a written guide for goal-oriented nursing action.
✓ provides the written framework necessary for individualized care and third-party reimbursement.
✓ includes a client profile, instructions for meeting basic needs, aspects of the medical plan to be implemented by the nurse, and a nursing care plan for the client's nursing diagnoses and collaborative problems.
✓ may combine both standardized and individualized approaches.
✓ supports conventional ethical principles of nursing and the moral principle of justice.

Skill-Building Activities

Practice in Critical Thinking: Recognizing Correct Information

Everyone must know and use various kinds of information. For example, we must know certain information to unlock a combination lock. To use this kind of lock you must remember a pattern of numbers and which direction to turn the dial on the lock. You must know the combination exactly; if you make any mistakes, the lock will not open. In nursing you must know and use many different types of information. There are many ways to know and use information. One way is to remember the information (you know your telephone number by memory). Another way is to be able to identify incorrect information. This skill is related to the skill of remembering, but it is somewhat different.

Learning the Skill

Sometimes when we do not remember how to spell a word, we try writing it out in different spellings until we recognize the correct spelling. Even when you are not sure you can remember the correct spelling, you can recognize the difference between the correct and incorrect spellings. You can also recognize incorrect grammar, even though you certainly have not memorized all possible sentences. We often recognize an incorrect sentence and then try to think of the grammar rule that applies to the situation.

Example A Some of the following sentences contain grammar errors. Indicate whether the grammar is correct or incorrect. If it is incorrect, tell why you think so.

1. Marta and Luis, both good athletes, runs every day.

2. My nursing class is so interesting that I think about it often!

3. The dean of our school told Jason and me to be sure to complete our program plans.

Example B In this activity you will be given a physician's order for IV fluids. There *may* be a mistake in some of this information. Your task is to recognize whether the information is correct or incorrect. If it is incorrect, you are to correct the mistake and explain briefly why the original information is incorrect.

Orders: Intravenous fluids, 5% Dextrose, 1000 mg to run over 8 hours

Applying the Skill

1. Some of the information in the following examples of norms contains errors. Make changes where you need to in order to make the information correct. Indicate your reasons for making the changes.

   a. The average B/P in the young adult is 120/80 mm H_2O.

   b. A normal pulse rate is 60–100 beats per minute.

   c. A normal white-blood-cell count is in the range of 4,500–11,000/mg.

   d. A normal red-blood-cell count for men is 4.6–6.2/ml.

   e. Normal range of pH for urine is 4.6–8.0.

2. In this activity, some of the information about the NANDA diagnostic labels may be incorrect. Make changes as needed to correct the information. Give your reasons for making the changes.

   a. Altered Nutrition: Less Than Body Requirements is the state in which an individual is experiencing an intake of nutrients that exceeds metabolic needs.

   b. High Risk for Infection has no defining characteristics.

   c. Hypothermia is the state in which an individual's body temperature is reduced below normal range.

   d. The major defining characteristic for Hyperthermia is an increase in body temperature above normal range.

   e. The major defining characteristics for Perceived Constipation are decreased frequency; hard, dry stool; straining at stool; painful defecation; abdominal distention; palpable mass.

---

* Adapted from *Critical Thinking Worksheets,* a supplement of *Addison-Wesley Chemistry,* by Wilbraham et al. (Menlo Park, CA: Addison-Wesley Publishing Company, 1990).

Applying the Nursing Process

(Answer Key, p. 385)

1. On the following form, construct a care plan (for one problem only) by placing the defining characteristics, nursing diagnosis, predicted outcomes, and nursing orders in the correct columns. Choose from the following scrambled list of items:

> Verbally denies he is ill.
> Pt. will adhere to activity limitations.
> Observed out of bed in spite of medical order for bedrest.
> Encourage to express feelings and concerns about being hospitalized.
> Give positive reinforcement for compliance (e.g., staying in bed, taking meds).
> Refused to take his 3 P.M. medication.
> Patient will acknowledge consequences of not complying with treatment regimen.
> Patient will agree to follow plans for care (e.g., medications, bedrest).
> Noncompliance (medical treatment plan) r/t denial of illness.
> Develop a written contract with patient regarding bedrest and meds.
> Evaluate patient's support system and need for emotional support from staff.

Defining Characteristics	Nursing Diagnosis	Predicted Outcomes	Nursing Orders

2. Use the "Guidelines for Writing Comprehensive Care Plans" in Box 9–2 to evaluate the nursing care plan in Figure 9–12. Use the following form. Comment on whether the care plan meets each of the guidelines (met/not met), or whether the guideline does not apply. If the guideline is not met, discuss or give an example to show how you arrived at that conclusion.

For Figure 9–12: Care Plan for Nikki Winters

Guideline 1:
Guideline 2:
Guideline 3:
Guideline 4:
Guideline 5:
Guideline 6:
Guideline 7:
Guideline 8:
Guideline 9:
Guideline 10:
Guideline 11:

3. Create a care plan for Mr. Cain, using the information in (*a*) through (*f*) and the instructions that follow (*f*).

   a. Use the Patient Kardex (Figure 9–15) for the patient profile, basic care needs, and collaborative aspects of care.

   b. Use the blank Nursing Care Plan (Figure 9–16) for your patient's complete problem list.

   c. You have the following information from the patient's data base.

Name: Harvey Cain   Age: 78   Birth date: 1/25/13
Marital Status: Married
Home Phone: 631-1098   Religion: Catholic: Wife's Name: Mildred Cain
                                  Father Wise, 842-0097   Vital Signs: Temp 100°F
Allergies: Codeine; states no   No special rites.   BP 100/60, Pulse 90,
   food allergies   Resp. 20

Mr. Cain is a thin, elderly male being admitted to Room 426 for an intestinal obstruction and dehydration. He has not had a bowel movement for five days. His abdomen is distended and painful; bowel sounds are absent. He has been vomiting large amounts of green fluid. His skin turgor is poor; his sacrum and heels are reddened, but the skin is intact. His tongue and mouth are dry, and he complains he is a little bit thirsty. He says, "I really feel awful. Am I going to die?" He appears too weak to manage his own hygiene needs. He is oriented to place and person and able to follow second-level commands, but is drowsy and lethargic.

---

   d. The physician, Elton Hobbs, M.D., has left the following orders:

   IV D₅Lactated Ringers, 125 cc/hr   Lab: CBC, Electrolytes, SMA12
   NPO   X ray: Flat plate of Abdomen, Barium enema
   Nasoenteric tube to Gomco suction   Call Dr. Martin Botha for consult
   Foley catheter to dependent drainage   Save any stools
   Hourly urine measurements   Bedrest
   Upper GI

   e. Your nursing unit has the following resources available:

   Standards of Care: *Standardized Care Plans:*
      Anorectal Abscess   Altered Oral Mucous Membrane
      Appendicitis   Bowel Incontinence
      Cholecystitis   Impaired Verbal Communication
      Intestinal Obstruction   Pain
      Peritonitis

The IV order should be written as IV D_5 Lactated Ringers, 125 cc/hr.

Protocols for Care of Patients having:
  Barium Enema
  Cholecystography
  Fiberoptic Colonoscopy
  Liver Biopsy
  Paracentesis

Policies and Procedures:
  Intravenous Therapy
  Nasoenteric Intubation and Suction

f. Mr. Cain's complete problem list has already been developed for you:

Potential Complications of Bowel Obstruction:
  Dehydration
  Electrolyte Imbalance
  Hypovolemic Shock
  Necrosis → Infection
High Risk for Altered Tissue Integrity (Pressure Ulcer) r/t decreased mobility, poor nutritional status, and poor skin turgor 2° dehydration
Abdominal Pain r/t abdominal distention
Altered Oral Mucous Membrane r/t fluid loss from vomiting 2° intestinal obstruction
Possible Fear of Dying r/t unknown outcome of illness and lack of information
Possible Fear or Anxiety r/t hospital environment, diagnostic tests, equipment & procedures
Potential Complications of IV Therapy: Phlebitis, Infiltration
Potential Complications of Nasoenteric Intubation: Ulceration → Hemorrhage
Potential Complications of Upper GI: Perforation, Aspiration
Potential Complications of Barium Enema

INSTRUCTIONS FOR PREPARING THE NURSING CARE PLAN

(Refer to "Content of the Comprehensive Care Plan" and Step 5 of the Care Planning Guide.)

1. Put the client profile information on the Kardex (Figure 9–15).

2. Put the instructions for meeting basic needs (hygiene, etc.) on the Kardex.

3. Incorporate the medical orders on the Kardex.

4. On the blank form (Figure 9–16), write the problems in the appropriate columns. Write them in order of priority, the most urgent one first, or assign priority numbers, with 1 being most urgent.

5. Indicate where the nursing interventions for each problem are to be found (review Figure 9–5 to see how this is done). Some of the problems would require the nurse to write the goals and nursing interventions. You do not need to do this; just write "Nurse will develop plan" beside those problems.

REFERENCE

Carpenito, L. (1991). *Nursing Care Plans and Documentation: Nursing Diagnoses and Collaborative Problems*. Philadelphia: J. B. Lippincott.

SHAWNEE MISSION MEDICAL CENTER

Date ord.	Radiology	Date Sch	D O N E	Date ord.	Laboratory	Date Sch	D O N E	Date ord.	Special Procedures	Date Sch	D O N E
									Daily Tests		
	Ancillary Consults										
									Daily Weight		

Diet:

Food Allergies:

Hold:

Feeding/Fluids

☐ Self
☐ Assist
☐ Feeder
☐ Force
☐ Restrict

	meal	Ext	IV
7-3			
3-11			
11-7			

☐ I&O
☐ IV
☐ Other_____

Safety Measures

☐ Siderails
☐ Restraints
☐ Other_____

Activities

☐ Bedrest
☐ BRP
☐ Dangle
☐ Chair
☐ Commode
☐ Up ad Lib
☐ Turn
☐ Ambulate

Transportation

per _____
_____

Hygiene

☐ Bedbath
☐ Assist
☐ Self Bath
☐ Shower
☐ Tub
☐ Vanity
☐ Oral Care

Bowel/Bladder

☐ Foley   IN _____
               OUT _____
☐ Cath care Bid
☐ Incontinent
☐ Colostomy
☐ Ileostomy
☐ Urostomy

Communication

Physical Therapy	Date	Treatments
Cardio-Pulmonary		

Drug Allergies:

Isolation: In   Out

Emergency Instructions: Religious Rites: Code Blue
Relatives: Clergy:
Phone: Religion:

Diagnosis: Surgery & Dates: Consults & Dates

Room	Name	Adm Date	Age	Physician

Figure 9–15. Patient Kardex. Courtesy of Shawnee Mission Medical Center, Merriam, KS.

PROBLEM LIST FOR HARVEY CAIN		
Date and Initials	Nursing Diagnoses/Problems	Source for Goals and Nursing Orders

Figure 9–16. Nursing Care Plan (Problem List) Form

1. The nurse provides services with respect for human dignity and the uniqueness of the client, unrestricted by considerations of social or economic status, personal attributes, or the nature of health problems.

2. The nurse safeguards the client's right to privacy by judiciously protecting information of a confidential nature.

3. The nurse acts to safeguard the client and the public when health care and safety are affected by the incompetent, unethical, or illegal practice of any person.

4. The nurse assumes responsibility and accountability for individual nursing judgments and actions.

5. The nurse maintains competence in nursing.

6. The nurse exercises informed judgment and uses individual competence and qualifications as criteria in seeking consultation, accepting responsibilities, and delegating nursing activities to others.

7. The nurse participates in activities that contribute to the ongoing development of the profession's body of knowledge.

8. The nurse participates in the profession's efforts to implement and improve standards of nursing.

9. The nurse participates in the profession's efforts to establish and maintain conditions of employment conducive to high-quality nursing care.

10. The nurse participates in the profession's effort to protect the public from misinformation and misrepresentation and to maintain the integrity of nursing.

11. The nurse collaborates with members of the health professions and other citizens in promoting community and national efforts to meet the health needs of the public.

Nursing Assessment Form Based on Roy's Adaptation Model

PATIENT HISTORY

PLEASE COMPLETE THE FOLLOWING QUESTIONS.

1. What are the reasons or symptoms that brought you to the hospital?
_____
_____

2. What major illnesses, previous hospitalizations & surgeries have you had?
_____
_____
_____
_____
_____
_____

3. Has there been any recent stress or crisis in your life (death, illness, divorce, family problems)? _____
_____

4. Are you allergic to any drugs, foods, tapes, environmental substances?
    No _____   Yes _____

List allergies	Describe Reactions

5. List all medications that you are currently taking. Include prescription, over-the-counter, and recreational drugs such as marijuana, cocaine, etc.

Medications	Amount Taken	Time Last Taken

6. What is your occupation? _____
    Are you: ____ Married ____ Single ____ Separated ____ Widowed
    ____ Divorced

7. Do you have any children? _____

8. To what race or ethnic group do you belong? _____

9. Who can help you when you return home? _____
    Do you plan to return to your present address after hospitalization?
_____

10. Who can we contact in case of emergency? _____
    Phone number: _____

11. Do you have any religious practices that will affect your care while in the hospital? _____

12. Do you feel you will require post-discharge assistance? _____

13. Is there any additional information that would assist us in caring for you?
_____

PLEASE CONTINUE ON BACK OF PAGE

Shawnee Mission Medical Center
NURSING ASSESSMENT FORM

Courtesy of Shawnee Mission Medical Center, Merriam, KS.

ADMISSION DATA (TO BE COMPLETED BY NURSE)

Date: _____   Arrive Time on Unit: _____
Accompanied by: _____
Mode of Transport: _____

Valuables: Sent home _____   Retained _____
List _____
Informed of Valuable Policy: Yes _____   No _____

Assistive Devices:
    Contact Lenses _____   Glasses _____
    Dentures: Upper _____   Lower _____   Partial _____
    Hearing Aid: _____
    Other _____   None _____

Ambulating Device:
    Cane _____   Crutches _____
    Walker _____   W/C _____
    Brace _____
    Other _____   None _____

Oriented to:
    Call light _____
    Bathroom _____
    Bed Control _____
    Patient Information Booklet _____

ID Bracelet: Correct _____   Replaced _____

VS: Temp _____   P _____   R _____   BP _____
    Height _____   Weight _____

NURSING ASSESSMENT

Appears:
Calm _____	Oriented _____	Confused _____
Fearful _____	Cooperative _____	Anxious _____
Agitated _____	Withdrawn _____	Well-
Language	Combative _____	groomed _____
Barrier _____		
Other _____		

Self Care Needs: None _____   Needs help with:
_____
_____
_____

Family Present: Yes _____   No _____
Who: _____
Potential Problems: Yes _____   No _____
Describe: _____

Discharge Planning Needs Identified:
    Yes _____   No _____   Describe: _____

IF YOU ARE EXPERIENCING A PROBLEM IN THE AREAS BELOW, PLEASE CHECK ( ) APPROPRIATE BLANK(S). IF YOU HAVE NO PROBLEMS, CHECK THE NO PROBLEM BLANK.

EXERCISE/REST:
Walking _____ Pain with exercise _____
Weakness _____ Insomnia _____
Breathlessness with exertion _____
Use of sleeping aids: _____
No Problems _____

PHYSICAL ASSESSMENT: (TO BE COMPLETED BY NURSE)
No Problems Identified _____
Unsteady Gait _____ Paralysis _____ Limited ROM _____
Joint Deformity _____
Describe: _____
_____
_____

NUTRITION/FLUIDS:
Special Diet: _____
Recent weight gain _____ weight loss _____
Swallowing/chewing difficulty _____
Food dislikes/likes _____
Alcohol use: Type _____
How often _____
No Problem _____

No Problems Identified _____
Nausea _____ Vomiting _____
Describe last food/drink & time taken _____
_____
Describe problems: _____
_____

ELIMINATION:
Constipation _____ Diarrhea _____
Ostomy _____ Type: _____
Use of laxatives/stool softeners/enemas _____
Urinary frequency _____ Burning _____
Blood in urine _____ Urinary infection _____
Urinating during night _____
No problem _____

No Problems Identified _____
Incontinence _____ Foley in place _____ Diversions _____
Stomas _____
Bowel Sounds: Present _____ Absent _____
Abdomen: Soft _____ Tender _____ Flat _____ Distended _____
Date of last bowel movement: _____
Describe: _____

OXYGENATION:
Shortness of breath _____ Wheeze _____ Cough _____
Pain with breathing _____ Blood in sputum _____
Home oxygen _____
Smoking: Packs/day _____ How long have you smoked? _____
Have you quit recently? _____
No problem _____

No Problems Identified _____
Irregular respirations _____ SOB _____ Using oxygen _____
Breath Sounds: Clear _____ Crackles _____ Wheezes _____
Cough: Productive _____ Non-productive _____
Describe: _____
_____

CIRCULATORY:
Heart Problems _____ Chest pain _____
High blood pressure _____ Varicose Veins _____
Swelling _____ Pacemaker _____ Shunts _____
Catheters _____
Have you ever had a blood transfusion: Yes _____ No _____
When? _____
No Problem _____

No Problems Identified _____
Peripheral Pulses: Normal _____ Slightly Impaired _____
Moderately Impaired _____ Absent _____
Edema: Present _____ Where _____
Heart Sounds: _____
C-V Devices Present _____ Where _____
Describe: _____

TEMPERATURE/SKIN:
With this illness, do you have:
Chills _____ Fever _____ Rashes _____ Bruises _____
Cuts _____ Open Sores _____
Have you travelled out of the USA in the last year?
Yes _____ No _____
No problem _____

No Problems Identified _____
Skin Color: Pink _____ Pale _____ Flushed _____ Mottled _____
Cyanotic _____ Jaundiced _____ Other _____
Temperature: Warm _____ Hot _____ Cool _____ Dry _____
Moist _____ Diaphoretic _____
Condition: Bruises _____ Rash _____ Open Sores _____
Describe: _____

NEURO/SENSORY:
Pain _____ Location: _____
Dizziness _____ Fainting _____ Seizures _____
Numbness/tingling _____ Difficulty with speech _____
Sight _____ Hearing _____ Taste _____
Memory loss _____
No Problem _____

No Problems Identified _____
LOC: Alert _____ Lethargic _____ Unresponsive _____
Disoriented _____ Unconscious _____ Memory Deficit _____
Speech: Slurred _____ Aphasic _____
Pain: Type _____ Severity _____ Duration _____
Pupil Reaction _____ Hand Grip _____
Describe: _____

ENDOCRINE/REPRODUCTIVE:
Menstrual problems _____ Bleeding _____ Cramping _____
Abnormal vaginal/penile discharge _____
Pelvic infection _____ Genital Lesions _____
Thyroid disorder _____
Diabetes _____ Duration of Diabetes _____
No Problem _____

No Problems Identified _____
Vaginal Bleeding _____ Amount _____
Pregnancy _____ gravida _____ Para _____
Blood Sugar Monitoring _____
Describe: _____

Patient/Family Signature: _____

RN Signature: _____ Time: _____
DR. notified: Date _____ Time _____

Patient Admission Assessment

Name: _____ Age: _____

Prefer to be called: _____ Date: _____

Next of Kin: _____ Relationship: _____ Phone: _____

Other contact person: _____ Phone: _____

Primary Language, if other than English: _____ Person completing form: _____

Why are you being admitted to the hospital? _____

NO NEED TO COMPLETE THIS SECTION IF THE PRE-OPERATIVE QUESTIONNAIRE IS COMPLETED

List any previous hospitalizations and/or surgeries: _____
_____
_____

Do you have any of these health problems (please check)

___Alzheimers	___Dizziness	___Hepatitis	___Asthma	___Chest Pain
___Epilepsy	___High Blood Pressure	___Hiatal Hernia	___Cough	___Heart Flutter
___Seizures	___Diabetes	___Arthritis	___Mucous Production	___Congestive Heart Failure
___Numbness	___Thyroid	___Back Injury	___Shortness of Breath on Activity	___Heart Pounding
___Tingling	___Swelling		___Difficulty Breathing	___Pacemaker
			___Emphysema	___No Problems

If yes, please explain: _____

Are there any other medical problems of which we should be aware? _____
_____

Do you have any eyesight and/or hearing difficulties?   Yes ☐   No ☐

If yes, indicate use of: glasses   contacts   hearing aid   other: _____

Do you wear dentures? Yes ☐   No ☐   If yes, what kind?   Upper   Lower   Partial   Full

Are you on a special diet?   Yes ☐   No ☐   If yes, what kind: _____

ALLERGIES

Do you have any allergies to: Food: _____ Type of Reaction: _____

Medications: _____ Type of Reaction: _____

Anesthesia: _____ Type of Reaction: _____

Other (wool, tape, pollens): _____ Type of Reaction: _____

It is important that we are aware of the use of any of the following substances in order to keep you comfortable and to avoid interaction with other medication/anesthetic that might be prescribed. Do you use any of the following? (Please circle)

Alcohol	Tobacco	Amphetamines (uppers)	Barbiturates (downers)	Tranquilizers
Marijuana	Heroin	Cocaine	Caffeine (tea, coffee, pop)	Other:_____

MEDICATIONS

Are you currently taking _any_ medications? Yes ☐ No ☐   Did you bring them with you? Yes ☐ No ☐

Are you taking your medications as ordered by your physician? Yes ☐ No ☐

Please list below, any medications you are taking (including prescription and over the counter medications)

MEDICATION	DOSE	HOW OFTEN	REASON	PRESCRIBING PHYSICIAN

Form No. 102A   (Revised 9/89)   PATIENT ADMISSION ASSESSMENT

Courtesy of Bronson Methodist Hospital, Kalamazoo, MI.

PATIENT ADMISSION ASSESSMENT
continued—Page 2

NUTRITION/ METABOLIC

Any recent weight loss or gain?: Yes ☐ No ☐   If yes, how much:_____ ☐ Gain   ☐ Loss

Do you have?: (Please circle)   Nausea/Vomiting   Stomach Pains   Poor Appetite

Difficulty Chewing or Swallowing   Heartburn   No Problems

Comments:_____

ELIMINATION

Last bowel movement: _____

What is your usual bowel pattern?   Daily   Twice a day   Every other day   Other:_____

Do you have?   Constipation   Diarrhea   Hemorrhoids Other: _____

Indicate any laxatives/enemas or "home remedies" that you use:_____

Have you been experiencing any urinary problems?:   Burning   Frequency   Urgency

Bed Wetting   Bloody Urine   Problems holding urine   Difficulty starting to urinate   Last void: _____

No Problems   Other:_____

How often do you urinate?:_____   Describe color: _____

Comments:_____

SEXUAL/ REPRODUCTIVE

FEMALE: Have you been through menopause?: Yes ☐ No ☐   Please explain your normal menstrual pattern:_____

Any recent problems or changes in your menstrual pattern?:   Yes ☐   No ☐   If yes, please explain:_____

Date of last normal period:_____   Could you be pregnant?: Yes ☐   No ☐

Do you take birth control pills?: Yes ☐ No ☐   Do you perform a monthly breast exam?: Yes ☐   No ☐

MALE: Have you experienced any?: (Please circle) Prostate problems   Sores on your penis   Testicular problems   Bleeding   Discharge

Do you perform a monthly testicular exam?:   Yes ☐   No ☐   No problems

---

SLEEP

How long do you sleep?:_____p.m. to_____a.m.   Is it adequate?: Yes ☐   No ☐   Do you nap? Yes ☐   No ☐

Do you have difficulty sleeping?:   Yes ☐   No ☐   If yes, what do you do to help yourself fall asleep?:_____

COGNITIVE/ PERCEPT

Do you have a history of chronic pain?:   Yes ☐   No ☐   If yes, please explain:_____

What do you do to relieve pain?:_____

How do you learn best?: (Please circle)   Reading   Listening   Demonstration

---

SELF-PERCEPT

How are you feeling about being hospitalized?:   Frightened   Calm   Angry   Worried   Relieved   Sad   Hopeful

Other:_____

ROLE/ RELATIONSHIP

Marital status: (Please circle)   Single   Married   Separated   Divorced   Widowed

Do you have children?:   Yes ☐   No ☐   List ages:_____

Are you presently employed?:   Yes ☐   No ☐   Occupation:_____

Are you presently in school?:   Yes ☐   No ☐   Will illness interfere?   Yes ☐   No ☐

Upon discharge, if needed, will you be able to afford: Medicine Yes ☐ No ☐   Supplies Yes ☐ No ☐   Medical Care Yes ☐ No ☐

COPING/ STRESS

Are you experiencing any stressful situations other than your illness/hospitalization?:   Yes ☐   No ☐

If yes, please describe:_____

How do you usually cope with tension or stress?:_____

VALUE/ BELIEF

Will illness/hospitalization interfere with any of the following?: (Please circle)

Spiritual or Religious Practice   Family Traditions   Cultural Beliefs or Practice   Will not interfere

If yes, please explain:_____

Would you like your Clergy or Hospital Chaplain to be contacted?:   Yes ☐   No ☐

If yes, state name and number:_____

Appendix D
Collaborative Problems Organized by Body System

Potential Complication: Gastrointestinal-Hepatic

PC: Paralytic Ileus/Small-Bowel Obstruction
PC: Hepatorenal Syndrome
PC: Hyperbilirubinemia
PC: Evisceration
PC: Hepatosplenomegaly
PC: Curling's Ulcer
PC: Ascites
PC: G.I. Bleeding

Potential Complication: Metabolic/Immune

PC: Hypoglycemia
PC: Hyperglycemia
PC: Negative Nitrogen Balance
PC: Electrolyte Imbalances
PC: Thyroid Dysfunction
PC: Hypothermia (severe)
PC: Hyperthermia (severe)
PC: Sepsis
PC: Acidosis/Alkalosis
PC: Diabetes
PC: Anasarca
PC: Hypo/Hyperthyroidism
PC: Allergic Reaction
PC: Donor-Tissue Rejection
PC: Adrenal Insufficiency

Potential Complication: Neurologic/Sensory

PC: Increased Intracranial Pressure
PC: Stroke
PC: Seizures
PC: Spinal Cord Compression
PC: Autonomic Dysreflexia
PC: Birth Injuries
PC: Hydrocephalus
PC: Microcephalus
PC: Meningitis
PC: Cranial Nerve Impairment
PC: Paresis/Paresthesia/Paralysis
PC: Peripheral Nerve Impairment
PC: Increased Intraocular Pressure
PC: Corneal Ulceration
PC: Neuropathies

Potential Complication: Cardiovascular

PC: Dysrhythmias
PC: Congestive Heart Failure
PC: Thromboemboli/Deep-Vein Thrombosis
PC: Hypovolemic Shock
PC: Peripheral Vascular Insufficiency
PC: Hypertension
PC: Congenital Heart Disease
PC: Thrombocytopenia
PC: Polycythemia
PC: Anemia
PC: Compartmental Syndrome
PC: Disseminated Intravascular Coagulation
PC: Endocarditis
PC: Sickling Crisis
PC: Embolism (air, fat)
PC: Spinal Shock
PC: Ischemic Ulcers

Potential Complication: Respiratory

PC: Atelectasis/Pneumonia
PC: Asthma
PC: C.O.P.D.
PC: Pulmonary Embolism
PC: Pleural Effusion
PC: Tracheal Necrosis
PC: Ventilator Dependency
PC: Pneumothorax
PC: Laryngeal Edema

Potential Complication: Renal/Urinary

PC: Acute Urinary Retention
PC: Renal Failure
PC: Bladder Perforation

Potential Complication: Reproductive

PC: Fetal Compromise
PC: Uterine Atony
PC: Pregnancy-Induced Hypertension
PC: Eclampsia
PC: Hydramnios
PC: Hypermenorrhea
PC: Polymenorrhea
PC: Syphilis
PC: Tetanic Uterine Contractions
PC: Placenta Previa; Abruptio Placenta
PC: Uterine Rupture
PC: Dysfunctional Labor

Potential Complication: Muscular/Skeletal

PC: Stress Fractures
PC: Osteoporosis
PC: Joint Dislocation
PC: Joint Inflammation
PC: Muscle Atrophy
PC: Osteomyelitis

Adapted with permission from L. J. Carpenito (1989), *Nursing Diagnosis: Application to Clinical Practice,* 3rd ed (Philadelphia: J. B. Lippincott), pp. 871–73.

This *Nursing Diagnosis Guide* consists of information provided in NANDA's *Taxonomy I — Revised, 1990,* unless otherwise specified. The diagnostic labels, definitions, defining characteristics, and risk and related factors are those approved at the Tenth Conference of the North American Nursing Diagnosis Association in 1992. The guide provides a quick reference in the clinical setting. The author's discussion and recommendations for using diagnoses are identified by the phrase *Author's Note*. The pointing-finger symbol (☞) indicates a comment in related labels.

Choosing a problem label: To use this guide, first identify your client's problem and its cue cluster (signs and symptoms). Using the list of NANDA labels organized by your chosen framework (inside front and back cover of your text), locate the labels that seem to describe the problem. Find these labels in this guide. Use the label that has defining characteristics that best match your client's cue cluster to describe the *problem* part of your nursing diagnosis.

Writing the etiology: A complete nursing diagnosis consists of *Problem + Etiology*. You may find the etiology under "related factors" or "risk factors," or it may be one of the other diagnostic labels. Because etiologies vary greatly among individuals, you will often need to write the etiology in your own words.

Alphabetical organization: Diagnostic labels are listed in the Guide in alphabetical order. Look for the noun, or main thought, rather than the modifier. For example, Ineffective Airway Clearance is found under *A* rather than *I*. The client has an *airway* problem, not an *ineffective* problem.

ACTIVITY DEFICIT, DIVERSIONAL
(*see* Diversional Activity Deficit)

ACTIVITY INTOLERANCE
Definition: A state in which an individual has insufficient physiological or psychological energy to endure or complete required or desired daily activities.

Defining Characteristics: Abnormal heart rate or blood pressure response to activity; exertional discomfort or dyspnea; electrocardiographic changes reflecting arrhythmias or ischemia. **Critical** — Verbal report of fatigue or weakness.

Related Factors: Bedrest/immobility; generalized weakness; sedentary life-style; imbalance between oxygen supply/demand.

Author's Note: Use this label only if the client has verbally reported fatigue or weakness in response to activity. Activity Intolerance is often caused by medical conditions (e.g., heart disease or peripheral arterial disease); however, a diagnostic statement such as Activity Intolerance r/t coronary artery disease is not useful for planning nursing care, since the nurse cannot effect change on either side of the statement.

Activity Intolerance is often the etiology of other problems, such as Self-Care Deficit, Social Isolation or Sexual Dysfunction, and it is probably used most effectively in this manner. Gordon (1987, p. 147) suggests that Activity Intolerance be specified by levels of endurance:

Level I: Walks regular pace on level ground but becomes more short of breath than normal when climbing one or more flights of stairs.

Level II: Walks one city block 500 feet on level or climbs one flight of stairs slowly without stopping.

Level III: Walks no more than 50 feet on level without stopping and is unable to climb one flight of stairs without stopping.

Level IV: Dyspnea and fatigue at rest.

An example of a resulting diagnostic statement is Self-care Deficit (Total) r/t Activity Intolerance (Level IV). Do not use Activity Intolerance if it is not possible to increase the client's endurance.

☞ *See also* Fatigue, Self-Care Deficit.

ACTIVITY INTOLERANCE, HIGH RISK FOR
Definition: A state in which an individual is at risk of experiencing insufficient physiological or psychological energy to endure or complete required or desired daily activities.

Defining Characteristics: Presence of risk factors such as history of previous intolerance; deconditioned status; presence of circulatory/respiratory problems; inexperience with the activity.

Related Factors: *See* the risk factors listed in Defining Characteristics.

Author's Note: Discriminate between Activity Intolerance, Fatigue, and Self-Care Deficit. Do not use Activity Intolerance if it is not possible to increase the client's endurance. *See* the note for Activity Intolerance.

ADJUSTMENT, IMPAIRED

Definition: The state in which the individual is unable to modify his/her life-style/behavior in a manner consistent with a change in health status.

Defining Characteristics: *Major* — Verbalization of nonacceptance of health status change; nonexistent or unsuccessful ability to be involved in problem solving or goal setting. *Minor* — Lack of movement toward independence; extended period of shock, disbelief, or anger regarding health-status change; lack of future-oriented thinking.

Related Factors: Disability requiring change in life-style; inadequate support systems; impaired cognition; sensory overload; assault to self-esteem; altered locus of control; incomplete grieving.

☛ *See also* Coping, Ineffective Individual.

AIRWAY CLEARANCE, INEFFECTIVE

Definition: A state in which an individual is unable to clear secretions or obstructions from the respiratory tract to maintain airway patency.

Defining Characteristics: Abnormal breath sounds (crackles, wheezes); changes in rate or depth of respiration; tachypnea; cough, effective/ineffective, with or without sputum; cyanosis; dyspnea.

Related Factors: Decreased energy/fatigue; tracheobronchial infection, obstruction, secretion; perceptual/cognitive impairment; trauma.

☛ Discriminate between this label and Impaired Gas Exchange, Ineffective Breathing Pattern, and High Risk for Aspiration.

ANTICIPATORY GRIEVING

(*see* Grieving, Anticipatory)

ANXIETY

Definition: A vague uneasy feeling whose source is often nonspecific or unknown to the individual.

Defining Characteristics: *Subjective* — Increased tension; apprehension; painful and persistent increased helplessness; uncertainty; fearful; scared; regretful; overexcited; rattled; distressed; jittery; feelings of inadequacy; shakiness; fear of unspecific consequences; expressed concerns regarding change in life events; worried; anxious. *Objective* —

Restlessness; insomnia; glancing about; poor eye contact; trembling/hand tremors; extraneous movement (foot shuffling, hand/arm movements); facial tension; voice quivering; focus on self; increased wariness; increased perspiration. **Critical** — Sympathetic stimulation: cardiovascular excitation, superficial vasoconstriction, pupil dilation.

Related Factors: Unconscious conflict about essential values/goals of life; threat to self-concept; threat of death; threat to or change in health status; threat to or change in role functioning; threat to or change in environment; threat to or change in interaction patterns; situational/maturational crises; interpersonal transmission/contagion; unmet needs.

Author's Note: Anxiety must be clearly differentiated from Fear because the nursing interventions are different. When a client is fearful, the focus is on removing or helping him to deal with the specific fear. When a client is anxious, the nurse helps him identify the cause of the anxiety; because the source of Anxiety cannot always be identified, however, nursing care may also focus on helping the client explore and express anxious feelings — not an effective approach when dealing with Fear.

The Anxious person cannot define, or does not know, the source of his anxiety. The only critical defining characteristic is stimulation of the sympathetic nervous system. A variety of other subjective and objective signs and symptoms can be used to help identify Anxiety (e.g., increased tension, worry, restlessness, poor eye contact, trembling). In contrast, Fear is specifically defined as "a feeling of dread related to an identifiable source which the person validates." People experience any number of physical and psychological reactions to fear; however, the only defining characteristic needed to make the diagnosis is *ability to identify the object of fear.*

Because the level of anxiety determines the nursing interventions, you should indicate whether anxiety is moderate, severe, or panic-level. Panic may require collaborative interventions, such as medication. Mild Anxiety should not be used at all, since it is a normal condition present in all human beings. Diagnose Anxiety only for clients who require special nursing interventions. Mild anxiety before surgery is a normal, healthy response. You would, in fact, wonder about the mental status of someone who felt absolutely no anxiety before surgery. Taylor et al. (1989, p. 137) use these four levels of anxiety:

Mild anxiety: Present in day-to-day living, mild anxiety increases alertness and perceptual fields. It motivates learning and growth.

Moderate anxiety: Narrows the person's perceptual fields so that the focus is on immediate concerns, with inattention to other communications and details.

Severe anxiety: Creates a very narrow focus on specific detail. All behavior is geared toward getting relief.

Panic: The person has loss of control and experiences dread and terror. The resulting disorganized state results in increased physical activity, distortion of perceptions and relationships, and loss of rational thought. This level of anxiety can lead to exhaustion and death.

Fear and Anxiety present diagnostic difficulty because they are not mutually exclusive. That is, a person who is afraid is usually anxious as well. Furthermore, many of the same signs and symptoms are present in both Fear and Anxiety, for example, increased heart and respiratory rate, dilated pupils, diaphoresis, muscle tension, and fatigue. Remember that in Fear the person can identify the threat; in Anxiety he usually cannot.

Anxiety	*Fear*
Vague uneasy feeling	Feeling of dread
Source of feeling unknown by person	Source of feeling is known by person
Threat is vague, nonspecific	Threat is specific, identifiable
Threat usually psychological (e.g., to self-image)	Threat often physical (e.g., to safety)
A variety of defining characteristics, both verbal and autonomic	Defining characteristic: Ability to identify object of fear

☛ Fear is a related diagnosis.

ASPIRATION, HIGH RISK FOR

Definition: The state in which an individual is at risk for entry of gastrointestinal secretions, oropharyngeal secretions, or solids or fluids into tracheobronchial passages.

Defining Characteristics: Presence of risk factors such as reduced level of consciousness; depressed cough and gag reflexes; presence of tracheostomy or endotracheal tube; incomplete lower esophageal sphincter; GI tubes; tube feedings; medication administration; situations hindering elevation of upper body; increased intragastric pressure; increased gastric residual; decreased GI motility; delayed gastric emptying; impaired swallowing; facial/oral/neck surgery or trauma; wired jaws.

Related Factors: *See* the risk factors above.

Author's Note: Use the most specific label for which the patient has the necessary defining characteristics.

☛ Related labels: Ineffective Airway Clearance, High Risk for Suffocation, High Risk for Injury, and High Risk for Trauma.

BATHING/HYGIENE SELF-CARE DEFICIT

(*see* Self-Care Deficit, Bathing/Hygiene)

BODY IMAGE DISTURBANCE

Definition: Disruption in the way one perceives one's body image.

Defining Characteristics: Critical — *A or B* must be present to justify the diagnosis of Body Image Disturbance. (*A*) verbal response to actual or perceived change in structure and/or function; (*B*) nonverbal response to actual or perceived change in structure and/or function. *Other* — The following clinical manifestations may be used to validate the presence of *A* or *B*. *Objective:* Missing body part; actual change in structure and/or function; not looking at body part; not touching body part; hiding or overexposing body part (intentional or unintentional); trauma to nonfunctioning part; change in social involvement; change in ability to estimate spatial relationship of body to environment. *Subjective:* Verbalization of change in life-style; fear of rejection or of reaction by others; focus on past strength, function, or appearance; negative feelings about body; and feelings of helplessness, hopelessness, or powerlessness; preoccupation with change or loss; emphasis on remaining strengths, heightened achievement; extension of body boundary to incorporate environmental objects; personalization of part or loss by name; depersonalization of part or loss by impersonal pronouns; refusal to verify actual change.

Related Factors: Biophysical; cognitive/perceptual; psychosocial; cultural or spiritual.

Author's Note: This label is related to Self-Esteem Disturbance and includes negative feelings about one's body or body parts. While Body Image Disturbance is often caused by loss of a body part or actual body changes, the change in structure or function can be perceived rather than actual. Clients on prolonged bedrest or who are dependent on machines (e.g., dialysis, respirator) may experience distortion of body image.

☛ *See also* Self-Esteem Disturbance.

BODY TEMPERATURE, HIGH RISK FOR ALTERED

Definition: The state in which the individual is at risk for failure to maintain body temperature within normal range.

Defining Characteristics: Presence of risk factors such as extremes of age; extremes of age or weight; exposure to cold/cool or warm/hot environments; dehydration; inactivity or vigorous activity; medications causing vasoconstriction/

vasodilation; altered metabolic rate; sedation; inappropriate clothing for environmental temperature; illness or trauma affecting temperature regulation.

Related Factors: *See* risk factors above.

☛ Differentiate between Altered Body Temperature, Hypo- or Hyperthermia, and Ineffective Thermoregulation.

BOWEL INCONTINENCE
(*see* Incontinence, Bowel)

BREASTFEEDING, EFFECTIVE
Definition: The state in which a mother-infant dyad/family exhibits adequate proficiency and satisfaction with breastfeeding process.

Defining Characteristics: *Major* — Mother able to position infant at breast to promote a successful latch-on response; infant is content after feeding; regular and sustained suckling/swallowing at the breast; appropriate infant weight patterns for age; effective mother/infant communication patterns (infant cues, maternal interpretation and response). *Minor* — Signs and/or symptoms of oxytocin release (let down or milk ejection reflex); adequate infant elimination patterns for age; eagerness of infant to nurse; maternal verbalization of satisfaction with the breastfeeding process.

Related Factors: Basic breastfeeding knowledge; normal breast structure; normal infant oral structure; infant gestational age greater than 34 weeks; support sources; maternal confidence.

BREASTFEEDING, INEFFECTIVE
Definition: The state in which a mother, infant, or child experiences dissatisfaction or difficulty with the breastfeeding process.

Defining Characteristics: *Major* — Unsatisfactory breastfeeding process. *Minor* — Actual or perceived inadequate milk supply; infant inability to attach onto maternal breast correctly; no observable signs of oxytocin release; observable signs of inadequate infant intake; nonsustained suckling at the breast; insufficient emptying of each breast per feeding; persistence of sore nipples beyond the first week of breastfeeding; insufficient opportunity for suckling at the breast; infant exhibiting fussiness and crying within the first hour after breastfeeding; unresponsive to other comfort measures; infant arching and crying at the breast; resisting latching on.

Related Factors: Prematurity; infant anomaly; maternal breast anomaly; previous breast surgery; previous history of breastfeeding failure; infant receiving supplemental feedings with artificial nipple; poor infant sucking reflex; nonsupportive partner/family; knowledge deficit; interruption in breastfeeding; maternal anxiety or ambivalence.

BREATHING PATTERN, INEFFECTIVE
Definition: The state in which an individual's inhalation and/or exhalation pattern does not enable adequate pulmonary inflation or emptying.

Defining Characteristics: Dyspnea, shortness of breath, tachypnea, fremitus, abnormal arterial blood gas, cyanosis, cough, nasal flaring, respiratory depth changes, assumption of 3-point position, pursed-lip breathing/prolonged expiratory phase, increased anteroposterior diameter, use of accessory muscles, altered chest excursion.

Related Factors: Neuromuscular impairment; pain, musculoskeletal impairment; perception/cognitive impairment; anxiety; decreased energy/fatigue.

Author's Note: Use this label with caution. If the condition cannot be treated by independent nursing actions, write it as a collaborative problem. Consider, too, that the ineffective breathing pattern may be merely a symptom of another problem, such as Anxiety.

☛ Compare this label to Activity Intolerance, Ineffective Airway Clearance, and Impaired Gas Exchange.

CARDIAC OUTPUT, DECREASED
Definition: A state in which the blood pumped by an individual's heart is sufficiently reduced that it is inadequate to meet the needs of the body's tissues.

Defining Characteristics: Variations in blood-pressure readings; arrhythmias; fatigue; jugular vein distention; color changes, skin and mucous membranes; oliguria; decreased peripheral pulses; cold, clammy skin; rales; dyspnea, orthopnea; restlessness. *Other Possible Characteristics:* Change in mental status; shortness of breath; syncope; vertigo; edema; cough; frothy sputum; gallop rhythm; weakness.

Author's Note: Author recommends that you do not use this label. The nurse can neither conclusively diagnose nor definitively treat this problem. When the client has Actual Decreased Cardiac Output, use a statement in which the problem is described as a human response to this pathophysiology (e.g., Activity Intolerance r/t decreased cardiac output). If the client is at risk of developing complications, write them as collaborative

problems (e.g., Potential Complication of M.I.: Cardiogenic Shock).
☛ Activity Intolerance, Self-Care Deficit.

CHRONIC LOW SELF-ESTEEM
(*see* Self-Esteem, Chronic Low)

CHRONIC PAIN
(*see* Pain, Chronic)

COMMUNICATION, IMPAIRED VERBAL
Definition: The state in which an individual experiences a decreased or absent ability to use or understand language in human interaction.

Defining Characteristics: Critical — Unable to speak dominant language; speaks or verbalizes with difficulty; does not or cannot speak. *Other* — Stuttering; slurring; difficulty forming words or sentences; difficulty expressing thought verbally; inappropriate verbalization; dyspnea; disorientation.
Related Factors: Decrease in circulation to brain; brain tumor; physical barrier (tracheostomy, intubation); anatomical defect, cleft palate; psychological barriers (psychosis, lack of stimuli); cultural difference; developmental or age-related.
Author's Note: This label should be used for those who desire to communicate but are having difficulty (Carpenito, 1991).

CONFLICT, DECISIONAL
(*see* Decisional Conflict)

CONSTIPATION
Definition: A state in which an individual experiences a change in normal bowel habits characterized by a decrease in frequency and/or passage of hard, dry stools.

Defining Characteristics: Decreased activity level; frequency less than usual pattern; hard, formed stools; palpable mass; reported feeling of pressure in rectum; reported feeling of rectal fullness; straining at stool. Other possible characteristics: Abdominal or back pain; decreased appetite; headache; interference with daily living; use of laxatives.
☛ Other labels to consider: Colonic Constipation, Perceived Constipation.

CONSTIPATION, COLONIC
Definition: The state in which an individual's pattern of elimination is characterized by hard, dry stool which results from a delay in passage of food residue.

Defining Characteristics: *Major* — Decreased frequency; hard, dry stool; straining at stool; painful defecation; abdominal distention; palpable mass. *Minor* — Rectal pressure; headache, decreased appetite; abdominal pain.
Related Factors: Less than adequate dietary, fluid, or fiber intake; inadequate physical activity; immobility; lack of privacy; emotional disturbances; chronic use of laxatives and/or enemas; stress; change in daily routine; metabolic problems (e.g., hypothyroidism, hypocalcemia, hypokalemia).
☛ *See also* Constipation and Perceived Constipation.

CONSTIPATION, PERCEIVED
Definition: The state in which an individual makes a self-diagnosis of constipation and ensures a daily bowel movement through abuse of laxatives, enemas, and suppositories.

Defining Characteristics: *Major* — Expectation of a daily bowel movement with the resulting overuse of laxatives, enemas, and suppositories; expected passage of stool at same time every day.
Related Factors: Cultural/family health beliefs; faulty appraisal; impaired thought processes.
☛ *See also* Constipation and Colonic Constipation.

COPING, DEFENSIVE
Definition: The state in which an individual repeatedly projects falsely positive self-evaluation based on a self-protective pattern which defends against underlying perceived threats to positive self-regard.

Defining Characteristics: *Major* — Denial of obvious problems/weaknesses; projection of blame/responsibility; rationalizes failures; hypersensitive to slight/criticism; grandiosity. *Minor* — Superior attitude toward others; difficulty establishing/maintaining relationships; hostile laughter or ridicule of others; difficulty in reality-testing perceptions; lack of follow-through or participation in treatment or therapy.
☛ Related labels: Ineffective Individual Coping, Ineffective Denial, Impaired Adjustment.

COPING, INEFFECTIVE FAMILY: COMPROMISED

Definition: A usually supportive primary person (family member or close friend) is providing insufficient, ineffective, or compromised support, comfort, assistance, or encouragement which may be needed by the client to manage or master adaptive tasks related to his or her health challenge.

Defining Characteristics: *Subjective* — Client expresses or confirms a concern or complaint about significant other's response to his or her health problem; significant person describes preoccupation with personal reaction (e.g., fear, anticipatory grief, guilt, anxiety) to client's illness, disability, or to other situational or developmental crises; significant person describes or confirms an inadequate understanding or knowledge base which interferes with effective assistive or supportive behaviors. *Objective* — Significant person attempts assistive or supportive behaviors with less than satisfactory results; significant person withdraws or enters into limited or temporary personal communication with the client at the time of need; significant person displays protective behavior disproportionate (too little or too much) to the client's abilities or need for autonomy.

Related Factors: Inadequate or incorrect information or understanding by a primary person; temporary preoccupation by a significant person who is trying to manage emotional conflicts and personal suffering and is unable to perceive or act effectively in regard to client's needs; temporary family disorganization and role changes; other situational or developmental crises or situations the significant person may be facing; little support provided by client, in turn, for primary person; prolonged disease or disability progression that exhausts supportive capacity of significant people.

☛ *See also* Ineffective Family Coping: Disabling, Altered Family Processes, Altered Parenting, and Parental Role Conflict.

COPING, INEFFECTIVE FAMILY: DISABLING

Definition: Behavior of significant person (family member or other primary person) that disables his or her own capacities and the client's capacities to effectively address tasks essential to either person's adaptation to the health challenge.

Defining Characteristics: Neglectful care of the client in regard to basic human needs and/or illness treatment; distortion of reality regarding the client's health problem, including extreme denial about its existence or severity; intolerance; rejection; abandonment; desertion; carrying on usual routines, disregarding client's needs; psychosomaticism; taking on illness signs of client; decisions and actions by family which are detrimental to economic or social well-being; agitation, depression, aggression, hostility; impaired restructuring of a meaningful life for self, impaired individualization, prolonged overconcern for client; neglectful relationships with other family members; client's development of helpless, inactive dependence.

Related Factors: Significant person with chronically unexpressed feelings of guilt, anxiety, hostility, despair, etc.; dissonant discrepancy of coping styles for dealing with adaptive tasks by the significant person and client or among significant people; highly ambivalent family relationships; arbitrary handling of family's resistance to treatment, which tends to solidify defensiveness as it fails to deal adequately with underlying anxiety.

☛ *See also* Ineffective Family Coping: Compromised, Altered Family Processes, Altered Parenting.

COPING, FAMILY: POTENTIAL FOR GROWTH

Definition: Effective managing of adaptive tasks by family member involved with the client's health challenge, who now is exhibiting desire and readiness for enhanced health and growth in regard to self and in relation to the client.

Defining Characteristics: Family member attempting to describe growth impact of crisis on his or her own values, priorities, goal, or relationships; family member moving in direction of health-promoting and enriching life-style which supports and monitors maturational processes, audits and negotiates treatment programs, and generally chooses experiences which optimize wellness; individual expressing interest in making contact on a one-to-one basis or on a mutual-aid group basis with another person who has experienced a similar situation.

Related Factors: Needs sufficiently gratified and adaptive tasks effectively addressed to enable goals of self-actualization to surface.

COPING, INEFFECTIVE INDIVIDUAL

Definition: Impairment of adaptive behaviors and problem-solving abilities of a person in meeting life's demands and roles.

Defining Characteristics: *Major* — Verbalization of inability to cope or inability to ask for help; inability to problem-solve. *Other* — Inability to meet role expectations; inability to meet basic needs; alteration in societal participation; destructive behavior toward self or others; inappropriate use of defense mechanisms; change in usual communication patterns; verbal manipulation; high illness rate; high rate of accidents.

Related Factors: Situational crises; maturational crises; personal vulnerability.

☛ Related labels: Defensive Coping, Impaired Adjustment.

DECISIONAL CONFLICT (SPECIFY)

Definition: The state of uncertainty about course of action to be taken when choice among competing actions involves risk, loss, or challenge to personal life values.

Defining Characteristics: *Major* — Verbalized uncertainty about choices; verbalization of undesired consequences of alternative actions being considered; vacillation between alternative choices; delayed decision making. *Minor* — Verbalized feeling of distress while attempting a decision; self-focusing; physical signs of distress or tension (increased heart rate, increased muscle tension, restlessness, etc.); questioning personal values and beliefs while attempting a decision.

Related Factors: Unclear personal values/beliefs; perceived threat to value system; lack of experience or interference with decision making; lack of relevant information; support system deficit; multiple or divergent sources of information.

Author's Note: Differentiate between this label, Spiritual Distress, and the inability to problem-solve associated with Ineffective Individual Coping.

DEFENSIVE COPING

(*see* Coping, Defensive)

DENIAL, INEFFECTIVE

Definition: The state of a conscious or unconscious attempt to disavow the knowledge or meaning of an event to reduce anxiety/fear to the detriment of health.

Defining Characteristics: *Major* — Delays seeking or refuses health-care attention to the detriment of health; does not perceive personal relevance of symptoms or danger. *Minor* — Uses home remedies (self-treatment) to relieve symptoms; does not admit fear of death or invalidism; minimizes symptoms; displaces source of symptoms to other organs; unable to admit impact of disease on life pattern; makes dismissive gestures or comments when

speaking of distressing events; displaces fear of impact of the condition; displays inappropriate affect.

Author's Note: Do not use to describe the denial that occurs as a part of the normal grief process.

☛ Discriminate between this label and Ineffective Individual Coping, Altered Health Maintenance, Noncompliance, and Dysfunctional Grieving.

DIARRHEA

Definition: A state in which an individual experiences a change in normal bowel habits characterized by the frequent passage of loose, fluid, unformed stools.

Defining Characteristics: Abdominal pain; cramping; increased frequency; increased frequency of bowel sounds; loose liquid stools; urgency. *Other Possible Characteristics:* Change in color.

☛ *See also* Bowel Incontinence.

DISUSE SYNDROME, HIGH RISK FOR

Definition: A state in which an individual is at risk for deterioration of body systems as the result of prescribed or unavoidable musculoskeletal inactivity.

(Complications from immobility can include pressure ulcer, constipation, stasis of pulmonary secretions, thrombosis, urinary tract infection/retention, decreased strength/endurance, orthostatic hypotension, decreased range of joint motion, disorientation, body image disturbance, and powerlessness.)

Defining Characteristics: Presence of risk factors such as paralysis; mechanical immobilization; prescribed immobilization; severe pain; altered level of consciousness.

Related Factors: *See* risk factors above.

Author's Note: This label describes potential complications of immobility. It is not necessary to write separate high risk diagnoses such as High Risk for Impaired Skin Integrity or High Risk for Activity Intolerance when the risk factor is immobility. These more specific labels should be used only if an actual problem develops (Carpenito, 1991) or if the risk factor is other than immobility.

DIVERSIONAL ACTIVITY DEFICIT

Definition: The state in which an individual experiences a decreased stimulation from or interest or engagement in recreational or leisure activities.

Defining Characteristics: Patient's statements regarding boredom, wish there was something to do, to read, etc.; usual hobbies cannot be undertaken in hospital.

Related Factors: Environmental lack of diversional activity, as in long-term hospitalization, frequent lengthy treatments.

DRESSING-GROOMING SELF-CARE DEFICIT
(*see* Self-Care Deficit, Dressing-Grooming)

DYSFUNCTIONAL GRIEVING
(*see* Grieving, Dysfunctional)

DYSREFLEXIA
Definition: The state in which an individual with a spinal cord injury at T7 or above experiences a life-threatening, uninhibited sympathetic response of the nervous system to a noxious stimulus.

Defining Characteristics: *Major*—Paroxysmal hypertension (sudden periodic elevated B/P, where systolic pressure is over 140 mmHg and diastolic is above 90 mmHg); bradycardia or tachycardia (pulse rate < 60 or > 100 beats per minute); diaphoresis (above the injury); red splotches on skin (above the injury); pallor (below the injury); headache (a diffuse pain in different portions of the head and not confined to any nerve-distribution area). *Minor*—Chilling; conjunctival congestion; Horner's Syndrome (contraction of the pupil, partial ptosis of the eyelid, enophthalmos and sometimes loss of sweating over the affected side of the face); paresthesia; pilomotor reflex (gooseflesh formation when skin is cooled); blurred vision; chest pain; metallic taste in mouth; nasal congestion.

Related Factors: Bladder distention; bowel distention; skin irritation; lack of patient and caregiver knowledge.

Author's Note: Dysreflexia exists as a potential problem for the patient with high spinal cord injury. If it occurs as an actual problem, and nursing interventions do not immediately resolve it, medical treatment is necessary. It cannot continue as an actual nursing diagnosis. Therefore, High Risk for Dysreflexia is a more useful label (Carpenito, 1991).

ELIMINATION, URINARY
(*see* Urinary Elimination, Altered Patterns)

FAMILY COPING, INEFFECTIVE
(*see* Coping, Ineffective Family)

FAMILY COPING: POTENTIAL FOR GROWTH
(*see* Coping, Family: Potential for Growth)

FAMILY PROCESSES, ALTERED
Definition: The state in which a family that normally functions effectively experiences a dysfunction.

Defining Characteristics: Family system unable to meet physical, emotional, or spiritual needs of its members; parents do not demonstrate respect for each other's views on child-rearing practices; inability to express/accept wide range of feelings; inability to express/accept feelings of members; family unable to meet security needs of its members; inability of the family members to relate to each other for mutual growth and maturation; family uninvolved in community activities; inability to accept/receive help appropriately; rigidity in function and roles; a family not demonstrating respect for individuality and autonomy of its members; family unable to adapt to change/deal with traumatic experience constructively; family failing to accomplish current/past developmental task; unhealthy family decision-making process; failure to send and receive clear messages; inappropriate boundary maintenance; inappropriate/poorly communicated family rules, rituals, symbols; unexamined family myths; inappropriate level and direction of energy.

Related Factors: Situation transition and/or crises; developmental transition and/or crisis.

Author's Note: This label describes a family that normally functions effectively but is experiencing a stressor that alters its functioning. The stressors causing Altered Family Processes tend to be situational or developmental transitions and crises like the following:

Serious illness of a family member	Loss of job
Death of a family member	Divorce
Infidelity	

This label is different from Ineffective Family Coping: Compromised, in which the stressor is withdrawal of support by a significant other. The family coping problem is caused by a change in the relationship between the family members — not necessarily by an external stressor such as death or divorce. Compromised Family Coping involves the client and a significant other, whereas Altered Family Processes involves the entire family.

Altered Family Processes describes a family that has the resources for effectively coping with stressors, in contrast with Ineffective Family Coping: Disabling, which describes a family that demonstrates destructive behaviors. If stressors are not effectively resolved, Altered Family Processes can progress to Ineffective Family Coping.

To differentiate between these three labels, carefully examine the defining characteristics and related factors of each in your *Nursing Diagnosis Guide*.

☞ *See also* Ineffective Family Coping, Parental Role Conflict, and Altered Parenting.

FATIGUE

Definition: An overwhelming sustained sense of exhaustion and decreased capacity for physical and mental work.

Defining Characteristics: *Major* — Verbalization of an unremitting and overwhelming lack of energy; inability to maintain usual routines. *Minor* — Perceived need for additional energy to accomplish routine tasks; increase in physical complaints; emotionally labile or irritable; impaired ability to concentrate; decreased performance; lethargic or listless; disinterest in surroundings/introspection; decreased libido; accident-prone.

Related Factors: Decreased/increased metabolic energy production; overwhelming psychological or emotional demands; increased energy requirements to perform activity of daily living; excessive social and/or role demands; states of discomfort; altered body chemistry (e.g., medications, drug withdrawal, chemotherapy).

Author's Note: Do not use this label to describe temporary tiredness resulting from lack of sleep. Fatigue describes a chronic condition; the client's previous energy levels and capabilities cannot be restored.

☞ *See also* Activity Intolerance, Self-Care Deficit, and Sleep Pattern Disturbance.

FEAR

Definition: Feeling of dread related to an identifiable source which the person validates.

Defining Characteristics: Ability to identify object of fear.
Author's Note: Differentiate between Fear and Anxiety.
☞ *See* Anxiety note.

FEEDING SELF-CARE DEFICIT

(*see* Self-Care Deficit, Feeding)

FLUID VOLUME DEFICIT (1)

Definition: The state in which an individual experiences vascular, cellular, or intracellular dehydration.

Defining Characteristics: *Major* — Dilute urine; increased urine output; sudden weight loss. *Minor* — Possible weight gain; hypotension; decreased venous filling; increased pulse rate; decreased skin turgor; decreased pulse volume/pressure; increased body temperature; dry skin; dry mucous membranes; hemoconcentration; weakness; edema; thirst.

Related Factors: Failure of regulatory mechanisms.
Author's Note: Use this label for clients experiencing vascular, cellular, or intracellular dehydration. Use cautiously, because many problems with fluid balance require a collaborative approach. Do not use this label routinely, even as a potential problem, for patients who are NPO. Independent nursing treatments for Fluid Volume Deficit aim to prevent fluid loss (e.g., diaphoresis) and encourage oral fluids. For a diagnosis such as High Risk for Fluid Volume Deficit r/t NPO order, there are no independent nursing actions to prevent or treat either side of the diagnostic statement.

Do not use High Risk for Fluid Volume Deficit to describe clients who are hemorrhaging or at risk of hemorrhaging; these situations usually represent collaborative problems.

> *Incorrect:* High Risk for Fluid Volume Deficit r/t postpartum hemorrhage
> *Correct:* Potential Complication of Childbirth: Postpartum Hemorrhage; High Risk for Postpartum Hemorrhage r/t retained placental fragments

This label can sometimes be used effectively as a nursing diagnosis; for example, Fluid Volume Deficit r/t decreased desire for fluids 2° altered taste caused by chemotherapy. An *actual* fluid volume deficit may be the etiology for other nursing diagnoses, such as Altered Oral Mucous Membranes r/t fluid volume deficit 2° fluid loss from severe vomiting and diarrhea.

☞ Differentiate between this label and Fluid Volume Deficit (2).

FLUID VOLUME DEFICIT (2)

Definition: The state in which an individual experiences vascular, cellular, or intracellular dehydration.

Defining Characteristics: *Major* — Decreased urine output; concentrated urine; output greater than intake; sudden weight loss; decreased venous filling; hemoconcentration, increased serum sodium. *Minor* — Hypotension; thirst; increased pulse rate; decreased skin turgor; decreased pulse volume/pressure; change in mental state; increased body temperature; dry skin; dry mucous membranes; weakness.

Related Factors: Active loss.
Author's Note: *See* note for Fluid Volume Deficit (1).
☞ Differentiate between this label and Fluid Volume Deficit (1).

FLUID VOLUME DEFICIT, HIGH RISK FOR

Definition: The state in which an individual is at risk of experiencing vascular, cellular, or intracellular dehydration.

Defining Characteristics: Presence of risk factors such as extremes of age or weight; excessive losses through normal routes (e.g., diarrhea); loss of fluid through abnormal routes (e.g., indwelling tubes); deviations affecting access to or intake or absorption of fluids (e.g., physical immobility); factors influencing fluids needs (e.g., hypermetabolic state); knowledge deficit related to fluid volume; medications (e.g., diuretics).

Related Factors: *See* risk factors above.

Author's Note: *See* note for Fluid Volume Deficit (1). Do not use routinely for patients who are NPO.

FLUID VOLUME EXCESS

Definition: The state in which an individual experiences increased fluid retention and edema.

Defining Characteristics: Edema; effusion; anasarca; weight gain; shortness of breath, orthopnea; intake greater than output; S3 heart sound; pulmonary congestion (chest X ray); abnormal breath sounds, crackles; change in respiratory pattern; change in mental status; decreased hemoglobin and hematocrit; blood-pressure changes; central venous pressure or pulmonary artery pressure changes; jugular vein distention; positive hepatojugular reflex; oliguria; specific gravity changes; azotemia; altered electrolytes; restlessness and anxiety.

Related Factors: Compromised regulatory mechanism; excess fluid intake; excess sodium intake.

Author's Note: Be sure you use this label to describe a condition that nurses can prevent or treat with independent actions. The main type of Fluid Volume Excess that nurses can treat independently is peripheral, dependent edema, which can be symptomatically relieved by elevating the client's affected limbs. If the client requires medical intervention to resolve the fluid imbalance, use a collaborative problem such as Potential Complication of Renal Failure: Generalized Edema. Fluid Volume Excess can also be the cause of complications, such as Potential Complication of Fluid Volume Excess: Pulmonary Edema.

Examples:

Incorrect: Fluid Volume Excess r/t decreased cardiac output

Correct: Potential Complication of Decreased Cardiac Output: Fluid Volume Excess

Correct: Potential Complication of Heart Failure: Pulmonary Edema

Correct: High Risk for Impaired Skin Integrity r/t fluid volume excess A.M.B. generalized edema

☛ This label is related to Decreased Cardiac Output, which also tends to be a collaborative problem rather than a nursing diagnosis.

FUNCTIONAL INCONTINENCE (URINARY)

(*see* Incontinence, Functional Urinary)

GAS EXCHANGE, IMPAIRED

Definition: The state in which the individual experiences a decreased passage of oxygen and/or carbon dioxide between the alveoli of the lungs and the vascular system.

Defining Characteristics: Confusion; somnolence; restlessness; irritability; inability to move secretions; hypercapnea; hypoxia.

Related Factors: Ventilation perfusion imbalance.

Author's Note: Author does not recommend using this label. Decreased passage of gases between the alveoli of the lungs and the vascular system can only be discovered by means of a medically prescribed diagnostic test: blood gas analysis. The defining characteristics offer little help. A client might easily have most of them without actually having impaired alveolar gas exchange. Since nurses can neither diagnose nor treat this condition, you should use a diagnostic statement that describes oxygen-related problems the nurse *can* treat (e.g., Activity Intolerance). If the client is *at risk* for Impaired Gas Exchange, you should write a collaborative problem, such as Potential Complication of Thrombophlebitis: Pulmonary Embolus.

☛ *See also* Activity Intolerance, Ineffective Airway Clearance, Ineffective Breathing Pattern.

GRIEVING, ANTICIPATORY

Definition: To be developed.

Defining Characteristics: Potential loss of significant object; expression of distress at potential loss; denial of potential loss; guilt; anger; sorrow; choked feelings; changes in eating habits; alterations in sleep patterns; alterations in activity level; altered libido; altered communication patterns.

Related Factors: To be developed.

Author's Note: Anticipatory Grieving may be a normal, not necessarily maladaptive, response. It occurs *before* the loss.

☛ *See also* Dysfunctional Grieving.

GRIEVING, DYSFUNCTIONAL

Definition: To be developed.

Defining Characteristics: Verbal expression of distress at loss; denial of loss; expression of guilt; expression of unresolved issues; anger; sadness; crying; difficulty in expressing loss; alterations in eating habits, sleep patterns, dream patterns, activity level, libido; idealization of lost object; reliving of past experiences; interference with life functioning; developmental regression; labile affect; alterations in concentration and/or pursuits of tasks.

Related Factors: Actual or perceived object loss (object loss is used in the broadest sense); objects may include people, possessions, a job, status, home, ideals, parts and processes of the body.

Author's Note: Most of the defining characteristics may also be present in the normal grief process. Grieving is dysfunctional only if it is prolonged (perhaps a year after the loss), or if the symptoms are unusually numerous or severe.

GROWTH AND DEVELOPMENT, ALTERED

Definition: The state in which an individual demonstrates deviations in norms from his/her age group.

Defining Characteristics: *Major*— Delay or difficulty in performing skills (motor, social, or expressive) typical of age group; altered physical growth; inability to perform self-care or self-control activities appropriate for age. *Minor*— Flat affect; listlessness, decreased responses.

Related Factors: Inadequate caretaking; indifference, inconsistent responsiveness, multiple caretakers; separation from significant others; environmental and stimulation deficiencies; effects of physical disability; prescribed dependence.

Author's Note: Author does not recommend use of this label. It is too broad to suggest nursing interventions. There are many nursing diagnoses that could be considered alterations in growth and development or that could be caused by altered growth and development (e.g., Self-Care Deficit, Urinary Incontinence, Impaired Verbal Communication, and Altered Parenting). When possible, these more specific labels should be used. Because growth and development are routinely assessed in nursing care of children, a diagnostic statement is usually not required for that application (it is usually included in pediatric standards of care).

HEALTH MAINTENANCE, ALTERED

Definition: Inability to identify, manage, and/or seek out help to maintain health.

Defining Characteristics: Demonstrated lack of knowledge regarding basic health practices; demonstrated lack of adaptive behaviors to internal/external environmental changes; reported or observed inability to take responsibility for meeting basic health practices in any or all functional pattern areas; history of lack of health-seeking behavior; expressed interest in improving health behaviors; reported or observed lack of equipment, financial and/or other resources; reported or observed impairment of personal support systems.

Related Factors: Lack of or significant alteration in communication skills (written, verbal, and/or gestural); lack of ability to make deliberate and thoughtful judgments; perceptual/cognitive impairment (complete/partial lack of gross and/or fine motor skills); ineffective individual coping; dysfunctional grieving; unachieved developmental tasks; ineffective family coping; disabling spiritual distress; lack of material resources.

Author's Note: Altered Health Maintenance should be used for clients who *wish* to change an unhealthy life-style or who *lack knowledge* of their disease or condition. It should not be used to describe clients who are not motivated to change or learn.

☞ *See also* Impaired Adjustment, Health-Seeking Behaviors, Knowledge Deficit, Noncompliance.

HEALTH-SEEKING BEHAVIORS (SPECIFY)

Definition: A state in which an individual in stable health is actively seeking ways to alter personal health habits, and/or the environment in order to move toward a higher level of health. (Stable health status is defined as age-appropriate illness-prevention measures achieved, client reports good or excellent health, and signs and symptoms of disease, if present, are controlled.)

Defining Characteristics: *Major*— Expressed or observed desire to seek a higher level of wellness. *Minor*— Expressed or observed desire for increased control of health practice; expression of concern about current environmental conditions on health status; stated or observed unfamiliarity with wellness community resources; demonstrated or observed lack of knowledge in health-promotion behaviors.

Author's Note: This label should be used for well clients who wish information about disease prevention or health promotion.

☞ *See also* Altered Health Maintenance.

HOME MAINTENANCE MANAGEMENT, IMPAIRED

Definition: Inability to independently maintain a safe, growth-promoting immediate environment.

Defining Characteristics: Critical — Household members express difficulty in maintaining their home in a comfortable fashion; household requests assistance with home maintenance; household members describe outstanding debts or financial crises; unwashed or unavailable cooking equipment, clothes, or linen; accumulation of dirt, food wastes, or hygienic wastes; overtaxed family members (e.g., exhausted, anxious; repeated hygienic disorders, infestations, or infections). *Other* — Disorderly surroundings; offensive odors; inappropriate household temperature; presence of vermin or rodents.

Related Factors: Individual/family member disease or injury; insufficient family organization or planning; insufficient finances; unfamiliarity with neighborhood resources; impaired cognitive or emotional functioning; lack of knowledge; lack of role modeling; inadequate support system.

☛ *See also* High Risk for Injury.

HOPELESSNESS

Definition: A subjective state in which an individual sees limited or no alternatives or personal choices available and is unable to mobilize energy on own behalf.

Defining Characteristics: *Major* — Passivity, decreased verbalization; decreased affect; verbal cues (despondent content, "I can't," sighing). *Minor* — Lack of initiative; decreased response to stimuli; decreased affect; turning away from speaker; closing eyes; shrugging in response to speaker; decreased appetite; increased/decreased sleep; lack of involvement in care/passively allowing care.

Related Factors: Prolonged activity restriction creating isolation; failing or deteriorating physiological condition; long-term stress; abandonment; lost belief in transcendent values/God.

Author's Note: Differentiate between this label and Powerlessness. Hopelessness implies that the person believes there *is* no solution to his problem ("no way out"). In Powerlessness, the person may know of a solution to his problem, but believe it is beyond his control to achieve the solution.

HYPERTHERMIA

Definition: A state in which an individual's body temperature is elevated above his/her normal range.

Defining Characteristics: *Major* — Increase in body temperature above normal range. *Minor* — Flushed skin, warm to touch, increased respiratory rate, tachycardia, seizures/convulsions.

Related Factors: Exposure to hot environment; vigorous activity; medications/anesthesia; inappropriate clothing; increased metabolic rate; illness or trauma; dehydration; inability or decreased ability to perspire.

Author's Note: If it is written as high-risk nursing diagnosis, the nurse can prescribe interventions to prevent and monitor for development of this condition. As an actual diagnosis, it presents difficulties. For many patients, an elevated temperature is not a problem, but merely a symptom of a disease process, which is treated by a medication such as acetaminophen or aspirin. Many (maybe most) hyperthermias require no independent nursing actions. Mild sustained elevation or reduction of body temperature because of external factors (*actual* Hyper- or Hypothermia) can be treated by nursing interventions such as adding or removing clothing. However, severe Hyper- or Hypothermia is a life-threatening condition requiring both medical and nursing intervention; it would be a collaborative problem, not a nursing diagnosis.

☛ *See also* High Risk for Altered Body Temperature, Ineffective Thermoregulation.

HYPOTHERMIA

Definition: The state in which the individual's temperature is reduced below normal range.

Defining Characteristics: *Major* — Reduction in body temperature below normal range; shivering (mild); cool skin; pallor (moderate). *Minor* — Slow capillary refill; tachycardia; cyanotic nail beds; hypertension; piloerection.

Related Factors: Exposure to cool or cold environment; illness or trauma; damage to hypothalamus; inability or decreased ability to shiver; malnutrition; inadequate clothing; consumption of alcohol; medications causing vasodilation; evaporation from skin in cool environment; decreased metabolic rate, inactivity; aging.

Author's Note: *See* Hyperthermia note.

☛ *See also* High Risk for Altered Body Temperature, Ineffective Thermoregulation.

IDENTITY DISTURBANCE, PERSONAL
(*see* Personal Identity Disturbance)

INCONTINENCE, BOWEL

Definition: A state in which an individual experiences a change in normal bowel habits characterized by involuntary passage of stool.

Defining Characteristics: Involuntary passage of stool.
Related Factors: To be developed.
☛ Discriminate between this label and Diarrhea.

INCONTINENCE, FUNCTIONAL (URINARY)

Definition: The state in which an individual experiences an involuntary, unpredictable passage of urine.

Defining Characteristics: *Major* — Urge to void or bladder contractions sufficiently strong to result in loss of urine before reaching an appropriate receptacle.
Related Factors: Altered environment; sensory, cognitive, or mobility deficits.
☛ *See also* Reflex Incontinence, Stress Incontinence, Total Incontinence, Urge Incontinence, and Altered Patterns of Urinary Elimination.

INCONTINENCE, REFLEX (URINARY)

Definition: The state in which an individual experiences an involuntary loss of urine, occurring at somewhat predictable intervals when a specific bladder volume is reached.

Defining Characteristics: *Major* — No awareness of bladder filling; no urge to void or feelings of bladder fullness; uninhibited bladder contraction/spasm at regular intervals.
Related Factors: Neurological impairment (e.g., spinal cord lesion which interferes with conduction of cerebral messages above the level of the reflex arc).
☛ *See also* Functional Incontinence, Stress Incontinence, Total Incontinence, Urge Incontinence, and Altered Patterns of Urinary Elimination.

INCONTINENCE, STRESS (URINARY)

Definition: The state in which an individual experiences a loss of urine of less than 50 ml occurring with increased abdominal pressure.

Defining Characteristics: *Major* — Reported or observed dribbling with increased abdominal pressure. *Minor* — Urinary urgency; urinary frequency (more often than every 2 hours).
Related Factors: Degenerative changes in pelvic muscles and structural supports associated with increased age; high intra-abdominal pressure (e.g., obesity, gravid uterus); incompetent bladder outlet; overdistention between voidings; weak pelvic muscles and pelvic supports.

☛ *See also* Functional Incontinence, Total Incontinence, Reflex Incontinence, Urge Incontinence, and Altered Patterns of Urinary Elimination.

INCONTINENCE, TOTAL (URINARY)

Definition: The state in which an individual experiences a continuous and unpredictable loss of urine.

Defining Characteristics: *Major* — Constant flow of urine occurs at unpredictable times without distention or uninhibited bladder contractions/spasm; unsuccessful incontinence refractory treatments; nocturia. *Minor* — Lack of perineal or bladder-filling awareness; unawareness of incontinence.
Related Factors: Neuropathy preventing transmission of reflex indicating bladder fullness; neurological dysfunction causing triggering of micturition at unpredictable times; independent contraction of detrusor reflex due to surgery; trauma or disease affecting spinal cord nerves; anatomic (fistula).
☛ *See also* Functional Incontinence, Stress Incontinence, Reflex Incontinence, Urge Incontinence, and Altered Patterns of Urinary Elimination.

INCONTINENCE, URGE (URINARY)

Definition: The state in which an individual experiences involuntary passage of urine occurring soon after a strong sense of urgency to void.

Defining Characteristics: *Major* — Urinary urgency; frequency (voiding more often than every 2 hours); bladder contracture/spasm. *Minor* — Nocturia (more than two times per night); voiding in small amounts (less than 100 cc) or in large amounts (more than 550 cc); inability to reach toilet in time.
Related Factors: Decreased bladder capacity (e.g., history of PID, abdominal surgeries, indwelling urinary catheter); irritation of bladder stretch receptors causing spasm (e.g., bladder infection); alcohol; caffeine; increased fluids; increased urine concentration; overdistention of bladder.
☛ See also Functional Incontinence, Reflex Incontinence, Stress Incontinence, Total Incontinence, and Altered Patterns of Urinary Elimination.

INDIVIDUAL COPING, INEFFECTIVE
(*see* Coping, Ineffective Individual)

INFECTION, HIGH RISK FOR

Definition: The state in which an individual is at increased risk for being invaded by pathogenic organisms.

Defining Characteristics: Presence of risk factors such as inadequate primary defenses (broken skin, traumatized tissue, decrease in ciliary action, stasis of body fluids, change in pH secretions, altered peristalsis); inadequate secondary defenses (e.g., decreased hemoglobin, leukopenia, suppressed inflammatory response) and immunosuppression; inadequate acquired immunity; tissue destruction and increased environmental exposure; chronic disease; invasive procedures; malnutrition; pharmaceutical agents; trauma; rupture of amniotic membranes; insufficient knowledge to avoid exposure to pathogens.

Related Factors: *See* risk factors above.

☛ *See also* Altered Protection.

INJURY, HIGH RISK FOR

Definition: A state in which the individual is at risk of injury as a result of environmental conditions interacting with the individual's adaptive and defensive resources.

Defining Characteristics: Presence of risk factors such as the following. *Internal* — biochemical, regulatory function (sensory dysfunction, integrative dysfunction, effector dysfunction, tissue hypoxia); malnutrition; immune/autoimmune; abnormal blood profile (leukocytosis/leukopenia; altered clotting factors; thrombocytopenia; sickle cell, Thalassemia; decreased hemoglobin); physical (broken skin, altered mobility); developmental age (physiological, psychosocial); psychological (affective, orientation). *External* — biological (immunization level of community, microorganism); chemical (pollutants, poisons, drugs, pharmaceutical agents, alcohol, caffeine, nicotine, preservative, cosmetics and dyes); nutrients (vitamins, food types); physical (design, structure, and arrangement of community, building, and/or equipment); mode of transport/transportation; people/provider (nosocomial agents, staffing patterns, cognitive, affective, and psychomotor factors).

Related Factors: *See* risk factors above.

Author's Note: This is a broad title that includes internal risk factors such as altered clotting factors and decreased hemoglobin. NANDA has not identified any critical defining characteristics for this title, so it is important to identify only those clients who are at high risk for this problem. Everyone has at least some risk for accidents and injury, but the label should be used only for those who require nursing intervention to prevent injury.

This label consists of five subcategories that describe *injury* more specifically: High Risk for Suffocation, Poison-

ing, Trauma, Aspiration, and Disuse Syndrome. When possible, use these more specific labels instead of High Risk for Injury, because they provide clearer direction for nursing care. None of the subcategories needs further specification except High Risk for Trauma, which includes wounds, burns, and fractures, and an unlimited number of risk factors.

☛ Related labels: High Risk for Aspiration, Poisoning, Suffocation, Trauma, Infection, or Altered Protection.

KNOWLEDGE DEFICIT (SPECIFY)

Definition: To be developed.

Defining Characteristics: Verbalization of the problem; inaccurate follow-through of instruction; inaccurate performance of test; inappropriate or exaggerated behaviors (e.g., hysterical, hostile, agitated, apathetic).

Related Factors: Lack of exposure; lack of recall; information misinterpretation; cognitive limitation; lack of interest in learning; unfamiliarity with information resources.

Author's Note: Author does not recommend use of this label, except as an etiology. Although this label was accepted in 1980, NANDA has not yet developed a definition or critical defining characteristics for it. At least two studies show Knowledge Deficit is one of the diagnoses most frequently used by nurses (Gordon, 1985; Lambert and Jones, 1989). This seems to be due at least in part to premature diagnosing: it is easy to recognize a knowledge deficit, label it as a problem, and not look beyond that to the human *response* to the lack of knowledge. It also happens because of the mistaken belief that information-giving is effective in changing human behavior.

For the following reasons, Knowledge Deficit should not, as a rule, be used to label the problem side of your diagnostic statement:

1. Knowledge Deficit is not truly a human response. *Response* suggests a behavior or action; Knowledge Deficit is simply a state of being.

2. Knowledge Deficit does not necessarily describe a *health* state.

3. Knowledge Deficit does not necessarily describe a *problem.* Nursing diagnoses should reflect altered functioning; but Knowledge Deficit simply means the person does not have some needed knowledge, not that his functioning is changed as a result of that. A client might not have any knowledge at all about the Basic Four Food Groups; but that does not necessarily mean he has impaired nutritional status.

Knowledge Deficit can contribute to any number of responses, including Anxiety, Altered Parenting, Self-Care Deficit, or Impaired Coping. Therefore, it may be used effectively as the etiology of a nursing diagnosis.

Examples: High Risk for Injury (Trauma) r/t lack of knowledge of proper application of seat-belts when pregnant

Anxiety r/t lack of knowledge of procedures involved in bone marrow aspiration.

If Knowledge Deficit is used as a problem, the goal must be "Patient will acquire knowledge about . . ." This causes the nurse to focus on giving information rather than on the behaviors caused by the patient's lack of knowledge. Using Knowledge Deficit as a problem label reinforces the belief that giving information will change behavior and solve the problem. On the other hand, when Knowledge Deficit is used as the etiology, it focuses attention on behaviors that indicate self-doubt, decisional conflict, anxiety, and so on. Note the different nursing care suggested by these statements:

Knowledge Deficit (Bone Marrow Aspiration) r/t lack of prior experience

Anxiety r/t knowledge deficit (bone marrow aspiration)

Patient teaching is an important intervention for most patients and for all the diagnostic labels (e.g., Constipation, Ineffective Breastfeeding, Altered Nutrition). It is not necessary, or even desirable, to have a Knowledge-Deficit diagnosis on every patient's care plan. You should simply include teaching as one of the nursing interventions for the other diagnoses you have made.

Some patients, such as a newly diagnosed diabetic, require a great deal of teaching in order to acquire necessary self-care skills. Such special teaching plans should be a part of the routine care on standardized care plans for these patients, and should not require an individualized diagnosis. However, if the agency does not use standardized care plans or protocols, you would need to write individualized orders for the teaching. If so, the best approach is still to use Knowledge Deficit as the etiology rather than the problem. If the patient does not have the necessary knowledge, she may not be able to manage her own health-care needs. The human response is not lack of knowledge, but high risk for decreased ability for maintaining health.

Example: High Risk for Altered Health Maintenance (Diabetes Management) r/t knowledge deficit (medication, diet, exercise, and skin care) r/t new diagnosis

Knowledge Deficit, if used, should describe conditions in which the patient needs new or additional knowledge. It should not be used for problems involving the patient's ability to learn (as in Knowledge Deficit r/t severe anxiety about outcome of surgery). Rakel and Bulechek (1990) propose a diagnosis of "Situational Learning Disabil-

ity: Impaired Ability to Learn" or "Situational Learning Disability: Lack of Motivation to Learn" for such conditions; however, these are not yet NANDA-approved labels.

LOW SELF-ESTEEM, CHRONIC
(*see* Self-Esteem, Chronic Low)

LOW SELF-ESTEEM, SITUATIONAL
(*see* Self-Esteem, Situational Low)

MOBILITY, IMPAIRED PHYSICAL
Definition: A state in which the individual experiences a limitation of ability for independent physical movement.

Defining Characteristics: Inability to purposefully move within the physical environment, including bed mobility, transfer, and ambulation; reluctance to attempt movement; limited range of motion; decreased muscle strength, control, and/or mass; imposed restrictions of movement, including mechanical, medical protocol; impaired coordination.

Related Factors: Intolerance to activity/decreased strength and endurance; pain/discomfort; perceptual/cognitive impairment; neuromuscular impairment; musculoskeletal impairment; depression/severe anxiety.

Suggested Functional-Level Classification:

0 = Completely independent

1 = Requires use of equipment or device

2 = Requires help from another person for assistance, supervision, or teaching.

3 = Requires help from another person and equipment or device.

4 = Dependent; does not participate in activity.

The preceding code is adapted from E. Jones et al., *Patient Classification for Long-Term Care: Users' Manual,* HEW, Publication No. HRA-74-3107, November 1974, as quoted in NANDA Taxonomy I — Revised, 1990.

Author's Note: Use this label for individuals with limited ability for independent physical movement, such as decreased ability to move arms or legs or generalized muscle weakness, when nursing interventions will focus on restoring mobility and function or preventing further deterioration.

Example: Impaired Physical Mobility r/t ineffective management of chronic pain 2° rheumatoid arthritis

Do not use Impaired Physical Mobility to describe temporary immobility that cannot be changed by the nurse (e.g., traction, prescribed bedrest, or permanent paralysis). It can, in these and many other instances, be used effectively as the etiology of other problems.

> **Examples:** Impaired Tissue Integrity (Decubitis Ulcer) r/t impaired physical mobility +4
>
> Diversional Activity Deficit r/t prescribed bedrest

☞ *See also* High Risk for Disuse Syndrome, High Risk for Injury and Self-Care Deficit.

MUCOUS MEMBRANE, ALTERED ORAL

(*see* Oral Mucous Membrane, Altered)

NONCOMPLIANCE (SPECIFY)

Definition: A person's informed decision not to adhere to a therapeutic recommendation.

Defining Characteristics: Critical — Behavior indicative of failure to adhere (by direct observation or by statements of patient or significant others). *Other* — Objective tests (physiological measures, detection of markers); evidence of development of complications; evidence of exacerbation of symptoms; failure to keep appointments; failure to progress.

Related Factors: Patient value system: health beliefs, cultural influences, spiritual values; client-provider relationships.

Author's Note: According to NANDA, Noncompliance should be diagnosed when a client makes an informed decision *not* to adhere to a therapeutic recommendation; for instance, when a medication has unpleasant side effects. Nursing intervention might then be directed at convincing the client of the value of continuing with the therapy, but the nurse should balance this with respect for the client's autonomy when a truly informed decision has been made. Remember that a decision to refuse therapy can be as rational as a decision to have therapy.

> **Example:** Noncompliance with Low-Calorie Diet r/t desire not to change eating habits A.M.B. "I realize being overweight is bad for my heart, but I'm far too old to change my ways. If eating what I like means I don't live as long, that's okay; these last few years won't be much fun anyway if I have to eat boiled eggs and lettuce."

The client in the above example knows the relationship between calories, obesity, and heart problems and has *chosen* not to comply with the prescribed diet. It is not clear how the nurse should intervene in this type of diagnosis.

You could try to persuade the client that she may enjoy life even more if she is thin, or that low-calorie foods can taste just as good as her usual diet; however, it may be that neither of these is true.

Gordon's (1987) definition is more useful. She defines Noncompliance as failure to adhere to a therapeutic recommendation after have made an informed decision *to* do so, and after expressing intention to do so. If the client is informed and *intends* to follow instructions, then nursing intervention can be directed at finding and removing the factors that keep him from doing so. In the following example, the client would like to comply with her diet, but situational factors are making it difficult. This diagnosis does suggest nursing intervention.

> **Example:** Noncompliance with Low-Calorie Diet r/t inconvenience of preparing special foods A.M.B. "My husband doesn't need to lose weight, and he loves fried food and pastries. He just won't eat the diet foods, and I really don't have time to cook one meal for myself and one for the rest of the family."

Following is a comparison of the NANDA and Gordon definitions of Noncompliance:

NANDA Definition of Noncompliance
> Client has the necessary information
> Client chooses not to comply

Gordon's Definition of Noncompliance
> Client has the necessary information
> Client has said he intends to comply
> Does not comply

Noncompliance should not be used in cases where the client is unable to follow instructions (e.g., too weak, cognitive disability) or lacks necessary information. If lack of ability or information is causing the noncompliance, Altered Health Maintenance is preferred.

Some nurses feel Noncompliance has a negative connotation. When using this label, be sure to express the etiology in neutral, nonjudgmental terms. You might prefer to use the term Nonadherence (Geissler, 1991), although it is not a NANDA-approved label.

☞ *See* Altered Health Maintenance.

NUTRITION, ALTERED: LESS THAN BODY REQUIREMENTS

Definition: The state in which an individual experiences an intake of nutrients insufficient to meet metabolic needs.

Defining Characteristics: Loss of weight with adequate food intake; body weight 20% or more under ideal; reported inadequate food intake less than recommended daily allowance; weakness of muscles required for swallowing or mastication; reported or evidence of lack of food; aversion to eating; reported altered taste sensation; satiety immediately after ingesting food; abdominal pain with or without pathology; sore, inflamed buccal cavity; capillary fragility; abdominal cramping; diarrhea and/or steatorrhea; hyperactive bowel sounds; lack of interest in food; perceived inability to ingest food; pale conjunctival and mucous membranes; poor muscle tone; excessive loss of hair; lack of information, misinformation; misconceptions.

Related Factors: Inability to ingest or digest food or absorb nutrients due to biological, psychological, or economic factors.

Author's Note: Use this label for clients who are able to eat, but unable to ingest, digest, or absorb nutrients adequate to meet metabolic needs. Inadequate ingestion might occur because of decreased appetite, nausea, being too poor to buy food, or any number of situations. Examples of clients unable to digest food or absorb particular nutrients are those with allergies, diarrhea, lactose intolerance, or poorly fitting dentures. NANDA does not specify which defining characteristics must be present in order to use this label. The author recommends using this label only if one of the following cues is present:

Body weight 20% under ideal
Observed or reported food intake less than recommended daily allowance (RDA) — either total calories or specific nutrients
Observed or reported food intake less than metabolic needs — either total calories or specific nutrients
Weight loss with adequate food intake

Do not use this label routinely for persons who are NPO or for those completely unable to ingest food for other reasons (e.g., unconscious patients). Nurses cannot prescribe independent nursing interventions for a diagnosis such as Altered Nutrition: Less Than Body Requirements r/t NPO — they cannot give the missing nutrients, and they cannot change the NPO order. Additionally, the patient is often NPO for only a short time before and after surgery; thus, any lack of nutrients is temporary and is resolved without nursing intervention. Long-term NPO status is a risk factor for other nursing diagnoses, such as High Risk for Fluid Volume Deficit or High Risk for Altered Oral Mucous Membrane, and for collaborative problems such as Potential Electrolyte Imbalance.

The client can have a total nutritional deficit, or she might be deficient in only one nutrient. When the deficit is less than total, it should be specified as follows:

> **Example:** Altered Nutrition: Less Than Body Requirements *for Protein* r/t lack of knowledge of Basic Four and limited budget for food

NUTRITION, ALTERED: MORE THAN BODY REQUIREMENTS

Definition: The state in which an individual is experiencing an intake of nutrients which exceeds metabolic needs.

Defining Characteristics: Weight 10% over ideal for height and frame; sedentary activity level; reported or observed dysfunctional eating pattern: pairing food with other activities; concentrating food intake at the end of day; eating in response to external cues such as time of day, social situation; eating in response to internal cues other than hunger (e.g., anxiety). **Critical** — Weight 20% over ideal for height and frame; triceps skin fold greater than 15 mm in men, 25 mm in women.

Related Factors: Excessive intake in relation to metabolic need.

NUTRITION, ALTERED: HIGH RISK FOR MORE THAN BODY REQUIREMENTS

Definition: The state in which an individual is at risk of experiencing an intake of nutrients which exceeds metabolic needs.

Defining Characteristics: Reported use of solid food as major food source before 5 months of age; observed use of food as reward or comfort measure; reported or observed higher baseline weight at beginning of each pregnancy; dysfunctional eating patterns: pairing food with other activities; concentrating food intake at end of day; eating in response to external cues such as time of day, social situation; eating in response to internal cues other than hunger, such as anxiety. **Critical** — Reported or observed obesity in one or both parents; rapid transition across growth percentiles in infants or children.

Related Factors: *See* risk factors above.

ORAL MUCOUS MEMBRANE, ALTERED

Definition: The state in which an individual experiences disruptions in the tissue layers of the oral cavity.

Defining Characteristics: Oral pain/discomfort; coated tongue; xerostomia (dry mouth); stomatitis; oral lesions or ulcers; lack of or decreased salivation; leukoplakia; edema; hyperemia; oral plaque; desquamation; vesicles; hemorrhagic gingivitis, carious teeth, halitosis.

Related Factors: Pathological conditions — oral cavity (radiation to head or neck); dehydration; trauma (chemical, e.g., acidic foods, drugs, noxious agents, alcohol; mechanical, e.g., ill-fitting dentures, braces, endotracheal/nasogastric tubes, surgery in oral cavity); NPO for more than 24 hours; ineffective oral hygiene; mouth breathing; malnutrition; infection; lack of or decreased salivation; medication.

☞ *See also* Impaired Tissue Integrity.

PAIN

Definition: A state in which an individual experiences and reports the presence of severe discomfort or an uncomfortable sensation.

Defining Characteristics: *Subjective* — Communication (verbal or coded) of pain descriptors. *Objective* — Guarding behavior, protective; self-focusing; narrowed focus (altered time perception, withdrawal from social contact, impaired thought process); distraction behavior (moaning, crying, pacing, seeking out other people and/or activities; restlessness); facial mask of pain (eyes lack luster, "beaten look," fixed or scattered movement, grimace); alteration in muscle tone (may span from listless to rigid); autonomic responses not seen in chronic stable pain (diaphoresis, blood pressure and pulse change, pupillary dilation, increased or decreased respiratory rate).
Related Factors: Injury agents (biological, chemical, physical, psychological).
Author's Note: There are no critical defining characteristics, but Pain can be diagnosed on the patient's verbal report alone, since that is sometimes the only sign of pain. None of the other defining characteristics taken alone would be sufficient to diagnose Pain. The related factors that NANDA lists, injury agents (biological, chemical, physical, psychological), indicate that a client can suffer both physical and psychological pain. The diagnosis is more useful if you use qualifiers to indicate the severity, location, and nature of the pain.

> *Examples:* Severe, stabbing chest **Pain** r/t fractured ribs
>
> Mild frontal **headache** r/t sinus congestion
>
> Moderate chronic **Pain** in knee joints (aching) r/t exercise 2° arthritis

It is important to differentiate between Pain and Chronic Pain because the nursing focus is different for each. Acute Pain, such as postoperative incision pain, is usually a collaborative problem that is managed primarily by administering narcotic analgesics. There are a few helpful independent nursing interventions, such as supporting the client during ambulation or teaching the client to splint the incision while moving about, but these alone would not provide adequate pain relief. The nurse can take a more active role in teaching the client self-management of Chronic Pain. When Pain is acute or caused by a stressor

that is not amenable to nursing intervention (e.g., a surgical incision), you may prefer to use it as an etiology rather than a problem.

> *Examples:* Ineffective Airway Clearance r/t weak cough r/t **pain** 2° chest incision
>
> High Risk for Disuse Syndrome r/t **severe pain** 2° metastasized cancer
>
> Sexual Dysfunction r/t partner's **severe chronic pain** 2° arthritis
>
> Sleep-Pattern Disturbance r/t **aching pain** in legs

☞ *See also* Pain, Chronic.

PAIN, CHRONIC
Definition: A state in which the individual experiences pain that continues for more than 6 months in duration.

Defining Characteristics: *Major* — Verbal report or observed evidence of pain experienced for more than 6 months. *Minor* — Fear of re-injury; physical and social withdrawal; altered ability to continue previous activities; anorexia; weight changes; changes in sleep patterns; facial mask; guarded movement.
Related Factors: Chronic physical-psychosocial disability.
☞ *See also* Pain.

PARENTAL ROLE CONFLICT
Definition: The state in which a parent experiences role confusion and conflict in response to crisis.

Defining Characteristics: *Major* — Parent(s) express(es) concerns/feelings of inadequacy to provide for child's physical and emotional needs during hospitalization or in the home; demonstrated disruption in caretaking routines; parent(s) express(es) concerns about changes in parental role, family functioning, communication, or health. *Minor* — Expresses concern about perceived loss of control over decisions relating to their child; reluctant to participate in usual caretaking activities even with encouragement and support; verbalize, demonstrate feelings of guilt, anger, fear, anxiety and/or frustrations about effect of child's illness on family process.
Related Factors: Separation from child due to chronic illness; intimidation with invasive or restrictive modalities (e.g., isolation, intubation), specialized care centers, policies; home care of a child with special needs (e.g., apnea monitoring, postural drainage, hyperalimentation); change in marital status; interruptions of family life due to home-care regimen (treatments, caregivers, lack of respite).

Author's Note: This label should be used when a situation, such as the child's illness, causes unsatisfactory role performance by previously effective parents.

☛ *See also* Altered Parenting, High Risk for Altered Parenting, Altered Family Processes.

PARENTING, ALTERED

(It is important to state as a preface to this diagnosis that adjustment to parenting in general is a normal maturational process that elicits nursing behaviors of prevention of potential problems and health promotion.)

Definition: The state in which a nurturing figure(s) experience(s) an inability to create an environment which promotes the optimum growth and development of another human being.

Defining Characteristics: Critical — Inattentive to infant/child needs; inappropriate caretaking behavior (toilet training, sleep/rest, feeding); history of child abuse or abandonment by primary caretaker. *Other* — Abandonment; runaway; verbalization, cannot control child; incidence of physical and psychological trauma; lack of parental attachment behaviors; inappropriate visual, tactile, auditory stimulation; negative identification of infant/child's characteristics; negative attachment of meanings to infant/child's characteristics; constant verbalization of disappointment in gender or physical characteristics of the infant/child; verbalization of resentment towards the infant/child; verbalization of role inadequacy; verbal disgust at body functions of infant/child; noncompliance with health appointments for self and/or infant/child; inappropriate or inconsistent discipline practices; frequent accidents; frequent illness; growth and development lag in the child; verbalizes desire to have child call him/herself by first name versus traditional cultural tendencies; child receives care from multiple caretakers without consideration for the needs of the infant/child; compulsively seeking role approval from others.

Related Factors: Lack of available role model; ineffective role model; physical and psychosocial abuse of nurturing figure; lack of support between/from significant other(s); unmet social/emotional maturation needs of parenting figures; interruption in bonding process (i.e., maternal, paternal, other); unrealistic expectation for self, infant, partner; perceived threat to own survival, physical and emotional; mental and/or physical illness; presence of stress (financial, legal, recent crisis, cultural move); lack of knowledge; limited cognitive functioning; lack of role identity; lack of or inappropriate response of child to relationship; multiple pregnancies.

Author's Note: This label represents a less healthy level of functioning than Parental Role Conflict.

☛ *See also* High Risk for Altered Parenting, Altered Family Processes, Ineffective Family Coping, and Parental Role Conflict.

PARENTING, HIGH RISK FOR ALTERED

(It is important to state as a preface to this diagnosis that adjustment to parenting in general is a normal maturational process that elicits nursing behaviors of prevention of potential problems and health promotion.)

Definition: The state in which a nurturing figure(s) is (are) at risk to experience an inability to create an environment which promotes the optimum growth and development of another human being.

Defining Characteristics: Critical — Inattentive to infant/child needs; inappropriate caretaking behavior (toilet training, sleep/rest, feeding); history of child abuse or abandonment by primary caretaker. *Other* — Lack of parental attachment behaviors; inappropriate visual, tactile, auditory stimulation; negative identification of infant/child's characteristics; negative attachment of meanings to infant/child's characteristics; constant verbalization of disappointment in gender or physical characteristics of the infant/child; verbalization of resentment towards the infant/child; verbalization of role inadequacy; verbal disgust at body functions of infant/child; noncompliance with health appointments for self and/or infant/child; inappropriate or inconsistent discipline practices; frequent accidents; frequent illness; growth and development lag in the child; verbalizes desire to have child call him/herself by first name versus traditional cultural tendencies; child receives care from multiple caretakers without consideration for the needs of the infant/child; compulsively seeking role approval from others.

Related Factors: Lack of available role model; ineffective role model; physical and psychosocial abuse of nurturing figure; lack of support between/from significant other(s); unmet social/emotional maturation needs of parenting figures; interruption in bonding process (i.e., maternal, paternal, other); unrealistic expectation for self, infant, partner; perceived threat to own survival, physical and emotional; mental and/or physical illness; presence of stress (financial, legal, recent crisis, cultural move); lack of knowledge; limited cognitive functioning; lack of role identity; lack of or inappropriate response of child to relationship; multiple pregnancies.

Author's Note: Critical Defining Characteristics are identical to *actual* Altered Parenting. If they are present, use Altered Parenting insted of this diagnosis.

☛ *See also* Altered Parenting, Altered Family Processes, Ineffective Family Coping, and Parental Role Conflict.

PERSONAL IDENTITY DISTURBANCE

Definition: Inability to distinguish between self and nonself.

Defining Characteristics: To be developed.

PHYSICAL MOBILITY, IMPAIRED
(*see* Mobility, Impaired Physical)

POISONING, HIGH RISK FOR

Definition: Accentuated risk of accidental exposure to or ingestion of drugs or dangerous products in doses sufficient to cause poisoning.

Defining Characteristics: Presence of risk factors such as the following. *Internal* (*individual*) — Reduced vision; verbalization of occupational setting without adequate safeguards; lack of safety or drug education; lack of proper precaution; cognitive or emotional difficulties; insufficient finances. *External* (*environmental*) — Large supplies of drugs in house; medicines stored in unlocked cabinets accessible to children or confused persons; availability of illicit drugs potentially contaminated by poisonous additives; flaking, peeling paint or plaster in presence of young children; chemical contamination of food and water; unprotected contact with heavy metals or chemicals; paint, lacquer, etc., in poorly ventilated areas or without effective protection; presence of poisonous vegetation; presence of atmospheric pollutants.

Related Factors: *See* risk factors above.

Author's Note: Use the most specific label for which defining characteristics are present.

☞ *See* High Risk for Injury, Impaired Home Maintenance Management, and High Risk for Trauma.

POST-TRAUMA RESPONSE

Definition: The state of an individual experiencing a sustained painful response to an overwhelming traumatic event(s).

Defining Characteristics: *Major* — Reexperience of the traumatic event which may be identified in cognitive, affective, and/or sensory motor activities (flashbacks, intrusive thoughts, repetitive dreams or nightmares, excessive verbalization of the traumatic event, verbalization of survival guilt or guilt about behavior required for survival). *Minor* — Psychic/emotional numbness (impaired interpretation of reality, confusion, dissociation or amne-

sia, vagueness about traumatic event, constricted affect); altered life-style (self-destructiveness, such as substance abuse, suicide attempt, or other acting-out behavior, difficulty with interpersonal relationship, development of phobia regarding trauma, poor impulse control/irritability and explosiveness).

Related Factors: Disasters, wars, epidemics, rape, assault, torture, catastrophic illness or accident.

☞ *See also* Rape-Trauma Syndrome.

POWERLESSNESS

Definition: Perception that one's own action will not significantly affect an outcome; a perceived lack of control over a current situation or immediate happening.

Defining Characteristics: *Severe* — Verbal expressions of having no control or influence over situation; verbal expressions of having no control or influence over outcome; verbal expressions of having no control over self-care; depression over physical deterioration which occurs despite patient compliance with regimens; apathy. *Moderate* — Nonparticipation in care or decision making when opportunities are provided; expressions of dissatisfaction and frustration over inability to perform previous tasks and/or activities; does not monitor progress; expression of doubt regarding role performance; reluctance to express true feelings; fearing alienation from caregivers; passivity; inability to seek information regarding care; dependence on others that may result in irritability, resentment, anger, and guilt; does not defend self-care practices when challenged. *Low* — Expressions of uncertainty about fluctuating energy levels; passivity.

Related Factors: Health-care environment; interpersonal interaction; illness-related regimen; life-style of helplessness.

Author's Note: Differentiate between this label and Hopelessness. Hopelessness implies that the person believes there *is* no solution to his problem ("no way out"). In Powerlessness, the person may know of a solution to his problem, but believe it is beyond his control to achieve the solution.

☞ *See also* High Risk for Disuse Syndrome.

PROTECTION, ALTERED

Definition: The state in which an individual experiences a decrease in the ability to guard the self from internal or external threats such as illness or injury.

Defining Characteristics: *Major* — Deficient immunity; impaired healing; altered clotting; maladaptive stress response; neuro-sensory alteration. *Minor* — Chilling; perspiring; dyspnea; cough; itching; restlessness; insomnia; fatigue; anorexia; weakness; immobility; disorientation; pressure sores.

Related Factors: Extremes of age; inadequate nutrition; alcohol abuse; abnormal blood profiles (leukopenia, thrombocytopenia, anemia, coagulation); drug therapies (antineoplastic, corticosteroid, immune, anticoagulant, thrombolytic); treatments (surgery, radiation), and diseases such as cancer and immune disorders.

Author's Note: When possible, use a more specific label, such as High Risk for Infection, Impaired Skin Integrity, Impaired Tissue Integrity, Altered Oral Mucous Membrane, or Fatigue.

☞ *See also* High Risk for Injury.

RAPE-TRAUMA SYNDROME

Definition: Forced, violent sexual penetration against the victim's will and consent. The trauma syndrome that develops from this attack or attempted attack includes an acute phase of disorganization of the victim's life-style and a long-term process of reorganization of life-style.

Defining Characteristics: *Acute Phase* — Emotional reactions (anger, embarrassment, fear of physical violence and death, humiliation, revenge, self-blame); multiple physical symptoms (gastrointestinal irritability, genitourinary discomfort, muscle tension, sleep-pattern disturbance). *Long-Term Phase* — Changes in life-style (change in residence; dealing with repetitive nightmares and phobias; seeking family support; seeking social network support).

☞ *See also* Rape-Trauma Syndrome: Compound Reaction and Rape-Trauma Syndrome: Silent Reaction.

RAPE-TRAUMA SYNDROME: COMPOUND REACTION

Definition: Forced, violent sexual penetration against the victim's will and consent. The trauma syndrome that develops from this attack or attempted attack includes an acute phase of disorganization of the victim's life-style and a long-term process of reorganization of life-style.

Defining Characteristics: *Acute Phase* — Emotional reactions (anger, embarrassment, fear of physical violence and death, humiliation, revenge, self-blame); multiple physical symptoms (gastrointestinal irritability, genitourinary discomfort, muscle tension, sleep-pattern disturbance); reactivated symptoms of such previous conditions (i.e., physical illness, psychiatric illness; reliance on alcohol and/or drugs). *Long-Term Phase* — Changes in life-style (change

in residence; dealing with repetitive nightmares and phobias; seeking family support; seeking social network support).

☞ *See also* Rape-Trauma Syndrome and Rape-Trauma Syndrome: Silent Reaction.

RAPE-TRAUMA SYNDROME: SILENT REACTION

Definition: Forced, violent sexual penetration against the victim's will and consent. The trauma syndrome that develops from this attack or attempted attack includes an acute phase of disorganization of the victim's life-style and a long-term process of reorganization of life-style.

Defining Characteristics: Abrupt changes in relationships with men; increase in nightmares; increased anxiety during interview (i.e., blocking of associations, long periods of silence, minor stuttering, physical distress); pronounced changes in sexual behavior; no verbalization of the occurrence of rape; sudden onset of phobic reactions.

☞ *See also* Rape-Trauma Syndrome and Rape-Trauma Syndrome: Compound Reaction.

REFLEX INCONTINENCE

(*see* Incontinence, Reflex)

RESPIRATORY FUNCTION

(*see* Airway Clearance, Ineffective; Breathing Patterns, Ineffective; Gas Exchange, Impaired)

ROLE CONFLICT, PARENTAL

(*see* Parental Role Conflict)

ROLE PERFORMANCE, ALTERED

Definition: Disruption in the way one perceives one's role performance.

Defining Characteristics: Change in self-perception of role; denial of role; change in others' perception of role; conflict in roles; change in physical capacity to resume role; lack of knowledge of role; change in usual patterns of responsibility.

Related Factors: To be developed.

Author's Note: This label is not well developed. When applicable, use the more specific Parental Role Conflict, Sexual Dysfunction, or Altered Family Processes. Carpenito

(1991) recommends considering role-performance disruptions as the etiology of other problems, such as Self-Concept Disturbance or High Risk for Impaired Home Maintenance Management.

SELF-CARE DEFICIT

Author's Note: This label describes a state in which a person experiences impaired ability to perform self-care activities. If the person is unable to perform any self-care activities, this is described as Total Self-Care Deficit. However the label is subdivided into more specific problems, each with its own critical defining characteristics which can exist in various combinations:

> Feeding Self-Care Deficit
> Bathing/Hygiene Self-Care Deficit
> Dressing/Grooming Self-Care Deficit
> Toileting Self-Care Deficit

Self-Care Deficits are frequently caused by Activity Intolerance, Impaired Physical Mobility, Pain, Anxiety, or Perceptual or Cognitive Impairment (e.g., Feeding Self-Care Deficit +2 r/t hyperactivity). As an etiology, Self-Care Deficit can cause Depression, Fear of becoming dependent, and Powerlessness (e.g., Fear of Becoming Totally Dependent r/t Total Self-Care Deficit +2 secondary to residual weakness from CVA).

In order to promote efforts to restore functioning, classify the patient's functional level using the following scale:

0 = Completely independent
1 = Requires use of equipment or device
2 = Requires help from another person, for assistance, supervision, or teaching
3 = Requires help from another person and equipment or device
4 = Dependent, does not participate in activity

This code adapted from E. Jones et al., *Patient Classification for Long-Term Care: Users' Manual,* HEW Publication No. HRA-74-3107, November 1974; as it appears in NANDA Taxonomy I — Revised, 1990.

☛ Related diagnostic labels: Activity Intolerance, Impaired Physical Mobility, Sensory-Perceptual Alterations, Altered Thought Processes. These are often etiologies of Self-Care Deficit.

SELF-CARE DEFICIT, BATHING/HYGIENE (SPECIFY LEVEL)

Definition: A state in which the individual experiences an impaired ability to perform or complete bathing/hygiene activities for self.

Defining Characteristics: Critical — Inability to wash body or body parts. *Other* — Inability to obtain or get to water source; inability to regulate temperature or flow.

Related Factors: Intolerance to activity, decreased strength and endurance; pain; discomfort; perceptual or cognitive impairment; neuromuscular impairment; musculoskeletal impairment; depression, severe anxiety.

Author's Note: Classify functional level (*see* Self-Care Deficit).

SELF-CARE DEFICIT, DRESSING/GROOMING (SPECIFY LEVEL)

Definition: A state in which the individual experiences an impaired ability to perform or complete dressing and grooming activities for self.

Defining Characteristics: Critical — Impaired ability to put on or take off necessary items of clothing. *Other* — Impaired ability to obtain or replace articles of clothing; impaired ability to fasten clothing; inability to maintain appearance at a satisfactory level.

Related Factors: Intolerance to activity, decreased strength and endurance; pain, discomfort; perceptual or cognitive impairment; neuromuscular impairment; musculoskeletal impairment; depression, severe anxiety.

Author's Note: Classify functional level (*see* Self-Care Deficit).

SELF-CARE DEFICIT, FEEDING (SPECIFY LEVEL)

Definition: A state in which the individual experiences an impaired ability to perform or complete feeding activities for self.

Defining Characteristics: Inability to bring food from a receptacle to the mouth.

Related Factors: Intolerance to activity, decreased strength and endurance; pain, discomfort; perceptual or cognitive impairment; depression, severe anxiety.

Author's Note: Classify functional level (*see* Self-Care Deficit).

SELF-CARE DEFICIT, TOILETING (SPECIFY LEVEL)

Definition: A state in which the individual experiences an impaired ability to perform or complete toileting activities for self.

Defining Characteristics: Critical — Unable to get to toilet or commode; unable to sit on or rise from toilet or commode; unable to manipulate clothing for toileting; unable to carry out proper toilet hygiene. *Other* — Unable to flush toilet or commode.

Related Factors: Impaired transfer ability; impaired mobility status; intolerance to activity, decreased strength and endurance; pain, discomfort; perceptual impairment; depression, severe anxiety.

Author's Note: Classify functional level (*see* Self-Care Deficit).

SELF-CARE DEFICIT, TOTAL

Author's Note: Use this label when patient has a self-care deficit in all areas: bathing/hygiene, dressing/grooming, feeding, and toileting. Specify level 0–4 (*see* Self-Care Deficit).

SELF-ESTEEM, CHRONIC LOW

Definition: Long-standing negative self-evaluation/feelings about self or own capabilities.

Defining Characteristics: *Major* — Self-negating verbalization; expressions of shame/guilt; evaluates self as unable to deal with events; rationalizes away/rejects positive feedback and exaggerates negative feedback about self; hesitant to try new things/situations. *Minor* — Frequent lack of success in work or other life events; overly conforming; dependent on others' opinions; lack of eye contact; nonassertive/passive; indecisive; excessively seeks reassurance.

☞ *See also* Situational Low Self-Esteem, Self-Esteem Disturbance, Hopelessness, Powerlessness.

SELF-ESTEEM DISTURBANCE

Definition: Negative self-evaluation/feelings about self or own capabilities, which may be directly or indirectly expressed.

Defining Characteristics: Self-negating verbalization; expressions of shame/guilt; evaluates self as unable to deal with events; rationalizes away/rejects positive feedback and exaggerates negative feedback about self; hesitant to try new things/situations; denial of problems obvious to others; projection of blame/responsibility for problems; rationalizing personal failures; hypersensitive to slight or criticism; grandiosity.

Author's Note: When you have adequate supporting clinical data, use the more specific labels, such as Chronic Low Self-Esteem.

☞ *See also* Body Image Disturbance, Personal Identity Disturbance, Chronic Low Self-Esteem, Situational Low Self-Esteem, Hopelessness, and Powerlessness.

SELF-ESTEEM, SITUATIONAL LOW

Definition: Negative self-evaluation/feelings about self which develop in response to a loss or change in an individual who previously had a positive self-evaluation.

Defining Characteristics: *Major* — Episodic occurrence of negative self-appraisal in response to life events in a person with previous positive self-evaluation; verbalization of negative feelings about the self (helplessness, uselessness). *Minor* — Self-negating verbalizations; expressions of shame/guilt; evaluates self as unable to handle situations/events; difficulty making decisions.

☞ *See also* Body Image Disturbance, Personal Identity Disturbance, Chronic Low Self-Esteem, Hopelessness, and Powerlessness.

SENSORY/PERCEPTUAL ALTERATIONS (SPECIFY): Auditory, Gustatory, Kinesthetic, Olfactory, Tactile, Visual

Definition: A state in which an individual experiences a change in the amount or patterning of incoming stimuli accompanied by a diminished, exaggerated, distorted, or impaired response to such stimuli.

Defining Characteristics: Disoriented in time, in place, or with persons; altered abstraction; altered conceptualization; change in problem-solving abilities; reported or measured change in sensory acuity; change in behavior pattern; anxiety; apathy; change in usual response to stimuli; indication of body-image alteration; restlessness; irritability; altered communication patterns. *Other Possible Characteristics* — Complaints of fatigue; alteration in posture; change in muscular tension; inappropriate responses; hallucinations.

Related Factors: Excessive or insufficient environmental stimuli; altered sensory reception, transmission and/or integration; chemical alterations: endogenous (electrolyte), exogenous (drugs, etc.); psychological stress.

Author's Note: This label may be more useful as the etiology of other problems. When High Risk for Sensory/Perceptual Alteration exists as a result of Immobility, consider using High Risk for Disuse syndrome.

When stated as a problem, the etiology is often a medical condition or pathophysiology that cannot be changed by nursing intervention. For Sensory-Perceptual Alteration (Auditory) r/t intracranial lesion, the nurse can do little to affect either the problem or the etiology. It would be better to diagnose something like Social Isolation r/t hearing loss. When possible, identify the client's specific response to the sensory-perceptual alteration.

> *Examples:* High Risk for Trauma (Burns) r/t **Tactile Alteration** A.M.B. numbness in fingers
>
> Self-Care Deficit (Total) r/t **Sensory-Perceptual Alteration** (Visual) A.M.B. ability to distinguish only light and dark.

☛ *See also* Altered Thought Processes and Unilateral Neglect.

SEXUAL DYSFUNCTION

Definition: The state in which an individual experiences a change in sexual function that is viewed as unsatisfying, unrewarding, or inadequate.

Defining Characteristics: Verbalization of problem; alterations in achieving perceived sex role; actual or perceived limitation imposed by disease and/or therapy; conflicts involving values; alteration in achieving sexual satisfaction; inability to achieve desired satisfaction; seeking confirmation of desirability; alteration in relationship with significant other; change of interest in self and others.

Related Factors: Biopsychosocial alteration of sexuality: ineffectual or absent role models; physical abuse; psychosocial abuse (e.g., harmful relationships); vulnerability; values conflict; lack of privacy; lack of significant other; altered body structure or function (pregnancy, recent childbirth, drugs, surgery, anomalies, disease process, trauma, radiation); misinformation or lack of knowledge.

Author's Note: If client data does not fit defining characteristics, consider the more general label, Altered Sexuality Patterns.

SEXUALITY PATTERNS, ALTERED

Definition: The state in which an individual expresses concern regarding his/her sexuality.

Defining Characteristics: *Major* — Reported difficulties, limitations, or changes in sexual behaviors or activities.

Related Factors: Knowledge/skill deficit about alternative responses to health-related transitions, altered body function or structure, illness or medical; lack of privacy; lack of significant other; ineffective or absent role models; conflicts

with sexual orientation or variant preferences; fear of pregnancy or of acquiring a sexually transmitted disease; impaired relationship with a significant other.

☛ *See also* Sexual Dysfunction, a more specific label.

SITUATIONAL LOW SELF-ESTEEM

(*see* Self-Esteem, Situational Low)

SKIN INTEGRITY, IMPAIRED

Definition: A state in which the individual's skin is adversely altered.

Defining Characteristics: Disruption of skin surface; destruction of skin layers; invasion of body structures.

Related Factors: *External* (*environmental*) — Hyper- or hypothermia; chemical substance; mechanical factors (shearing forces, pressure, restraint); radiation; physical immobilization; humidity. *Internal* (*somatic*) — Medication; altered nutritional state (obesity, emaciation); altered metabolic state; altered circulation; altered sensation; altered pigmentation; skeletal prominence; developmental factors; immunological deficit; alterations in turgor (change in elasticity).

Author's Note: Impaired Skin Integrity is rather nonspecific, even though it is at the sixth level of the taxonomy. A disruption of the skin surface might be a surgical incision, abrasion, blisters, or decubitus ulcers — to name only a few. When this label is used, the type of disruption should be specified in the problem, not the etiology. Note in the following example that dermal ulcer is a specific *type* of impaired skin integrity, not a cause of impairment.

> *Example:*
>
> *Correct:* Impaired Skin Integrity: **dermal ulcer** r/t complete immobility
>
> *Incorrect:* Impaired Skin Integrity r/t **dermal ulcer**

When an ulcer is deeper than the epidermis, use Impaired Tissue Integrity instead of Impaired Skin Integrity. Deeper ulcers may require a collaborative approach (e.g., surgical treatment).

Do not use Impaired Skin Integrity as a label for a surgical incision, since there are no independent nursing actions to treat this condition, and the condition is usually self-limiting. The usual nursing care for a surgical incision is to prevent and detect infection; therefore, a diagnosis of High Risk for Infection of Surgical Incision might be used instead of Impaired Skin Integrity. (Recall, also, that high-risk problems should be diagnosed only when the client is at higher risk than the general population; thus, even High Risk for Infection should not be used routinely for all surgery patients.)

SKIN INTEGRITY, HIGH RISK FOR IMPAIRED

Definition: A state in which the individual's skin is at risk of being adversely altered.

Defining Characteristics: *External (environmental)* — Hyper- or hypothermia; chemical substance; mechanical factors (shearing forces, pressure, restraint); radiation; physical immobilization; excretions; humidity. *Internal (somatic)* — Medication; altered nutritional state (obesity, emaciation); altered metabolic state; altered circulation; altered sensation; altered pigmentation; skeletal prominence; developmental factors; immunological deficit; alterations in turgor (change in elasticity).

Author's Note: This label should be used for clients who have no symptoms, but who are at risk of developing disruption of skin surface or destruction of skin layers. The presence of more than one risk factor increases the likelihood of skin damage. When High Risk for Impaired Skin Integrity occurs as a result of Immobility, and when other body systems are also at risk for impairment, Carpenito (1991) recommends using High Risk for Disuse Syndrome.

SLEEP-PATTERN DISTURBANCE

Definition: Disruption of sleep time causes discomfort or interferes with desired life-style.

Defining Characteristics: Critical — Verbal complaints of difficulty falling asleep; awakening earlier or later than desired; interrupted sleep; verbal complaints of not feeling well-rested. *Other* — Changes in behavior and performance (increasing irritability, restlessness, disorientation, lethargy, listlessness); physical signs (mild fleeting nystagmus, slight hand tremor, ptosis of eyelid, expressionless face, dark circles under eyes, frequent yawning, changes in posture); thick speech with mispronunciation and incorrect words.

Related Factors: Sensory alterations — internal (illness, psychological stress); external (environmental changes, social cues).

Author's Note: This label is used when disruption of sleep causes discomfort or interferes with the client's desired life-style. Do not confuse it with Fatigue.

Sleep-Pattern Disturbance is a rather general label. The etiological factors can sometimes make it specific enough to direct nursing intervention, as in *Sleep Pattern Disturbance related to frequent awakening of infant during the*

night. When possible, the specific type of Sleep Pattern Disturbance should be identified in order to better direct care.

> ***Examples:*** Sleep Pattern Disturbance (**Early Awakening**) r/t depression
>
> Sleep Pattern Disturbance (**Delayed Onset of Sleep**) r/t overstimulation prior to bedtime.

☛ *See also* Fatigue and Activity Intolerance.

SOCIAL INTERACTION, IMPAIRED

Definition: The state in which an individual participates in an insufficient or excessive quantity or ineffective quality of social exchange.

Defining Characteristics: *Major* — Verbalized or observed discomfort in social situations; verbalized or observed inability to receive or communicate a satisfying sense of belonging, caring, interest, or shared history; observed use of unsuccessful social interaction behaviors; dysfunctional interaction with peers, family and/or others. *Minor* — Family report of change of style or pattern of interaction.

Related Factors: Knowledge/skill deficit about ways to enhance mutuality; communication barriers; self-concept disturbance; absence of available significant others or peers; limited physical mobility; therapeutic isolation; sociocultural dissonance; environmental barriers; altered thought processes.

☛ *See also* Altered Thought Processes, Impaired Communication, and Social Isolation.

SOCIAL ISOLATION

Definition: Aloneness experienced by the individual and perceived as imposed by others and as a negative or threatened state.

Defining Characteristics: Critical — Absence of supportive significant other(s) (family, friends, group); expresses feelings of aloneness imposed by others; expresses feelings of rejection. *Other* — Sad, dull affect; inappropriate or immature interests/activities for developmental age/stage; uncommunicative, withdrawn, no eye contact; preoccupation with own thoughts; repetitive meaningless actions; projects hostility in voice, behavior; seeks to be alone, or exists in a subculture; evidence of physical/mental handicap or altered state of wellness; shows behavior unaccepted by dominant cultural group; experiences feelings of difference from others; inadequacy in or absence of significant purpose in life; inability to meet expectations of others; insecurity in public; expresses values acceptable to the subculture but unacceptable to the dominant cultural group; expresses interests inappropriate to the developmental age/stage.

Related Factors: Factors contributing to the absence of satisfying personal relationships, such as delay in accomplishing developmental tasks; immature interests; alterations in physical appearance; alterations in mental status; unaccepted social behavior; unaccepted social values; altered state of wellness; inadequate personal resources; inability to engage in satisfying personal relationships.

☛ *See also* Altered Thought Processes, Impaired Communication, and Impaired Social Interaction.

SPIRITUAL DISTRESS (DISTRESS OF THE HUMAN SPIRIT)

Definition: Disruption in the life principle which pervades a person's entire being and which integrates and transcends one's biological and psychosocial nature.

Defining Characteristics: Critical — Expresses concern with meaning of life/death and/or belief systems. *Other* — anger toward God; questions meaning of suffering; verbalizes inner conflict about beliefs; verbalizes concern about relationship with deity; questions meaning of own existence; unable to participate in usual religious practices; seeks spiritual assistance; questions moral/ethical implications of therapeutic regimen; gallows humor; displacement of anger toward religious representatives; description of nightmares/sleep disturbances; alteration in behavior/mood evidenced by anger, crying, withdrawal, preoccupation, anxiety, hostility, apathy, and so forth.

Related Factors: Separation from religious/cultural ties; challenged belief and value system (e.g., due to moral/ethical implications of therapy or intense suffering).

STRESS INCONTINENCE

(*see* Incontinence, Stress)

SUFFOCATION, HIGH RISK FOR

Definition: Accentuated risk of accidental suffocation (inadequate air available for inhalation).

Defining Characteristics: Presence of risk factors such as the following. *Internal (individual)* — Reduced olfactory sensation; reduced motor abilities; lack of safety education; lack of safety precautions; cognitive or emotional difficulties; disease or injury process. *External (environmental)* — Pillow placed in an infant's crib; propped bottle placed in an infant's crib; vehicle warming in closed garage; children playing with plastic bags or inserting small objects into their mouths or noses; discarded or unused refrigerators or freezers without removed doors; children left unattended in bathtubs or pools; household gas leaks; smoking in bed; use of fuel-burning heaters not vented to outside; low-strung clothesline; pacifier hung around infant's head; person who eats large mouthfuls of food.

Related Factors: *See* risk factors above.

Author's Note: Use the most specific label that matches the client's defining characteristics.

☛ *See also* Impaired Home Maintenance Management, High Risk for Injury, and High Risk for Trauma.

SWALLOWING, IMPAIRED

Definition: The state in which an individual has decreased ability to voluntarily pass fluids and/or solids from the mouth to the stomach.

Defining Characteristics: *Major* — Observed evidence of difficulty in swallowing (e.g., stasis of food in oral cavity, coughing/choking). *Minor* — Evidence of aspiration.

Related Factors: Neuromuscular impairment (e.g., decreased or absent gag reflex, decreased strength or excursion of muscles involved in mastication, perceptual impairment, facial paralysis); mechanical obstruction (e.g., edema, tracheostomy tube, tumor); fatigue; limited awareness; reddened, irritated oropharyngeal cavity.

☛ *See also* High Risk for Aspiration.

TEMPERATURE, BODY, HIGH RISK FOR ALTERED

(*see* Body Temperature . . .)

THERMOREGULATION, INEFFECTIVE

Definition: The state in which the individual's temperature fluctuates between hypothermia and hyperthermia.

Defining Characteristics: *Major* — Fluctuations in body temperature above or below the normal range. See also major and minor characteristics present in hypothermia and hyperthermia.

Related Factors: Trauma or illness; immaturity; aging; fluctuating environmental temperature.

Author's Note: This label is most appropriate for those who are especially vulnerable to environmental conditions (i.e., newborns and the elderly).

☞ *See also* High Risk for Altered Body Temperature, Hyperthermia, and Hypothermia.

THOUGHT PROCESSES, ALTERED

Definition: A state in which an individual experiences a disruption in cognitive operations and activities.

Defining Characteristics: Inaccurate interpretation of environment; cognitive dissonance; distractibility; memory deficit/problems; egocentricity; hyper- or hypovigilance. *Other Possible Characteristics:* Inappropriate non-reality-based thinking.

Related Factors: To be developed.

Author's Note: May be the etiology of other problems, such as Self-Care Deficit, Impaired Home Maintenance Management, or Impaired Social Interaction.

☞ *See also* Sensory/Perceptual Alterations.

TISSUE INTEGRITY, IMPAIRED

Definition: A state in which an individual experiences damage to mucous membrane, corneal, integumentary, or subcutaneous tissue.

Defining Characteristics: *Major*— Damaged or destroyed tissue (cornea, mucous membrane, integumentary, or subcutaneous).

Related Factors: Altered circulation; nutritional deficit/excess; fluid deficit/excess; knowledge deficit; impaired physical mobility; irritants, chemical (including body excretions, secretions, medications); thermal (temperature extremes); mechanical (pressure, shear, friction); radiation (including therapeutic radiation).

Author's Note: If tissue integrity is at risk because of immobility, and if other systems are also at risk, consider using High Risk for Disuse Syndrome.

☞ *See also* Altered Oral Mucous Membrane and Impaired Skin Integrity.

TISSUE PERFUSION, ALTERED (SPECIFY):
Cardiopulmonary, Cerebral, Gastrointestinal, Peripheral, Renal.

Definition: The state in which an individual experiences a decrease in nutrition and oxygenation at the cellular level due to a deficit in capillary blood supply.

Defining Characteristics:

A. Chances that characteristics will be present in given diagnosis.

B. Estimated sensitivities and specificities. Chances that characteristic will not be explained by any other diagnosis.

	A.	B.
Skin temperature: cold extremities	High	Low
Skin color, dependent: blue or purple	Moderate	Low
(**Critical**) Pale on elevation; color does not return on lowering of leg	High	High
(**Critical**) Diminished arterial pulsations	High	High
Skin quality: shining	High	Low
Lack of lanugo	High	Moderate
Round scars covered with atrophied skin; gangrene	Low	High
Slow-growing, dry, brittle nails	High	Moderate
Claudication	Moderate	High
Blood-pressure changes in extremities; bruits	Moderate	Moderate
Slow healing of lesions	High	Low

Related Factors: Interruption of flow, arterial; interruption of flow, venous; exchange problems; hypovolemia; hypervolemia.

Author's Note: Further work and development are required for the subcomponents, specifically cerebral, renal, and gastrointestinal. Unlike Altered Peripheral Tissue Perfusion, the qualifying labels Renal, Cerebral, Cardiopulmonary, and Gastrointestinal require medical intervention to improve tissue perfusion; they are useful primarily as etiologies for other problems. Even if potential rather than actual, these conditions usually represent collaborative problems. Nursing care should focus on interventions for specific *responses* to impaired perfusion, such as the following:

Altered Thought Processes r/t decreased cerebral tissue perfusion

Activity Intolerance r/t decreased cardiopulmonary tissue perfusion

Fluid Volume Excess r/t decreased renal tissue perfusion.

Altered *Peripheral* Tissue Perfusion is the only one of these labels that can be treated by independent nursing interventions. For that label, it is important to determine whether the altered tissue perfusion is venous or arterial.

☞ *See also* High Risk for Injury and High Risk for Disuse Syndrome.

TOILETING SELF-CARE DEFICIT
(see Self-Care Deficit, Toileting)

TOTAL INCONTINENCE
(see Incontinence, Total)

TRAUMA, HIGH RISK FOR

Definition: Accentuated risk of accidental tissue injury (e.g., wound, burn, fracture).

Defining Characteristics: Presence of risk factors such as the following. *Internal (individual)* — Weakness; poor vision; balancing difficulties, reduced temperature and/or tactile sensation; reduced large or small muscle coordination; reduced hand-eye coordination; lack of safety education; lack of safety precautions; insufficient finances to purchase safety equipment or effect repairs; cognitive or emotional difficulties; history of previous trauma. *External (environmental)* — Slippery floors (e.g., wet or highly waxed); snow or ice collected on stairs, walkways; unanchored rugs; bathtub without hand grip or antislip equipment; use of unsteady ladders or chairs; entering unlighted rooms; unsturdy or absent stair rails; unanchored electric wires; litter or liquid spills on floors or stairways; high beds; children playing without gates at the top of the stairs; obstructed passageways; unsafe window protection in homes with young children; inappropriate call-for-aid mechanisms for bed-resting client; pot handles facing toward front of stove; bathing in very hot water (e.g., unsupervised bathing of young children); potential igniting gas leaks; delayed lighting of gas burner or oven; experimenting with chemicals or gasoline; unscreened fires or heaters; wearing plastic apron or flowing clothes around open flame; children playing with matches, candles, cigarettes; inadequately stored combustible or corrosives (e.g., matches, oily rags, lye); highly flammable children's toys or clothing; overloaded fuse boxes; contact with rapidly moving machinery, industrial belts, or pulleys; sliding on coarse bed linen or struggling within bed restraints; faulty electrical plugs, frayed wires, or defective appliances; contact with acids or alkalis; playing with fireworks or gunpowder; contact with intense cold; overexposure to sun, sun lamps, radiotherapy; use of cracked dishware or glasses; knives stored uncovered; guns or ammunition stored unlocked; large icicles hanging from the roof; exposure to dangerous machinery; children playing with sharp-edged toys; high-crime neighborhood and vulnerable clients; driving a mechanically unsafe vehicle; driving after partaking of alcoholic beverages or drugs; driving at excessive speeds; driving without necessary visual aids; children riding in the front seat in car; smoking in bed or near oxygen; overloaded electrical outlets; grease waste collected on stoves; use of thin or worn potholders; misuse of necessary headgear for motorized cyclists; young children carried on adult bicycles; unsafe road or road-crossing conditions; play or work near vehicle pathways (e.g., driveways, laneways, railroad tracks); nonuse or misuse of seat restraints.

Related Factors: *See* risk factors above.

☛ *See also* High Risk for Injury, High Risk for Aspiration, High Risk for Poisoning, High Risk for Suffocation, and Impaired Home Maintenance Management.

UNILATERAL NEGLECT

Definition: A state in which an individual is perceptually unaware of and inattentive to one side of the body.

Defining Characteristics: *Major* — Consistent inattention to stimuli on an affected side. *Minor* — Inadequate self-care; positioning and/or safety precautions in regard to the affected side; does not look toward affected side; leaves food on plate on the affected side.

Related Factors: Effects of disturbed perceptual abilities (e.g., hemianopsia; one-sided blindness); neurologic illness or trauma.

☛ *See also* Self-Care Deficit and Sensory/Perceptual Alterations.

URGE INCONTINENCE
(see Incontinence, Urge)

URINARY ELIMINATION, ALTERED PATTERNS OF

Definition: The state in which the individual experiences a disturbance in urine elimination.

Defining Characteristics: Dysuria; frequency; hesitancy; incontinence; nocturia; retention; urgency.

Related Factors: Multiple causality, including anatomical obstruction, sensory motor impairment, urinary tract infection.

Author's Note: Use a more specific label when possible.

☛ *See also* Urinary Incontinence (Functional, Reflex, Stress, Total, and Urge) and Urinary Retention.

URINARY INCONTINENCE, FUNCTIONAL
(see Incontinence, Functional Urinary)

URINARY INCONTINENCE, REFLEX

(*see* Incontinence, Reflex Urinary)

URINARY INCONTINENCE, STRESS

(*see* Incontinence, Stress Urinary)

URINARY INCONTINENCE, TOTAL

(*see* Incontinence, Total Urinary)

URINARY INCONTINENCE, URGE

(*see* Incontinence, Urge Urinary)

URINARY RETENTION

Definition: The state in which the individual experiences incomplete emptying of the bladder.

Defining Characteristics: *Major*— Bladder distention; small, frequent voiding or absence of urine output. *Minor*— Sensation of bladder fullness; dribbling; residual urine; dysuria; overflow incontinence.

Related Factors: High urethral pressure caused by weak detrusor; inhibition of reflex arc; strong sphincter; blockage.

Author's Note: Do not use for temporary conditions (e.g., post-delivery) for which the only treatment is catheterization.

☞ *See also* Altered Patterns of Urinary Elimination.

VERBAL COMMUNICATION, IMPAIRED

(*see* Communication, Impaired Verbal)

VIOLENCE, HIGH RISK FOR: SELF-DIRECTED OR DIRECTED AT OTHERS

Definition: A state in which an individual experiences behaviors that can be physically harmful either to the self or others.

Defining Characteristics: Presence of risk factors such as body language (e.g., clenched fists, tense facial expression, rigid posture, tautness indicating effort to control); hostile threatening verbalizations (e.g., boasting to or prior abuse of others); increased motor activity (e.g., pacing, excitement, irritability, agitation); overt and aggressive acts (e.g., goal-directed destruction of objects in environment); possession of destructive means (e.g., gun, knife, or other weapon); rage; self-destructive behavior, active aggressive suicidal acts; suspicion of others, paranoid ideation, delusions, hallucinations; substance abuse/withdrawal. *Other Possible Characteristics:* Increasing anxiety levels; fear of self or others; inability to verbalize feelings; repetition of verbalizations (continued complaints, requests, or demands); anger; provocative behavior (e.g., argumentative, dissatisfied, overreactive, hypersensitive); vulnerable self-esteem; depression (specifically active, aggressive, suicidal acts).

Related Factors: Antisocial character; battered women; catatonic excitement; child abuse; manic excitement; organic brain syndrome; panic states; rage reactions; suicidal behavior; temporal lobe epilepsy; toxic reactions to medications.

REFERENCES

Carpenito, L. J. (1991). *Handbook of Nursing Diagnosis*, 4th ed. Philadelphia: J. B. Lippincott.

Geissler, E. (1991). Transcultural nursing and nursing diagnoses. *Nursing and Health Care, 12*(4): 190–92, 203.

Gordon, M. (1985). Practice based data set for a nursing information system. *Journal of Medical Systems, 9*: 43–55.

Gordon, M. (1987). *Nursing Diagnosis: Process and Application.* 2nd ed. New York: McGraw-Hill.

Janken, J. and Cullinan, C. (1991). Validation of the nursing diagnosis sensory/perceptual alteration: Auditory. In Carrol-Johnson, R., ed., *Classification of Nursing Diagnoses: Proceedings of the Ninth Conference*. North American Nursing Diagnosis Association. Philadelphia: J. B. Lippincott.

Lambert, M., and Jones, P. (1989). Nursing diagnoses recorded in nursing situations encountered in a Department of Public Health. In Carroll-Johnson, R., ed., *Classification of Nursing Diagnoses: Proceedings of the Eighth Conference*. North American Nursing Diagnosis Association. Philadelphia: J. B. Lippincott, 364–67.

Rakel, B., and Bulechek, G. (1990). Development of alterations in learning: Situational learning disabilities. *Nursing Diagnosis, 1*(4): 134–145.

Taylor, et al. (1989). *Fundamentals of Nursing.* Philadelphia: J. B. Lippincott.

ANSWER KEY for "Applying the Nursing Process"

CHAPTER 1   (pp. 16–19)

1. The appropriate phenomena of concern for the nurse are that Mr. Callaway
   a.   smokes two packs of cigarettes a day.
   b.   coughs a lot.
   c.   becomes short of breath when climbing stairs.
   Lesions on his lungs are clearly a medical concern. Biopsy, too, is most directly a medical concern. Nursing would deal with any fears, anxieties, or knowledge deficits, and so forth that Mr. Callaway had about the biopsy or the lesions.

2. The most important purpose of the nursing process is to improve the quality of patient care.

3.   1—c   4—d   7—d
        2—a   5—d   8—e
        3—c   6—a   9—b

4. The case illustrates that the nursing process is dynamic/cyclic and goal-directed. The nursing process has all the other qualities listed, but they are not clearly demonstrated by the example given in this case.

5.   a.   Interpersonal skills
        b.   Technical skills
        c.   Intellectual skills
        d.   Creativity and curiosity
        e.   Adaptability

6a.
   I—settled her comfortably in bed
   A—interviewed her
   A—obtained a temperature
   A—examined Ms. Boiko's chart
   I —applied oxygen
   A—performed the physical examination
   D—wrote a diagnosis

   P—set a goal
   P—wrote nursing orders for skin care
   I—bathed Ms. Boiko
   E—observed that her coccygeal area was still red (This could also be A for ongoing assessment.)
   E—concluded the goal had not been met
   E—decided to change the care plan

6b. The client data is as follows: Temp 101°, pulse 120, resp. 32, B/P 100/68, reddened area over coccyx, unable to move about in bed, coccyx still red, a small area of skin was peeling off, there was some serous drainage. (Juan also obtained data that Ms. Boiko had been turned every 2 hours except for 6 hours each night. This is data about care that was given to Ms. Boiko, but it is not data about human responses.)

6c. You should have circled the following as examples of reexamination of the nursing process steps:
   • *Juan concluded that the goal had not been met.* This shows that he went back and examined his original goal.
   • *He was sure his data was adequate and that his nursing diagnosis was accurate.* This demonstrates reexamination of the data base and the original nursing diagnosis.
   • *When asked, the other staff members assured Juan that the 2-hour turning schedule had been carried out.* This shows that Juan checked to see if the nursing orders were correctly implemented.
   • *He decided to change the order on the care plan.* This shows revision of the care plan.

6d. The nursing orders are
   •   Orders for skin care
   •   A schedule for turning every 2 hours except at night
   •   Orders for frequent, continued observation
   •   An order to turn every 2 hours around the clock
   Because your information states that Juan was bathing Ms. Boiko, you may have assumed he wrote a nursing order for that; however, the case study does not say this, and you must use only the information provided. Juan did perform some other nursing actions, such as settling the client in bed; however we do not know that they were written as nursing orders. Don't confuse nursing interventions (carried out) with nursing orders (written down).

6e. This is the most obvious example of overlapping of steps: "Two days later, when bathing Ms. Boiko, Juan observed that her coccygeal area was still red, a small area of skin was peeling off, and there was some serous drainage." In this example, Juan is implementing (bathing) at the same time he is assessing or evaluating (observing her coccygeal area).
   You might also have chosen: "Juan Apodaca, RN, settled her comfortably in bed and briefly interviewed her about her symptoms." *Settling* is implementation, while *interviewed* is assessment. As written, it isn't 100% clear that these occurred at the same time; however, if you think they did, then this, too, is a case of overlapping steps.

6f. Juan demonstrated the nursing qualities of creativity and adaptability by not continuing to use the turning schedule that was the routine on his unit. He was not content to do what was usually done, but reasoned that in this case something more was needed.

6g. The answer is (3)—individualized care.
   (1)   Any turning schedule assures continuity of care over shifts and caregivers. The pertinent information in the question is that this is not just any schedule. It is a special schedule.
   (2)   See comment (1).
   (4)   Nothing about the schedule encourages client participation.

CHAPTER 2   (pp. 35–37)

1. *Nursing is an applied discipline. C **is correct**.* The nurse applied principles of nursing to the care of a particular patient.
   D may match, too. The nurse probably used principles to make the decisions, although the case doesn't say so. She might have based her decisions on what the other nurses had been doing, on habit, on some rules she was aware of, and on her emotions. This case doesn't clearly demonstrate application of principles.
   In *A*, the nurse is active, but the case doesn't mention application of principles. In *B*, the nurse is acquiring knowledge but not applying it.
   Nursing draws on knowledge from other subjects and fields. ***B** **is correct**.* The nurse is acquiring knowledge from other subjects and fields: psychology, pharmacology, and physiology.
   In *A*, it appears the nurse will need knowledge from other subjects, but the case doesn't point out which fields, nor that such knowledge is actually being used.

373

C would be correct if the knowledge clearly came from a field other than nursing (such as physics). This case clearly demonstrates the application of principles, but it isn't clear which field the principles came from.

In *D*, the nurse may have used knowledge from other fields to make the decisions, although the case doesn't say so. She might have based her decisions on what the other nurses had been doing, on habit, on some rules she was aware of, on her emotions, etc.

Nurses deal with change in stressful environments. A **is the best example** of change: the client stopped breathing, he has 3 IVs to keep track of, the nurse had to interrupt her care to go to a meeting, the schedule for neuro checks was changed, and the patient's medication was changed. All of these changes are stressful, as would be the workload of 15-minute neuro checks and 3 IVs.

B does not necessarily indicate change or stress. This nurse may not find all that reading stressful. *C* indicates neither change or stress. Perhaps this is the only patient the nurse has to care for, and he finds it relaxing to deal with immobile patients.

D demonstrates that the nurse made several decisions, probably based on some principles. You might interpret these as stressful, but the situation doesn't make that clear. Nothing is said about change in the example.

Nurses make frequent, varied, and important decisions in their work. D **is correct.** It demonstrates a series of decisions the nurse made.

C represents only one decision made by the nurse, not "frequent and varied" decisions.

In *A* and *B* the nurse made no decisions.

2. *Nurse C* demonstrated critical thinking.
3. *Nurse A* did not have an attitude of inquiry. She blindly accepted the night nurse's advice for therapy (authority) without any evidence that Mr. Stewart was truly hypoglycemic. The description of Mr. Stewart given by the night nurse could have indicated almost anything—not necessarily diabetes. Nurse A may also have failed to be reflective, jumping to the conclusion that Mr. Stewart was hypoglycemic. *Nurse B* made the same thinking errors as Nurse A—even more so, since she had no plans of her own to assess Mr. Stewart (as far as we can tell from the case). She did not look up diabetes in a text in order to make her own judgments about Mr. Stewart's symptoms. She appears to have no confidence in her ability to make judgments. *Nurse D* did not reflect before giving the orange juice. She accepted the night nurse's advice to give orange juice without any evidence that it was needed. She certainly jumped to the conclusion that Mr. Stewart had a hypoglycemic reaction when she initiated a care plan without even assessing the patient.

4. a. Creative   c. Critical
   b. Directed   d. Associative
5. a. E   c. S
   b. E   d. P

Actually, (*a*) and (*b*) might demonstrate practice wisdom. In the absence of ethical knowledge, the nurse in (*a*) might have said what she did because her nursing instructor told her this was the proper behavior, or because agency policies specify that patient data is confidential. The nurse in (*b*) might have heard another nurse say that families should not look at the charts; if her action is based on this, it is practice wisdom. If it is based upon her understanding of the principles of autonomy and confidentiality, it is ethical knowledge.

CHAPTER 3   (pp. 70–75)

1. These meet standards and should have check marks: *a* and *d.*
   a. Demonstrates that data collection is "systematic, accessible, communicated, and recorded."
   d. Demonstrates that data collection is "accessible, communicated, and recorded."
   These are incorrect: *b* and *c.*
   b. Data collection is not "continuous."
   c. Data collection is not "systematic."
2. a. C   d. I   f. C
   b. C   e. C   g. I
   c. I

3.

Subjective Data	Objective Data	Primary Source	Secondary Source
f, j, n, r	a, b, c, d, e, g, h, i, k, l, m, o, p, q	c, e, f, i, j, k, l, m, n, o, q, r	a, b, d, g, h, p

4. Either way is correct. If you chose to read the chart first, your reasons should include the following:
   a. It would give me at least some information about her, so I would feel more comfortable.
   b. It might help me to formulate my initial questions.
   c. It would prevent me from repeating examinations or topics that had already been covered.
   d. It would assure that I review the chart early in the data-collection process. I might forget to do it later.
   If you chose not to read the chart first, your reasons should probably be as follows:
   a. I prefer not to have any preconceived ideas or biases about her when I interview her. It would help me to be more objective.
   b. I might not have time to read the chart and still be sure of getting the interview and examination all finished in time for surgery.
5. a. The nurse who recorded the B/P on the chart used examination(*E*). The nurse reading the chart really used none of these; you could say she used observation, since she used her sense of sight to read the number on the chart.
   b. I   e. E   h. E
   c. O   f. O   i. I
   d. O   g. I
   j. E (Auscultation does use the sense of hearing, but it is a special examination skill that requires the use of a stethoscope to aid that sense.)
   k. I (In a sense, the nurse obtained the data by interview [I] from the anesthetist; the anesthetist used the sense of touch, or observation [O].)
6. *B,* because it is best to start with nonthreatening, less personal material, saving the more delicate subjects until the nurse-patient relationship is better established.
7. a. C   d. O   g. O   i. O
   b. O   e. O   h. C   j. O
   c. C   f. C
8. Some examples of questions the nurse might ask follow:
   a. *Closed questions:* "Is it sharp or dull?" "Is it continuous, or does it come and go?" "How long have you had it?" "Do you take any medication for it?"
   b. *Open-ended questions:* "Tell me more about it." "Would you describe it for me?" "Tell me about how it began."

9. a. To *prepare* for the interview you should do the following:
      (1) Form your goals for the interview.
      (2) Decide on a time to do it. You will need 15–20 minutes when you do not have treatments and other tasks to do for other patients. You will need to be sure the patient isn't scheduled to leave the unit for tests or treatments, that it isn't too close to mealtime, and so on.
      (3) Ask her family to leave.
      (4) Ask her if she needs anything for pain, and allow enough time for the medication to work if you give it.
      (5) Be sure she has water; ask if she needs to go to the bathroom.
      (6) Assess her emotional status/anxiety level.
      (7) Turn down TV; turn off phone.
      (8) Pull the curtain around the bed.
      (Note: You should not have listed "review her chart," because this had already been done.)
   b. To elicit from Ms. Contini *her* understanding of "Reason for Hospitalization," you might say, "Tell me why you are here," or "Why did you come to the hospital?" Since the chart tells you she is here for knee surgery, it is more open and honest to say something like, "I see you're having knee surgery. I'd like to hear what brought you to that decision."
   c. In a comprehensive assessment you should ask the questions about sexual functioning. You cannot assume she is celibate or uninterested in sex because she is too old, single, or in too much pain. In fact, if the patient does have a sexual partner, one of the nurse's roles is to help the patient adapt to diseases/disabilities in order to preserve sexual functioning. This might be important to this patient, if her arthritis pain is interfering with her sexual functioning.

10. The data that should be validated are as follows:
    Because subjective and objective data do not match: *a, b, f*
    The subjective information is not the same at both times: *d*
    You will want to repeat the earlier data to be sure the client was giving reliable data. If he tells you the same thing both times, and he seems lucid, it is probably valid: *e*
    The data in item *c* does *not* need to be validated. You would expect some staining of the fingers and teeth from a heavy smoker.

11. The judgments/conclusions you should draw a line through are: *c, e, f, h, k, l, m.*

12. a. Neither. This action contributes to the patient's autonomy. Both veracity and confidentiality can affect the patient's autonomy, but neither of those is involved in this instance.
    b. Veracity
    c. Veracity
    d. Confidentiality
    e. Both veracity and confidentiality: Confidentiality, because the nurse does not intend to keep the information confidential; veracity, because she is being honest with the client about what she intends to do with the information.

13. a. Role-relationship (because it is about her family), or Coping/stress-tolerance (because as her main concern, it causes stress)
    b. Nutritional-metabolic

   c. Cognitive-perceptual
   d. Sleep-rest
   e. Self-perception
   f. Health-perception/health-management
   g. Health-perception/health-management

CHAPTER 4   (pp. 111–116)

1. 1 *b*   2. *c*   3. *a*   4. *a*
2. a. False. Nurses can identify nursing diagnoses, collaborative, and other problems. They should not all be labeled as nursing diagnoses.
   b. True.
   c. True.
   d. False. Problem status can be actual, potential (high-risk), or possible.
   e. True.
   f. False. Describes human responses to stressors such as medical conditions.
   g. True.
3. You might discuss with her how nursing diagnosis can accomplish the following:
   a. Help her to individualize her patient care
   b. Actually make care planning easier for her instead of "more work"
   c. Improve her care by providing a focus for planning goals and interventions
   d. Help her define her job to patients and other health-care professionals
   e. Help in staffing, budgeting, and work load
   f. Improve communication between nurses
   g. Increase her autonomy and accountability
   h. Help her prepare for the time when patient records will be computerized

   (Nursing diagnosis is also important for nursing education and research, but these are less relevant reasons to the staff nurse, whose most immediate concern is in providing quality patient care.)

4. The patient problems are *c, e, h,* and *i.*
   a. Appendicitis is a medical diagnosis. (Recall that a medical diagnosis can be the cause of a patient problem.)
   b. Catheter obstruction might be the etiology for a problem of urinary retention or infection. It is a nursing problem.
   d. Asthma is a medical diagnosis.
   f. Bowel resection surgery is a treatment. It may be the source of several medical patient problems.
   g. NPO is a medical order. It may cause thirst, dry mouth, and various other human responses.
   j. Skin care is stated as a need. The problem might be High risk for Impaired Skin Integrity.
   k. Low white-blood-cell count is a lab test value. It might be the symptom of a problem.
   l. Lack of cooperation is a problem for the nurse, not necessarily for the patient.
   m. Contant need for attention is a problem for the nurse, not necessarily for the patient. The problem is whatever is causing the patient to need constant attention (a symptom).

5. Stressors
   A blood clot in her right thigh.
   Intravenous catheter.

Heparin drip. While this is a therapy for the blood clot, it is also a stressor in other ways because of its possible side effects.

Complete bedrest. (If you are not aware of the physiological and psychological effects of immobility, ask your instructor to recommend some reading, or look under "Hazards of Immobility" in a fundamentals of nursing book.)

Responses

Thigh was swollen and warm; also slightly red.
She rang for the nurse several times.
Asking to have her leg checked.
Requesting pain medication.
She was observed reading her Bible . . .
Twenty-four hours later, her clotting time returned to normal.

6.

Response	Level	Dimension
Thigh swollen	Organic	Physical
Thigh warm	Organic	Physical
Thigh red	Organic	Physical
Rang for nurse several times	Whole-person	Interpersonal; probably caused by a psychological response (e.g., anxiety, fear)
Requesting pain medication	Whole-person	Interpersonal
Observed reading her Bible	Whole-person	Spiritual
Clotting time returned to normal	Systemic	Physical

7.

For a client with a medical diagnosis of	Problem	r/t Etiology
Fractured femur	a. Acute Pain	r/t edema and tissue trauma
	b. High risk for Impaired Skin Integrity: pressure sores or excoriation	r/t pressure from cast, immobility
Pneumonia	a. Ineffective Breathing Patterns	r/t obstructed airways and decreased chest excursion
	b. Activity Intolerance	r/t decreased oxygenation secondary to ineffective breathing patterns

8. a. *c*   c. *c*   e. *n*   g. *c*
     b. *n*   d. *c*   f. *c*   h. *n*

9. a. A (Actual pain)
     b. Pot (High Risk for Injury: falls)
     c. Pot   g. Pos
     d. Pot   h. Pot
     e. Pos   i. A
     f. A   j. Pos

k. A (She has signs and symptoms of pain.)
l. Pot (Her medical diagnosis and the signs of inflammation lead you to think she will develop pain if it is not already present. You might choose *possible*, but she really has no symptoms of pain.)
m. Pos (Limping is a sign of pain, but not enough for positive diagnosis, as it could be caused by weakness or joint stiffness.)

10. The nursing diagnoses are *b, c, d* and *e*.
   a. This is a collaborative problem; the nurse cannot independently treat or prevent either arrhythmia or myocardial infarction.

In the nursing diagnoses, the parts you should have circled follow:
   b. Low Self-Esteem and Perceived Sexual Inadequacy.
   c. High Risk for Skin Breakdown.
   d. Perineal Rash and Excoriation, and perhaps Urinary Incontinence. Whether or not the nurse can intervene independently would depend upon the cause of the incontinence.
   e. Confusion and Disorientation.

11.

Cluster 1	NANDA Pattern in Which Problem Occurs?
B/P 190/100	**Choosing** or Knowing
Hasn't been taking B/P pills because "don't make me feel any better."	
Forgets to take B/P pills	

Cluster 2	
50 lb overweight	**Exchanging (Nutrition)** or Moving (Activity)
Eats fast food; snacks a lot	
Sedentary job	
No physical exercise	
Eats out for fun	

Cluster 3	
B/P 190/100	**Exchanging (Regulation or Cardiac)** or Exchanging (Nutrition), or Choosing, or Moving (Activity)
Hasn't been taking B/P pills regularly	
50 lb overweight	
Sedentary job	
No physical exercise	
Eats fast food; snacks a lot	

There seem to be three themes running through these cues: her failure to take pills, her obesity, and her hypertension. Because hypertension is a medical problem, the best way to handle it would be to use it as one of the cues in the "pills" and "obesity" group. Students often identify it as a problem, so it is included as a cue group (Cluster 3) here to show you how to deal with it if you have done that.

Step 1. In this step, determine which patterns seem to be involved. In Cluster 1 the cue *they don't make me feel any better* represents a lack of knowledge about the medication (Knowing)—antihypertensive medications usually don't improve the way a patient feels, since you can't feel high blood pressure. The cue *forgets* also represents Knowing. The cue *hasn't been taking B/P pills* represents the selection of alternatives (Choosing).

In Cluster 2, the cues *50 lb overweight, eats fast food, snacks a lot* and *eats out for fun* all relate to Exchanging (Nutrition). The cues *sedentary job* and *no physical exercise* relate to Moving (Activity).

In Cluster 3, some of the cues relate to Choosing, some to Moving, and some to Exchanging.

Step 2. In this step you must tentatively identify both the problem and the etiology to be able to determine in which pattern the problem resides (a preliminary to labeling the problem).

In Cluster 1 the problem is that she hasn't been taking the pills (Choosing). This is because she lacks knowledge about whether they are helping her and because she forgets (Knowing).

In Cluster 2 the best explanation is that she is overweight because she consumes too many calories and burns too few with exercise. The problem is obesity (Exchanging: Nutrition).

In Cluster 3 the best explanation is that she is hypertensive. The exact etiology of essential hypertension is unknown, but obesity, improper diet, lack of exercise, and failure to take her pills are all contributing factors. The problem is a medical one: hypertension (Exchanging). It is not clear whether you should use Exchanging (Regulation) or Exchanging (Cardiac), but most available information points to classifying this as an Exchanging (Cardiac) problem. You can see how to classify this problem now, but you would not include it on your care plan, since it is a medical problem. For nurses, hypertension is merely a cue to other nursing diagnoses.

12. *Cluster 1*
Using your own terms you might have written something like "Failure to follow regimen for taking blood-pressure medications related to lack of knowledge about effects of the medication and forgetting."

Using NANDA labels you would write, "Noncompliance (blood-pressure medications) related to knowledge deficit (therapeutic effects) and forgetfulness."

Cluster 2
In your own words you might write, "Obesity related to improper eating habits and lack of exercise."
Using NANDA labels:
"Altered Nutrition: More than Body Requirements, related to improper eating habits and lack of exercise."

Cluster 3 is a medical diagnosis, hypertension.

13. a. Your explanations might be something like the following:
The client has a pressure sore on his sacrum because the paralysis keeps him from moving about in bed, and because his age causes his tissues to be fragile.

The client has broken skin on his sacrum because
1. he is old.
2. he is immobile secondary to being paralyzed on his left side.

You might have said, "Unable to move about in bed because of paralysis," but this is an incomplete explanation because it does not mention the broken skin.

b. Possible explanations:
Larry may become dehydrated because
1. he is losing fluids from diarrhea and vomiting, and
2. he cannot take in fluids because of the vomiting.

Possible fluid deficit because of excess fluid loss and inadequate fluid intake.

Insufficient fluids in body because of diarrhea and vomiting.

You might have said: "Losing fluids because of vomiting and diarrhea," but that is an incomplete explanation because it addresses only fluid loss and does not consider insufficient fluid intake nor the possible results of excess loss and inadequate intake (fluid deficit).

14. a. (3). The nurse might be generalizing from past experience; stereotypes are often based on very limited experience with members of a group. However, you cannot draw that conclusion because there is no information to indicate that.
b. (2).
c. (4) and (5). It could also be premature data collection—Susan could have asked, "Why is that?" It is not stereotyping, because stereotypes are based on *lack* of experience with a group.
d. (6). Actually, this case does not fully demonstrate that a diagnostic error was made. We are inferring that because the nurse was immobilized, she missed important diagnoses.

CHAPTER 5 (pp. 153–160)

1. 1973
2. a. Definition
   b. Defining characteristics
   c. Risk factors
   d. Critical defining characteristics (You could also use *major* defining characteristics here.)
   e. Title or label
   f. Related factors
3. a. Label   d. Qualifying term
   b. Risk factors   e. Related factors
   c. Label
4. a. 2   d. 3
   b. 1   e. 5
   c. 4
5. The correctly written diagnoses are *a, d, e, g, h.*
   b—Both parts of the statement mean the same thing.
   c—Elevated temperature is a symptom, not a combination of cues.
   f—Problem needs more specific descriptor; nurse cannot alter the problem or the etiology.
   i—Problem needs more specific descriptor; etiology is legally questionable.
   j—Crying is a symptom, not a problem.
6. Risk factors: possibility of going blind, post-op NPO
   Related factors: progressive loss of vision, effects of surgery, recent loss of job
7. a. Nonadherance to Medication Regimen r/t lack of understanding of effects of the medication and forgetting to take it. (This is not a NANDA label. See Nursing Diagnosis Guide, Noncompliance.)
   b. Impaired Skin Integrity: pressure sore on coccyx r/t inability to move about in bed (or r/t immobility)
   c. Altered Nutrition: More Than Body Requirements r/t irregular schedule, emotional eating pattern, and insufficient exercise
   or
   Altered Nutrition: More Than Body Requirements r/t excess calorie intake and inadequate exercise

d. Potential Complication of Hysterectomy: Hemorrhage
e. High Risk for Infection Transmission r/t communicable nature of the disease
or
Possible Self-Esteem Disturbance r/t social implications of the disease
or
High Risk for Altered Sexuality Patterns r/t pain, infectious nature of the disease, and implications for relationships

8. Altered Nutrition: More Than Body Requirements
Diarrhea   Constipation
High Risk for Infection   Altered Protection
High Risk for Aspiration   Activity Intolerance
Social Isolation

9. *a, c, d, e*

10. *Examples:*
a—Activity Intolerance **(Level II)**
c—Sensory-Perceptual Alteration **(Visual)**
d—**Moderate** Chronic **Back** Pain
e—Impaired Physical Mobility **(inability to sit up)**

11. a. Bowel Incontinence
    b. Diarrhea
    c. Ineffective Individual Coping
    d. High Risk for Aspiration
    e. Ineffective Airway Clearance

12. 1. *a*   4. *b*
    2. *c*   5. *e*
    3. *d*   6. *f*

13. a. Ineffective Denial
    b. Dressing/Grooming Self-Care Deficit +2
    c. Unilateral Neglect
    d. Stress Incontinence
    e. Urge Incontinence
    f. Altered Tissue Perfusion (Peripheral)
    g. High Risk for Fluid Volume Deficit
    h. Parental Role Conflict
    i. Decisional Conflict (whether to have an abortion)
    j. Activity Intolerance

14. Long-term stress
Loss of belief in God
Prolonged activity restriction creating isolation

15. a. Ms. Petrie
    b. Jill
    c. Mr. A.

16. a. Perceived Constipation r/t impaired thought processes A.M.B. overuse of laxatives and suppositories, and expectation of a daily bowel movement
    b. Colonic Constipation r/t unknown etiology
    c. Colonic Constipation r/t inadequate fluid and fiber intake and inadequate physical activity 2° weakness from chronic lung disease
    d. Ineffective Individual Coping r/t complex etiology A.M.B. verbalizing inability to cope and observed inability to problem-solve
    e. Potential Complication of IV Therapy: phlebitis, infiltration, infection
    f. Possible High Risk for Violence to Self, possibly r/t toxic reaction to medications
    g. Health-Seeking behaviors (exercise)

17. a. Low   c. High
    b. Low   d. Medium

e. High   g. Medium
f. Medium   h. Low

18. a. 4   e. 1
    b. 5   f. 3
    c. 1   g. 1
    d. 3

CHAPTER 6   (pp. 202–213)

1. The correct activities are *b, c, e, g, h, j.*
Activity *a* occurs in the assessment step; *d* occurs in the implementation step; *f* is data collection, and is usually considered a part of assessment, although it might be a part of evaluation; *i* is done in the diagnosis step.

2. a. Formal
    b. Informal
    c. Initial
    d. Ongoing
    e. Ongoing (definitely). This might be formal planning, but not all formal planning is done "as new information is obtained." Ongoing planning might include time-sequenced planning, and might also involve the client's discharge plan, but ongoing planning is the only kind that meets this definition under all conditions.
    f. Discharge. This defines discharge planning. Of course, it also includes formal planning; it could be done either as a part of the initial or ongoing plan.

3. You should have included four of the following:
    a. Gives direction for individualized care.
    b. Provides for continuity of care.
    c. Coordinates the client's care.
    d. Promotes efficient functioning of the nursing team.
    e. Directs documentation.
    f. Serves as a guide for staff assignments.
    g. Provides documentation for insurance reimbursement.
    h. Assures adequate discharge planning.

4. Client

5. The measurable goals are
Eats fruit at least   Rates pain as 3 on a 1–10
  3 times/day.   scale.
Skin warm and dry to   States less anxious than
  touch.   before exercise.
Temp. will be < 100.1°.   Will not have foul-smelling
States he feels more   lochia.
  confident.   Verbalizes understanding of
                                home-care instructions.

6. Some suggested opposite, normal responses are given below. You may have thought of others that are slightly different; they should be similar, however.
    b. Absence of redness or swelling at site. Skin intact. Wound edges intact if healing by primary intention. Granulation tissue present if healing by secondary and tertiary intention.
    c. Temperature at least 98.0° F. Skin warm, dry, and pink. No shivering.
    d. Able to dress self. Able to dress self without assistance.
    e. Mucous membranes pink, moist, without lesions (intact). No bleeding.

7. Examples of expected outcomes using the opposite responses in Exercise 6:

	Subject	Action Verb	Special Conditions	Performance Criteria
a.	(Client)	will have	(none)	regular, soft, formed B.M.
b.	Skin	will be	(none)	without redness or swelling at site.
	Skin	will be	(none)	intact.
	Wound edges	will be,	if healing by primary intention,	intact.
	Granulation tissue	will be,	if healing by secondary and tertiary intention,	present.
c.	Temp.	will be	(none)	at least 98.0°F.
	Skin	will be	(none)	warm, dry, and pink.
	(Client)	will not	(none)	shiver.
d.	(Client)	will dress	(unassisted)	self.
e.	Mucous membranes	will be	(none)	pink, moist, without lesions or bleeding.

8. *Back Pain r/t incision of recent spinal fusion and muscle stiffness from decreased mobility.*
Good predicted outcomes are individualized to fit the client. For instance, you would not say "VS—within normal limits," but would list the client's usual pulse, B/P, etc. Some ideas for outcome criteria follow:
  a. Experiences adequate pain relief, as evidenced by
   (1) Client will state pain is less than 3 on a 1–10 scale, within 20 minutes after receiving IM analgesic.
   (2) Will have no need for analgesics by day 7 postoperative.
   (3) After medication, will have no facial grimace or muscle tension; VS-WNL for client.
  b. Relief of muscle stiffness, as evidenced by
   (1) Client verbalizes he feels relaxed after being turned and repositioned.

9. Goals and nursing orders for High Risk for Impaired Skin Integrity (Pressure Ulcers) r/t long periods of lying in bed follow.

Goals/Predicted Outcomes	Nursing Orders
1. Maintain skin integrity, as evidenced by	1. Turn q2h around the clock.
a. No redness over bony prominences.	2. Assess skin over bony prominences with @ turning.
b. Skin intact, good turgor.	3. Encourage balanced diet, with protein and Vit. C.
	4. Use egg-crate mattress or foam-&-fatty-pad.
	5. Keep sheets taut and wrinkle-free; check bed @ turning for foreign objects.
	6. Don't use soap to bathe (skin is dry). Use lotion & light massage after bath.

10.
a. G	d. N	g. G	j. G
b. G	e. N	h. N	
c. N	f. G	i. N	

11. The action verbs are *apply, demonstrate, verbalize.*

12. Student care plans should be sure to include short-term goals. Students usually do not care for a client long enough to evaluate progress toward long-term goals. Short-term goals enable them to evaluate the results of the care they give the client. If appropriate, students should also write long-term goals so that other nurses can evaluate long-term progress after the student leaves.

13.
a.	P	e.	A
b.	C	f.	P
c.	A	g.	C
d.	C	h.	P

14. The correctly written goals are *b, c, f, i, m, n,* and *o.* Errors are as follows:

	Predicted Outcome	Errors (Guideline Violated)
a.	Client will develop adequate leg strength by 9/1.	*Develop* is not measurable; *adequate* is not observable/measurable. Should not write *client.*
b.	. . . VS-WNL, Hct and Hbg WNL.	"Within normal limits (WNL)" is not specific; but we do not know who the patient is so we cannot individualize the norms.
d.	Will feel better by morning.	*Feel better* is not specific, observable, or measurable.
e.	Improved appetite.	No verb; no special conditions or performance criteria; not observable/measurable.
g.	(On a 30-bed unit with only 2 wheelchairs) Will spend 4 hours each day in a wheelchair.	Not realistic.
h.	Client will discuss expectations of hospitalization and will relate the effects of a high carbohydrate diet on blood-sugar levels with a basic knowledge of exchange diet for diabetes.	Should not write *client.* Too long and complex. Derived from more than one diagnosis (one relates to expectations of hospitalization, and one to diet).
j.	Injects self with insulin.	No performance criteria (e.g.,using sterile technique).
k.	Will state adequate pain relief from analgesics and will take at least 100 cc of p.o. fluids per hour.	Derived from more than one nursing diagnosis (pain & fluids).
l.	IV will remain patent and run at 125 cc/hr.	A nursing goal, not a statement of desired client response.

15. Independent: *a, b, e, f, g, h, i, j, k, l, m*
Dependent: *c, d*
Observation: *h, i; f* might be considered an observation order, since it states specifically *how* the observation is to be made.
Treatment: Orders *a, b, e, g,* and *m* could be either treatment or prevention, depending on the problem (*m* is most likely health promotion).
c, d are treatment only.

Prevention: Orders *a, b, e, g,* and *m* could be either prevention or treatment (*m* is most likely health promotion).
Orders *j, k, l* are prevention only.
Order *f* is preventive in the sense that it would prevent injury to rectal mucosa.

Health promotion: Order *b* might be considered health promotion, if Ms. Adkins's grief work is progressing normally, and she has no problem in that area. It would more likely be used to treat the etiology of some problem.
Order *k* could be considered health promotion if done in a family of well clients.
Order *m* is really the only nursing order that is clearly for health promotion.

Physical care: *c, d, f, g, h, i, j,* possibly *e*
Teaching: *a, k, m*
Counseling: *b;* possibly *l* if persuasion or help with decision-making is needed.

Referral: *l*
Environment management: *e, g, j*

16. In order of priority: *b, e, c, a, d*
  *b. <u>Chronic Pain</u> r/t inflammation of knees 2° rheumatoid arthritis
  *e. <u>High Risk for Noncompliance with NPO Order</u> r/t lack of understanding of its importance for anesthesia
  *c. <u>High Risk for Sleep-Pattern Disturbance</u> r/t strange environment and possible anxiety regarding surgery
  a. <u>High Risk for Low Situational Self-esteem</u> r/t unresolved feelings about inability to bear children after hysterectomy
  d. <u>Altered Nutrition: More Than Body Requirements for Calories</u> r/t excess calorie intake from "emotional eating"

Rationale:
<u>Diagnosis *b*</u> has to take first priority. The pain will need to be under control in order to accomplish *e* (teaching about importance of NPO), since pain interferes with learning, and *c* (hypnotics-sedatives do not work effectively to produce sleep in the presence of pain).

<u>Diagnosis *e*</u> would be second because you would not want to teach about NPO after you had taken measures to promote sleep.

<u>Diagnosis *c*</u> is a physiological need, which ordinarily comes before an esteem need (*a*). It is also a more immediate need. The client does need to sleep tonight; the self-esteem problem is only a potential problem, and there will be time to assess for that later. However, if these feelings actually develop and interfere with sleep during the evening, the priority might be changed.

<u>Diagnosis *a*</u> would probably come before *d* because (1) it may be more amenable to short-term intervention by the nurse, and (2) poor self-esteem might make the pattern of "emotional" eating worse. Teaching could be done for *d* while the client is in the hospital, but the problem does not seem to be caused by a lack of knowledge, so about all the nurse could do for this problem is make referrals.

17. See underlined nursing diagnoses in #16 above.
18. Examples of goals and nursing orders for the three top-priority nursing diagnoses follow. You may think of others that would be appropriate. (To save space, orders are not dated or signed.)

19.

Nursing Diagnoses	Goals and Predicted Outcomes	Nursing Orders
b. Chronic Pain r/t inflammation of knees 2° rheumatoid arthritis	Will be able to carry out ADLs prior to surgery. Will state that pain is within acceptable limits prior to O.R., at all times.	1. Assess intensity of pain before & after meds. 2. Ask client what she usually does to manage/relieve pain. 3. Provide assistance with ADLs and ambulation prn 4. Obtain medical order for analgesics prn 5. WMP to knees, on 15 min., off 15 min. prn 6. Teach guided imagery or other pain-management techniques, day 2 post-op.
e. High Risk for Noncompliance with NPO order r/t lack of understanding of its importance for anesthesia	Will remain NPO after midnight. After teaching, will relate side effects of anesthesia to need for NPO.	1. Assess client's knowledge of anesthesia and side effects, 3–11 today. 2. Teach rationale for NPO before anesthesia (3–11 R.N.). 3. Remove water pitcher and glasses from room after midnight. 4. Put NPO sign above bed/note on Kardex (2400).
c. High Risk for Sleep-Pattern Disturbance r/t strange environment & possible anxiety regarding surgery	Will be asleep by midnight and remain asleep until 0600 (daily). Will state in A.M. that she slept well and feels rested (daily). Will express anxiety prn. No signs of anxiety, e.g., restlessness, withdrawal, autonomic NS responses, excessive verbalization.	1. Observe for any signs of anxiety (on @ pt. contact). 2. Note client's usual sleep routines and observe them as far as possible, nights, daily. 3. If anxious, help to recognize & express anxiety & identify source. 4. Backrub at H.S. daily. 5. After adequate pain-relief measures (see med. orders), Nembutal 100 mg. p.o. at H.S. 6. Leave bathroom light on at night.

19. a. (1) Potential Complications of Hysterectomy: Hemorrhage, urinary retention, thrombo-phlebitis, trauma to the ureter or bladder, incision infection. (Complications of anesthesia are not included. Potential Urinary Tract Infection would be included either as a nursing diagnosis or as a Potential Complication of Indwelling Catheter.) Recall that etiologies are used only on student collaborative problems.

(2) Potential Complications of Hysterectomy:
Hemorrhage r/t failure of hemostasis
Urinary retention r/t edema, nerve trauma or temporary atony
Thrombophlebitis r/t decreased activity and increased tendency of blood to clot 2° body defenses in response to surgery
Surgical trauma to the ureter or bladder
Incision infection r/t portal of entry for pathogens 2° break in first line of defense (intact skin)
Abd. discomfort & distention r/t handling of viscera, decreased peristalsis 2° anesthesia

(3)

Potential Complications of Hysterectomy:	Predicted outcomes
Hemorrhage	1. Pulse and BP within normal limits for patient, within 4 hours post-op. Will not deviate more than 20% from baseline at any time.
	2. Saturates less than 1 vag. pad q2h. Minimal amounts on day 2.
	3. Abd. dressing dry at all times.
Urinary retention	1. Voids within 8 hrs p̄ removal of cath. at least 100 cc.
	2. Bladder will not be palpable at any time.
	3. Voids adequate amounts based on intake.
	4. States she feels she is emptying her bladder after voiding.
Thrombo-phlebitis	1. States no tenderness or calf pain.
	2. No edema of lower extremities.
	3. No redness of legs or along veins.
	4. Homan's sign negative.
Trauma to the ureter or bladder	1. Urine will be yellow/amber. No blood in urine.
	2. States no back or flank pain.
Incision infection	1. Temp. < 100.1 at all times; 98.6 by dismissal.
	2. Incision free of redness or drainage, edges approximated.
Abdominal discomfort & distention	1. Abd. soft, not distended.
	2. States no abd. discomfort.
	3. Bowel sounds auscultated in all 4 quads. by 24 hr post-op.
	4. States passing flatus by 24 hr post-op.

19. b. Care Plan for Potential Complications of Intravenous Therapy.
(1) Signs and symptoms:
Inflammation: Localized diffuse redness of skin around insertion site; tender to touch; skin warm at area of redness. Possibly pus at insertion site.
Phlebitis: Hardness along vein, usually above insertion site; redness of vein and surrounding vein; warmth and tenderness at insertion site and along vein.
Infiltration: Swelling at site; painful to touch or to infusion of fluids; absence of blood return when bag lowered or tubing aspirated; skin around site hard, cold, pale; fluid not running well.

(2) Predicted outcomes and nursing orders for each complication:

Sign/Symptom	Predicted Outcomes	Nursing Orders
Inflammation	1. No redness, warmth or pus at insertion site. 2. States not tender. 3. Temp.< 100°	1. Inspect site q4h for signs of inflammation. 2. Wash hands before IV care. 3. Teach pt. to avoid touching site. 4. Do not leave bottle hanging for > 8 hr. 5. Change dressing & tubing q24h, on 3–11 shift. Use aseptic technique per agency procedure. 6. Do not disconnect tubing to change gown, etc. 7. If symptoms noted, DC IV and notify physician.
Phlebitis	1. No hardness, redness or warmth along or around vein and site. 2. States not tender. 3. Pulse and temp. WNL.	1. Inspect site q4h for signs of phlebitis. 2. Check for tenderness. 3. Pulse and temp. q8h. Retake in 1 hr if elevated. 4. If symptoms occur, remove IV, restart at new site, and notify physician.
Infiltration	1. Skin not cool, pale, hard or swollen at insertion site. 2. States not tender to touch. 3. No c/o pain on infusion of fluid or meds. 4. Infusing at prescribed rate.	1. Inspect site hourly for signs of infiltration. 2. Check rate hourly. 3. If symptoms present, remove IV and restart at new site. 4. Teach pt. to call for help if any discomfort, if container nearly empty, or if flow changes.

CHAPTER 7 (pp. 250–257)

1. **Dependent Nursing Actions**
   Definition: Any action that requires a medical order.
   Examples: (a) Give Nembutal 100 mg. p.o. at HS (per medical order); (b) Obtain physician's order for analgesic if needed to relieve arthritis pain.

   Independent Nursing Actions
   Definition: Any action that does not require a physician's order.
   Examples: (a) Offer client a backrub at HS. (b) Find out what time client usually goes to sleep. Offer milk or other protein at HS. (c) Do pre-op teaching and routines early so client will have time to relax before HS.

   Interdependent Nursing Actions
   Definition: Require collaboration with other health-care professionals, such as a dietitian, visiting nurse, or social worker.
   Examples: (a) Refer client to Social Services Dept. if necessary for home help. (b) Refer client to home health agency if needed. (c) Interview client further to determine if there is a friend or someone who will be available to help her at home.

2. Ms. Atwell's privacy and dignity may be threatened by the enema, most obviously. However, the nurse should also respect her privacy when she takes the pHisohex shower. Ms. Atwell may be embarrassed that she has difficulty walking. She may be uncomfortable talking about her hysterectomy or loss of childbearing ability. She will have her hip exposed for the pre-op injection.

3. a. A possible collaborative nursing action might be to refer Ms. Atwell to a home health agency or a visiting nurse agency. Another possibility might be to arrange for outpatient physical therapy.
   b. A possible independent nursing action might be to talk with Ms. Atwell about alternative ways to manage household chores, such as sitting down to iron or not ironing at all.

4. She should look up pHisohex in the Hospital Formulary or call the pharmacist to ask what it is. She might also read the unit procedures for preoperative preparations. She should not instruct Ms. Atwell to take the shower until she knows what it is expected to accomplish and if there are any potential problems it could cause.

5. To prepare Ms. Atwell for implementation of the medical order, first assess whether she still needs a sleeping pill. If she is asleep, do not wake her to give her the pill. If she does need it, tell her what it is and what it is expected to do for her. Explain how she can make it more effective (e.g., by turning off the lights and staying in bed).

6. Therapeutic communication that might be needed by Ms. Atwell:

   You might talk with her to help her identify and relieve anxiety. She states she is not anxious about surgery, but she might have other anxieties (loss of childbearing function, how she will manage at home). Communication could help you identify whether she is grieving over loss of childbearing ability. You would need to communicate to assess her understanding of the importance of NPO and to do preoperative teaching.

7. a. *Determine that the action is appropriate. Assess for readiness.* The turning is postponed because one need takes priority over another, not because the action would be less successful if performed at this time. You might also have chosen *respects client dignity*—the client might not like to have her visitor see her in pain.
   b. *Be sure you know the rationale for the intervention. Question any actions that you do not understand. Improve your knowledge base.*
   c. *Provide for privacy and comfort.*
   Perform interventions according to professional standards. (The ANA Code of Ethics requires that you maintain client dignity.)
   d. *Perform interventions according to professional standards of care and agency policies.* Most agencies have a policy that requires insulin dosage to be checked by two professional nurses. The nurse in this case does not lack knowledge of the intervention; she is simply guarding against error.
   e. *Perform interventions according to professional standards* (which include safety).
   f. *Determine that the action is still needed and appropriate.* The antihypertensive medication may not be needed if the client's blood pressure is now lower than normal.

8. a. S   c. C   e. P
   b. P   d. S   f. C

   Items *c* and *f* are peculiar to computer systems; *a, b, d,* or *e* might also be true of computer records, depending upon the type of program used.

9. *If nurse was unable to chart until 8 P.M.:*
   12/6/92, 8:00 P.M.
   D—Says his head hurts and light makes his eyes hurt. Eyes shut tightly.
   A—Cool cloth placed on head; door closed. Tylenol #3, tabs i, given p.o. at 6 P.M. (see medication record). Plan: Disturb as little as possible, keep room dark, notify Dr. King if headache unrelieved after second dose of Tylenol #3.
   R—At 7 P.M., stated head still hurts.————L. Nye, RN.

   Alternatively, if charting was done at 6 and 7 P.M.:
   12/6/92, 6:00 P.M.
   D—Says his head hurts and light makes his eyes hurt. Eyes shut tightly.————
   A—Cool cloth placed on head; door closed. Tylenol #3, tabs i, given p.o. (see medication record).—L. Nye, RN.
   12/6/92, 7:00 P.M.
   R—States head still hurts.————
   A—Disturb as little as possible, keep room dark, notify Dr. King if headache unrelieved after second dose of Tylenol #3.————————L. Nye, RN.
   (Did you remember to date, time, and sign your entry, and to draw lines through blank spaces?)

10. See Figure 7–10.

11. 12/9/92 #2—High Risk for Noncompliance with Pre- and
    2100   Post-op Instructions r/t lack of knowledge.
    S—States she understands preoperative teaching, including need for NPO.
    O—Preoperative teaching done. Explained NPO after 2400, including rationale.————
    A—No knowledge deficit regarding pre-op procedures.————
    P—Remove water pitcher at 2400 today.———— When awake, remind her not to drink or eat anything.————L. Nye, RN.
    (Did you remember to date, time, and sign your entry?)

DATE 1-6-92	2300-0700	0700-1500	1500-2300
SIGNATURE			*L. Nye R.N.*
EXERCISE/REST — Type of activity / How far? How long? / Repositioned / ROM / Aides (walker, cane, crutches, etc.) / Sleep	___Bedrest ___Reposition q 2 hrs ___BRP/BSC ___Chair/WC ___Walk ___Sleeping ___Check q hr ___Request SR down ___Tx____hrs Patient Response	___Bedrest ___Reposition q 2 hrs ___BRP/BSC ___Walk ___Up ad lib ___Tx ___hrs Patient Response	___Bedrest ___Reposition q 2 hrs ___BRP/BSC ___Walk _X_Up ad lib ___Tx ___ hrs Patient Response *Walks erect. Steady gait.*
NUTRITION/ FLUID/ELEC — N/V / Feeding assistance / Tube feedings	___No Problems identified ___Not assessed/sleeping ___NPO	___No Problems identified ___Feed ___Assist Feed ___NPO	_X_No Problems Identified ___Feed ___Assist Feed ___NPO
ELIMINATION — Stool: freq/char / Urine: freq/char / Bowel sounds / flatus, distention	___No Problems Identified ___Urine ___Abd. status ___Stool ___Incontinent	___No Problems Identified ___Urine ___Abd. status ___Stool ___Incontinent	___No Problems Identified ___Urine ___Abd. status _2100_Stool *S. S. enema, c̄ large unformed stool.* ___Incontinent
OXYGENATION — Breathing pattern / Breath sounds / Chest tubes / Sputum / O_2 / Tissue perfusion	___Eupneic ___Lungs clear to auscultation ___O_2 ___IS c assist ___Cough/sputum	___Eupneic ___Lungs clear to auscultation ___O_2 ___IS c assist ___Cough/sputum	_X_Eupneic _X_Lungs clear to auscultation ___O_2 ___IS c assist ___Cough/sputum
CIRCULATION — Pulse quality/presence / Heart sounds / Edema	___No problems identified ___Pedal pulses ___Cap Refill ___Numbness/tingling ___Edema ___TED Hose ___R/L toes/fingers pink/pale & warm/cool	___No problems identified ___Pedal pulses ___Cap refill ___Numbness/tingling ___Edema ___TED Hose ___R/L toes/fingers pink/pale & warm/cool	___No problems identified _ƚ_Pedal pulses *= bil.* ___Cap refill ___Numbness/tingling _X_Edema *+1, Ⓛ ankle* ___TED Hose ___R/L toes/fingers pink/pale & warm/cool
TEMP REGUL/ SKIN INTEGRITY — Skin assessment / Wound/incision / Rash / Heparin Lock Site	___Hep Lock ___Dressing/incision Normal ___Warm/dry ___Cast dry/intact ___Brace/splint ___Checked q 2 hr for fit/position	___Hep Lock ___Dressing/incision normal ___Warm/dry ___Cast dry/intact ___Brace/splint ___Checked q 2 hr for fit/position	___Hep Lock ___Dressing/incision Normal _X_Warm/dry ___Cast dry/intact ___Brace/splint ___Checked q 2 hr for fit/position

PATIENT DAILY ASSESSMENT SUMMARY FLOW SHEET

2 NORTH (PILOT)

Figure 7–10. Patient Daily Assessment Summary Flowsheet—Completed. Courtesy of Shawnee Mission Medical Center.

	DATE	2300-0700	0700-1500	1500-2300
	SIGNATURE			*L. Nye, R.N.*
SENSORY/ NEURO	Visual/hearing aid Communication aid Perceptual ability Pain Neuro assessment Level of conscious.	__Alert/oriented __No c/o pain __C/o pain (Location) __See MAR __Dorsi/Plantar flex __Indicates pain relief	__Alert/oriented __No c/o pain __C/o pain (Location) __See MAR __Dorsi/Plantar flex __Indicates pain relief	X Alert/oriented __No c/o pain X C/o pain *abd cramps* (Location) X See MAR __Dorsi/Plantar flex __Indicates pain relief
ENDOCRINE	Uterine/prostate status Menstrual/lactation Pregnancy Endocrine status	___NA ___No s/s hypo/hyper glycemia ___See Diabetic Record	___NA ___No s/s hypo/hyper glycemia ___See Diabetic Record	X NA ___No s/s hypo/hyper glycemia ___See Diabetic Record
SELF CONCEPT/ INTERDEPENDENCE	Emotional status Coping mechanisms Role of S.O.	__Cooperative __Freq call lite use/ demands __Safety assessment min/mod/intense Posey/wrist restraints __Pt/family emotional support (Mod/intense	__Cooperative __Freq. call lite use/ demands __Safety assessment min/mod/intense Posey/wrist restraints __Pt/family emotional support (mod/intense	X Cooperative __Freq call lite use/ demands __Safety assessment min/mod/intense Posey/wrist restraints __Pt/family emotional support (Mod/intense)
ROLE FUNCTION	Knowledge deficit Learning abilities Discharge planning Adaptive difficulty to new roles	___Nursing cares/ procedures explained ___Special teaching: ___Pt. indicates understanding	___Nursing cares/ procedures explained ___Special teaching: ___Pt. indicates understanding	X Nursing cares/ procedures explained X Special teaching: *pre-op. See Ns. Prog. notes* X Pt. indicates understanding

	TIME	NURSING PROGRESS NOTES
	1800	Sensori-Neuro- *Ibuprofen given for c/o abd cramping. (See MAR.)* *L. Nye, R.N.*
	1900	Sensori-Neuro- *States, "I feel better now."* Role Function- *Pre-op teaching done, including NPO at midnight & rationale for NPO.* *L. Nye, R.N.*

Figure 7–10. Concluded.

CHAPTER 8 (pp. 283–288)

1. The specific, measurable or observable criteria are *b*, *c*, and *d*.

   a. "Safe" is not measurable. "Side rails up" would demonstrate this.

   e. "Adequate number" is not measurable. "Three w/c on each unit" is measurable.

   f. "Systematic" is not measurable. "A complete abdominal assessment is recorded in the client's chart once per shift" is measurable.

2. 1. *b* and *c*

    2. *a* (The data would come from the manual in structure evaluation. In process evaluation, one might note whether a nurse is following procedures, but the data itself would come from one's observation of the nurse's activities.)

    3. *c* (possibly *b*—client might report whether nurse has done required teaching, etc.)

    4. *c*

    5. *b*

    6. *a*

    7. *b*

    8. *a*

3. 1. *c*   5. *a*

    2. *b*   6. *a* (possibly *b*)

    3. *a*   7. *a*

    4. *c*

4. a. Possible outcome criteria:

    Oral mucosa pink, moist, intact

    States no oral pain

    No inflammation or ulcerations in oral cavity

    Able to swallow without difficulty (when no longer NPO)

   b. Examples of methods for obtaining data for the criteria:

    Examine the patient's oral cavity.

    Ask the client if his mouth is sore.

    Examine the parient's oral cavity.

    Observe the client swallowing, or ask him if he is having any difficulty.

    (If you were performing a retrospective audit, you would look for this evidence in the chart—probably in the progress notes.

5. a. The following are examples; you may have thought of other cues. Verbal cues that would indicate achievement of the objective:

    Ms. Atwell states, "I'm confident everything will go all right. I certainly don't have any experience with this kind of thing, but I know you will tell me what I need to know. I feel pretty relaxed, actually."

   b. Nonverbal cues that would indicate achievement of the objective:

    Client shows no facial tension.

    Hands folded loosely in lap.

    Sitting quietly; no fidgeting.

   c. Verbal cues that would indicate the objective has not been achieved:

    "I'd really rather not talk about it now."

    "I'm still pretty scared."

   d. Nonverbal cues that would indicate the objective has not been achieved:

Moving restlessly in bed	Tearful; pale
Perspiring heavily	Facial muscles tense
Not making eye contact	Wringing hands
Voice is shaky, tremulous	Pulse elevated

6. *High Risk for Anxiety.* Goal met. Ct. verbalizes understanding of procedure and effects of surgery; exhibits no physical signs of anxiety. (Could also quote progress notes verbatim as evidence of goal achievement.)

High Risk for Grief. Goal partially met. Client expressed feelings of relief at no longer having menses, but avoided discussion of inability to bear children. Will need to follow up after surgery.

High Risk for Noncompliance with NPO. Goal partially met. Client verbalized reasons for NPO and verbalized intent to comply with restriction; however, she did drink some water at 0230, stating "I forgot."

7. *High Risk for Anxiety* . . . You could discontinue this entire section of the plan: nursing diagnosis, goals, and nursing orders. The problem has been resolved.

High Risk for Grief . . . This is still a potential problem. You should keep the diagnosis and goal.

High Risk for Noncompliance . . . Because the goals are only partially met, you need to keep the diagnoses. You should mark off the first goal, because she has already done this.

8. a. retrospective audit

   b. is not

   c. ongoing

   d. criterion

9. b. Even though the client does not have Actual Impaired Skin Integrity, High Risk for Impaired Skin Integrity still exists. If the nursing interventions are discontinued, the client will undoubtedly develop Impaired Skin Integrity.

CHAPTER 9 (pp. 328–333)

1.

Defining Characteristics	Nursing Diagnosis	Predicted Outcomes	Nursing Orders
Verbally denies he is ill. Observed out of bed in spite of medical order for bedrest. Refused to take his 3 P.M. meds.	Noncompliance (Medical Treatment Plan) r/t denial of illness.	Pt will adhere to activity limitations. Pt will acknowledge consequences of not complying with treatment regimen. Pt will agree to follow plans for care (eg., meds, bedrest).	Encourage to express feelings & concerns about being hospitalized. Give positive reinforcement for compliance (e.g., staying in bed, taking meds). Develop a written contract with pt regarding bedrest and meds. Evaluate pt's support system and need for emotional support from staff.

2. *Figure 9–12. Care Plan for Nikki Winters*

Guideline 1: Does not apply. This care plan is for client problems only and is not intended to address the client's medical plan of care nor his routine basic needs. It does, however include some client-profile information (name, admitting date, and diagnosis).

Guideline 2: Not met. Problems are dated but not signed.

Guideline 3: Met. The problems are numbered in order of priority.

Guideline 4: Probably met. The plan does not indicate that the nursing orders are listed in order of priority, but they appear to be.

Guideline 5: Met, for the most part. Plan occasionally fails to abbreviate (e.g., uses *secondary to* instead of *2°*).

Guideline 6: Met. Written legibly, typed (not in ink).

Guideline 7: Met. Refers to other sources for detailed treatments (e.g., IV therapy).

Guideline 8: Partially met. Considers physiological and psychological (self-esteem) needs. Does not address sociocultural or spiritual needs. However, Ms. Winters's data base does not indicate that she has any special needs in these areas.

Guideline 9: The problem list is individualized. There is not enough data about Ms. Winters to adequately individualize her nursing orders. For instance, we do not know what kinds of fluids and fiber-foods she likes to eat.

Guideline 10: Some collaborative aspects are included e.g., IV Therapy, Heparin administration). Lab tests, X ray, and so forth would probably be in another section.

Guideline 11: This plan does not show any discharge planning. However, it may be included in the Standards of Care for Abdominal Hysterectomy or the Nursing Care Plan for Thrombophlebitis.

3. The care plan for Harvey Cain appears in Figures 9–17 and 9–18.

PATIENT CARDEX
SMMC-602839 (rev. 11/84)

SHAWNEE MISSION MEDICAL CENTER

Date ord.	Radiology	Date Sch	DONE	Date ord.	Laboratory	Date Sch	DONE	Date ord.	Special Procedures	Date Sch	DONE
1-1-92	Upper G I	1/1		1-1-92	CBC, Lytes	1-1	✔				
1-1-92	Flat plate abd	1/1			SMA₁₂						
									Daily Tests		
	Ancillary Consults										
									Daily Weight		

Diet: NPO

Food Allergies: none stated

Hold:

Feeding/Fluids NPO

☐ Self
☐ Assist
☐ Feeder
☐ Force
☐ Restrict

	meal	Ext	IV
7-3			
3-11			
11-7			

☒ I&O (hourly)
☒ IV D₅ LR 1250 c/hr
☐ Other_____

Safety Measures

☒ Siderails
☐ Restraints
☐ Other_____

Activities

☒ Bedrest
☐ BRP
☐ Dangle
☐ Chair
☐ Commode
☐ Up ad Lib
☒ Turn
☐ Ambulate

Transportation
per Cart

Hygiene

☒ Bedbath
☐ Assist
☐ Self Bath
☐ Shower
☐ Tub
☐ Vanity
☐ Oral Care

Bowel/Bladder

☒ Foley IN 1-1
         OUT
☒ Cath care Bid
☐ Incontinent
☐ Colostomy
☐ Ileostomy
☐ Urostomy

Communication

1-1-90 dark any stools

Physical Therapy	Date	Treatments
	1/1	Nasoenteric tube to Gomco
Cardio-Pulmonary		

Drug Allergies: Codeine

Isolation: In   Out

Emergency Instructions:
Relatives: Mildred Cain (wife)
Phone: 631-1098

Clergy: Fr. Wise 842-0097
Religion: Catholic

Religious Rites: No Special   Code Blue

Diagnosis: Intestinal Obstruction, Dehydration

Surgery & Dates:

Consults & Dates
Martin Botha, M.D. 1/1/90

Room	Name	Adm Date	Age	Physician
426	Cain, Harvey	1-1-92	78	ELTON HOBBS, M.D.

Figure 9–17. Kardex for Harvey Cain. Courtesy of Shawnee Mission Medical Center.

PROBLEM LIST FOR HARVEY CAIN

Date and Initials	Nursing Diagnoses/Problems	Source for Goals and Nursing Orders
1-1-92 JW	Potential Complications of Bowel Obstruction	Refer to Standards of Care for Intestinal Obstruction.
1-1-92 JW	Potential Altered Tissue Integrity (Pressure Ulcer) r/t decreased mobility, poor nutrition . . .	Nurse will develop goals and nursing orders.
1-1-92 JW	Abdominal Pain r/t abdominal distention	Refer to standardized care plan for Pain.
1-1-92 JW	Altered Oral Mucous Membranes r/t fluid loss from vomiting 2° intestinal obstruction	Refer to standardized care plan for altered Oral Mucous Membrane.
1-1-92 JW	Possible Fear or Anxiety r/t hospital environment, diagnostic tests, equipment, and procedures	Nurse will develop goals and nursing orders.
1-1-92 JW	Possible Fear of Dying r/t unknown outcome of illness and lack of information	Nurse will develop goals and nursing orders.
1-1-92 JW	Potential Complications of Upper GI: Perforation. . .	Nurse will develop goals and nursing orders.
1-1-92 JW	Potential Complications of IV Therapy . . .	See "Policies and Procedures for IV Therapy."
1-1-92 JW	Potential Complications of Nasoenteric Intubation: Ulceration —> Hemorrhage	See "Policies and Procedures for Nasoenteric Intubation and Suction."
1-1-92 JW	Potential Complications of Barium Enema	See "Protocol for Barium Enema."

Figure 9–18. Problem List for Harvey Cain

INDEX

patient-care plan, 292
Standard, defined, 259
Standard discharge planning, 306
Standards of care, 297
Standards of Nursing Practice, *12, 13, 48, 79, 275*
State board exams, 4
Stereotypes, 102
Stressful environments, dealing with, 24
Stress incontinence. *See Incontinence, stress urinary*
Stressors, 3
    human responses to, 83
Structure evaluation, 260
Subject, of goal statement, 171
Subjective data, 41, 233
Suffocation, high risk for, 368
    See also Home mainte-nance management, impaired; Injury, high risk for; Trauma, high risk for
Swallowing, impaired, 368
    See also Aspiration, high risk for
Synthesis, 91
Synthesizing ideas, 280

T
Tanner, C., 28
Taxonomy
    defined, 123
    NANDA, modifications of, 143
Taxonomy II, 119
Taxonomy I - Revised, 1990, 119
Teaching orders, as nursing intervention, 190
Teaching, patient. *See Patient teaching*
Teaching plans, formal, 194
Team nursing, 216
Technical skills, 10, 22, 222
Temperature, body, high risk for altered. *See Body temperature, high risk for altered*
Terminal evaluation, 263
Tests, diagnostic, patient's response to, 85

Theory, definition, 40
Thermoregulation, ineffective, 368-369
    See also Body temperature, high risk for altered; Hyperthermia; Hypothermia
Third party reimbursement, 224
Third party reimbursement, patient-care plan and, 292
Thought processes, altered, 369
    See also Sensory/perceptual alterations
Tissue integrity, impaired, 369
    See also Oral mucous membrane, altered; Skin integrity, altered
Tissue perfusion, altered, 369
    See also Disuse syndrome, high risk for; Injury, high risk for
Toileting self-care deficit. *See Self-care deficit, toileting*
Total incontinence. *See Incontinence, total urinary*
Trauma, high risk for, 370
    See also Aspiration, high risk for; Home maintenance manage-ment, impaired; Injury, high risk for; Poisoning, high risk for; Suffoca-tion, high risk for
Treatment
    diagnostic, patient's response to, 85
    orders, 187

U
Unilateral neglect, 370
    See also Self-care deficit; Sensory/perceptual alterations
Unitary Person Framework, 57, 311
Urge incontinence. *See Incontinence, urge urinary*

Urinary elimination, altered patterns of, 370
    See also Urinary retention
Urinary incontinence, functional. *See Incontinence, func-tional urinary*
    reflex. *See Incontinence, reflex urinary*
    stress. *See Incontinence, stress urinary*
    total. *See Incontinence, total urinary*
    urge. *See Incontinence, urge urinary*
Urinary retention, 371
    See also Urinary elimina-tion, altered patterns of

V
Validation, of data, 54
Veracity, 62
Verbal communication, impaired. *See Commu-nication, impaired verbal*
Violence, high risk for, 138
Violence, high risk for, self-directed or directed at others, 371

W
Warren, J., 81
Wellness
    in acute-care setting, 324-325
    assessment, 61-62
    nursing in, 4
    nursing process and, 13-15
Wellness diagnosis, 141-145
    goals for, 177-178
    labels, 141-145
    NANDA definition of, 86
    NANDA terminology in, 141-143
    non-NANDA labeling systems, 143-145
Werner, J., 274
Wiedenbach, E., 4

Z
Ziegler, S., 21, 23

NANDA Approved Diagnostic Labels*
Grouped by Roy's Adaptational Model (1992)

PHYSIOLOGICAL MODE**

1. Exercise/Rest (Activity)
Disuse syndrome, high risk for
Fatigue
Injury, high risk for
Mobility, impaired physical
Self-care deficit, bathing/hygiene
Sleep pattern disturbance

2. Nutrition
Breastfeeding, effective
Breastfeeding, ineffective
Breastfeeding, interrupted*
Infant feeding pattern, ineffective*
Infection, high risk for
Nutrition, altered: less than body
    requirements
Nutrition, altered: more than body
    requirements
Nutrition, altered: high risk for more
    than body requirements
Poisoning, high risk for
Self-care deficit, feeding (specify
    level)
Swallowing, impaired

3. Elimination
Constipation
Constipation, colonic
Constipation, perceived
Diarrhea
Incontinence, bowel
Incontinence, functional (urinary)
Incontinence, reflex (urinary)
Incontinence, stress (urinary)
Incontinence, total (urinary)
Incontinence, urge (urinary)
Self-care deficit, toileting (specify
    level)
Urinary elimination, altered
    patterns of
Urinary retention

4. Fluids and Electrolytes
Fluid volume deficit (1)
Fluid volume deficit (2)
Fluid volume deficit, high risk for
Fluid volume excess

5. Oxygenation/Circulation
Airway clearance, ineffective
Aspiration, high risk for

Cardiac output, decreased
Gas exchange, impaired
Suffocation, high risk for
Tissue perfusion, altered (specify):
    cardiopulmonary, cerebral,
    gastrointestinal, peripheral, renal
Ventilation, inability to sustain
    spontaneous*
Ventilatory weaning response,
    dysfunctional*

6. Endocrine Function/Temperature Regulation
Body temperature, high risk for
    altered
Hyperthermia
Hypothermia
Protection, altered
Thermoregulation, ineffective

7. Skin (and tissue) Integrity
Oral mucous membrane, altered
Peripheral neurovascular dysfunc-
    tion, high risk for*
Skin integrity, impaired
Skin integrity, high risk for impaired
Tissue integrity, impaired

8. Senses
Pain
Pain, chronic
Sensory/perceptual alterations
    (specify): auditory, gustatory,
    kinesthetic, olfactory, tactile,
    visual
Trauma, high risk for

9. Neurological Function
Dysreflexia
Unilateral neglect

SELF-CONCEPT MODE**
Anxiety
Body image disturbance
Coping, defensive
Decisional conflict (specify)
Denial, ineffective
Fear
Grieving, anticipatory
Grieving, dysfunctional
Health maintenance, altered

Health-seeking behaviors (specify)
Hopelessness
Noncompliance
Personal identity disturbance
Post-trauma response
Powerlessness
Rape-trauma syndrome: compound
    reaction
Rape-trauma syndrome: silent reaction
Self-care deficit, dressing/grooming
    (specify level)
Self-esteem, chronic low
Self-esteem, disturbance
Self-esteem, situational low
Self-mutilation, high risk for*
Spiritual distress (distress of the human
    spirit)
Thought processes, altered
Violence, potential for: self-directed

ROLE FUNCTION MODE**
Adjustment, impaired
Coping, ineffective individual
Diversional activity deficit
Home maintenance management,
    impaired
Knowledge deficit (specify)
Management of therapeutic regimen,
    ineffective
Parental role conflict
Parenting, altered
Parenting, high risk for altered
Role performance, altered
Verbal communication, impaired

INTERDEPENDENCE MODE**
Activity intolerance
Activity intolerance, high risk for
Caregiver role strain*
Caregiver role strain, high risk for*
Coping, ineffective family: compro-
    mised
Coping, ineffective family: disabling
Coping, family: potential for growth
Family processes, altered
Relocation stress syndrome
Sexual dysfunction
Sexuality patterns, altered
Social interaction, impaired
Social isolation
Violence, high risk for: directed at
    others

*Tenth Conference, 1992
**The diagnosis, *Altered Growth and Development*, can occur in any of the modes.